Skeletal Muscle Repair and Regeneration

Skeletal Muscle Repair and Regeneration

Editor: Keith Seibert

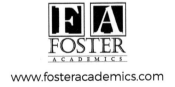

www.fosteracademics.com

www.fosteracademics.com

Cataloging-in-Publication Data

Skeletal muscle repair and regeneration / edited by Keith Seibert.
    p. cm.
Includes bibliographical references and index.
ISBN 978-1-64646-619-1
1. Muscles. 2. Musculoskeletal system. 3. Muscles--Diseases--Treatment.
4. Muscles--Wounds and injuries. 5. Muscles--Regeneration. I. Seibert, Keith.
QP321 .S543 2023
612.74--dc23

Foster Academics,
118-35 Queens Blvd., Suite 400,
Forest Hills, NY 11375, USA

ISBN 978-1-64646-619-1 (Hardback)

Contents

Preface

Skeletal muscles are organs found in the vertebrate muscular system that are usually connected to skeleton bones through tendons. It is the most abundant tissue in the human body and it is longer than other muscle tissues. It also has a strong innate ability to repair tissue damage occurred through an accident or degenerative illnesses, like muscular dystrophy, and regenerate new muscle fibers. Satellite cells and myogenic progenitors located between the muscle fiber membrane and the basal lamina are primarily responsible for regeneration. Skeletal muscles have the ability to regenerate and repair themselves following a trauma in a sophisticated and well-organized manner. This process requires the existence of varied cell populations, the up and down regulation of different gene expressions, along with the involvement of numerous growth agents. The topics in this book on the regeneration of skeletal muscles are of utmost significance and bound to provide incredible insights to readers. The readers would gain knowledge that would broaden their perspective in this area of orthopedics.

The information contained in this book is the result of intensive hard work done by researchers in this field. All due efforts have been made to make this book serve as a complete guiding source for students and researchers. The topics in this book have been comprehensively explained to help readers understand the growing trends in the field.

I would like to thank the entire group of writers who made sincere efforts in this book and my family who supported me in my efforts of working on this book. I take this opportunity to thank all those who have been a guiding force throughout my life.

Editor

Epigallocatechin Gallate Modulates Muscle Homeostasis in Type 2 Diabetes and Obesity by Targeting Energetic and Redox Pathways

Ester Casanova [1,*,†], **Josepa Salvadó** [1], **Anna Crescenti** [2] **and Albert Gibert-Ramos** [1,*,†]

[1] Nutrigenomics Research Group, Department of Biochemistry and Biotechnology, Universitat Rovira i Virgili (URV), Campus Sescelades, 43007 Tarragona, Spain; mariajosepa.salvado@urv.cat

[2] Technological Unit of Nutrition and Health, EURECAT-Technology Centre of Catalonia, Avinguda Universitat 1, 43204 Reus, Spain; anna.crescenti@eurecat.org

* Correspondence: ester.casanova@urv.cat (E.C.); albert.gibert@urv.cat (A.G.-R.);

† These authors contributed equally to this work.

Abstract: Obesity is associated with the hypertrophy and hyperplasia of adipose tissue, affecting the healthy secretion profile of pro- and anti-inflammatory adipokines. Increased influx of fatty acids and inflammatory adipokines from adipose tissue can induce muscle oxidative stress and inflammation and negatively regulate myocyte metabolism. Muscle has emerged as an important mediator of homeostatic control through the consumption of energy substrates, as well as governing systemic signaling networks. In muscle, obesity is related to decreased glucose uptake, deregulation of lipid metabolism, and mitochondrial dysfunction. This review focuses on the effect of epigallocatechin-gallate (EGCG) on oxidative stress and inflammation, linked to the metabolic dysfunction of skeletal muscle in obesity and their underlying mechanisms. EGCG works by increasing the expression of antioxidant enzymes, by reversing the increase of reactive oxygen species (ROS) production in skeletal muscle and regulating mitochondria-involved autophagy. Moreover, EGCG increases muscle lipid oxidation and stimulates glucose uptake in insulin-resistant skeletal muscle. EGCG acts by modulating cell signaling including the NF-κB, AMP-activated protein kinase (AMPK), and mitogen-activated protein kinase (MAPK) signaling pathways, and through epigenetic mechanisms such as DNA methylation and histone acetylation.

Keywords: epigallocatechin gallate; obesity; muscle; oxidative stress; cell signaling

1. Structure, Bioavailability and Metabolism of Epigallocatechin Gallate

Epigallocatechin gallate (EGCG) is a major constituent of green tea (7380 mg per 100 g of dried leaves). Smaller amounts of EGCG are found in apple skin, plums, onions, hazelnuts, pecans and carob powder (at 109 mg per 100 g) [1]. Green tea, from the *Camellia sinensis* L., contains very high levels of flavan-3-ols monomers, also known as catechins, and its main components are (−)-epicatechin (EC), (−)-epigallocatechin (EGC), (−)-epicatechin gallate (ECG), and (−)-epigallocatechin gallate (EGCG). Green tea leaves are steamed to reduce oxidation, however, during the production of black tea, the levels of flavan-3-ols drop. The reason behind is that tea leaves are processed in a specific way that includes fermentation, which converts these flavan-3-ols in theaflavins and thearubigins [2].

1.1. Molecular Structure

The structure of EGCG consists of four rings resulting from the esterification of EGC with gallic acid: the A and C rings constitute the benzopyran ring with a pyrogallol moiety at position 2, the B ring, with a gallate moiety at position 3, and the D ring (Figure 1). The presence of this ester carbon makes EGCG highly susceptible to nucleophilic attack [3]. The B and D rings of EGCG have vicinal 3', 4', 5' and 3", 4" and 5"-trihydroxy groups respectively, which give EGCG its anti-oxidative potential [3]. These ortho-dihydroxy pairings found in rings B and D account for EGCG's potent divalent metal chelating capacity [4]. EGCG has been found to be a more efficient radical scavenger than its structural analogues EGC, EC, and ECG, which all have fewer hydroxyl groups [4]. The EGCG molecule is less stable in neutral and alkaline media because the hydroxyl groups on the phenyl ring are attacked by the basic medium, leading to the formation of a more active phenoxide anion. This instability results in low bioavailability [3].

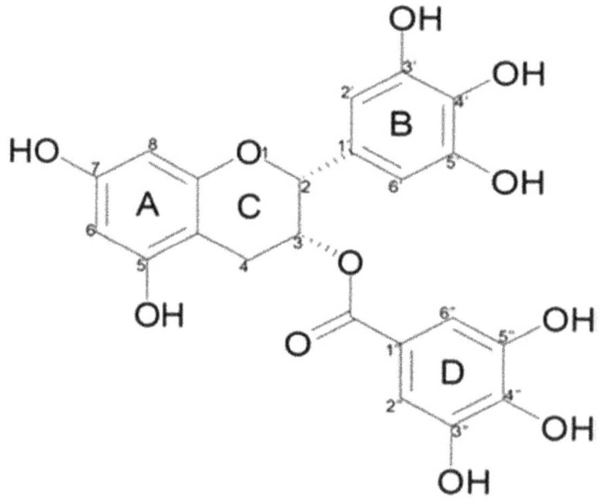

(-)-Epigallocatechin-3-gallate

Figure 1. Chemical structure of (−)-Epigallocatechin-3-gallate. The four rings resulting from the esterification of epigallocatechin (EGC) with gallic acid are indicated by letters (A, B, C and D) and each carbon from each ring is indicated by numbers (1–8).

1.2. Bioavailability and Metabolism

Many studies have shown a low systemic bioavailability of EGCG when it is taken orally. In an acute feeding study, healthy human subjects consumed 500 mL of green tea containing 648 μmol of flavan-3-ols, after which plasma and urine were collected over a 24-h period and analyzed by HPLC-MS [5]. The plasma contained a total of 10 metabolites in the form of O-methylated, sulfated, and glucuronide conjugates of EC and EGC, along with the native green tea flavan-3-ols EGCG and ECG [5]. The peak plasma concentration (Cmax) of unmetabolized EGCG was 55 nM and the time to reach Cmax (Tmax) was 1.6 h. Both the Tmax and the observed transformations are indicative of absorption in the small intestine [6]. The appearance of unmetabolized EGCG and ECG in plasma is unusual in dietary flavonoids and might be a consequence of the galloyl moiety inhibiting phase II metabolism [7,8].

While catechins are usually glucuronidated or sulfated in human plasma, EGCG can be found in free form and in high proportions (77–90%) [9–12]. Nevertheless, the fact remains that EGCG is poorly absorbed when administered orally due to its high solubility, resulting in low membrane permeability in human studies [4]. Moreover, EGCG is stable during gastric digestion at a low pH, but very unstable under duodenal conditions, in a more alkaline medium, which leads to low bioavailability.

The plasma levels of EGCG after intragastric administration of decaffeinated green tea to rats was found to be 0.1% [13]. Ullmann and colleagues reported that after the administration of 1600 mg EGCG to healthy volunteers, the Cmax was 3392 ng/mL [12]. Other human studies on the plasma kinetics of

EGCG and its conjugated metabolites indicated that the total mean of EGCG area under the plasma concentration time curve between 0-h to infinity (AUC (0–N)) ranged from 442 to 10,368 ng·h/mL, and the mean terminal elimination half-life (t1/2z) was from 1.9 to 4.6 h when purified and isolated EGCG was supplemented to healthy individuals [12]. In addition, another study examined the plasma kinetics of purified EGCG after administrations of 800 mg once per day and 400 mg twice per day for 4 weeks [9]. A peak in the serum levels of EGCG was observed after it had been administered at 400 and 800 mg [9]. An unexpected high amount of bound EGCG was found when the affinity of EGCG for human serum albumin was tested in physiological conditions. These results imply that almost all EGCG is transported in the blood bound to albumin, and explains the wide tissue distribution and chemical stability of EGCG in vivo [14]. EGCG kinetics have also been studied in rat and mouse models. Male Sprague Dawley rats that were given 0.6% green tea in their drinking water for 14 days had an EGCG concentration in the large intestine of 487.8 ± 121.5 ng/g, while its concentration in the bladder was approximately of 201.4 ± 154 ng/g EGCG [15]. A few studies have shown that EGCG does indeed cross the blood-brain barrier [16,17]. In particular, male and female mice administered orally with 200 µL of 0.05% EGCG solution containing 3.7 MBq [^{3}H]EGCG displayed 0.32% and 0.33%, respectively, of total radioactivity in the brain 24 h after uptake, which was comparable with most other organs [17]. Kohri et al. showed that after an oral administration of radioactive EGCG, its concentration in blood starts to increase after 8 h, shows a peak at 24 h, and then starts to decrease. In their study, they also show that major urinary excretion happened during the increase and peak periods, and that at 72 h its excretion was 32.1% of the oral dose, while its excretion in the feces during the following 72 h was 35.2% of the dose [18]. Kohri and colleagues also studied the metabolic fate of EGCG in rats supplemented with antibiotics and [4-^{3}H]EGCG, and found that the excretion levels were lower than in normal rats, and so, concluded that the radioactivity observed in the blood and urine came from EGCG degradation by the microbiota. Additionally, the authors report that a particular metabolite in the normal rats was purified and identified as 5-(5′-hydroxyphenyl)-γ-valerolactone 3′-O-β-glucuronide (M-2), while in feces, EGC (40.8% of the fecal radioactivity) and 5-(3′,5′-dihydroxyphenyl)-γ-valerolactone (M-1, 16.8%) were detected [18]. They propose that M-1 was absorbed in the body after EGCG was degraded by intestinal bacteria, yielding M-1 with EGC as an intermediate. Additionally, M-2 could have been formed from M-1 in the intestinal mucosa and/or liver, then entered the systemic circulation, and finally excreted in the urine [18].

Urine excreted 0 to 24 h after green tea consumption, contained a profile of flavan-3-ol conjugates similar to the plasma; however, ECG and EGCG were undetectable [18]. These outcomes indicate that the intact flavan-3-ols, ECG and EGCG do not undergo extensive metabolic modifications. Several researchers have observed that it is not possible to detect EGCG in urine, despite its presence in plasma [9,19,20], which is difficult to explain. It could be that the kidneys are unable to absorb EGCG from the plasma; however, if this is the case, there must be other mechanisms that produce its rapid decline after Cmax is reached [21]. Auger et al. [22] supplemented patients with an ileostomy with pure EGCG from green tea and analyzed the ileal fluid and urine over a period of 24 h. They did not find EGC or its metabolites in urine, thus establishing that degalloylation did not occur endogenously [21]. It has been hypothesized in animal studies that EGCG may be cleared from the plasma in the liver and returned to the small intestine through the bile [23,24]. Although this enterohepatic recirculation is not yet proven in humans, it might be possible that this EGCG from the bile is degallated by the gut microbiota, and then, if no more degradation happens, it is excreted in urine as EC and EGC metabolites [6].

Most of the consumed flavan-3-ols after green tea ingestion reach the large intestine where they are modified by the microbiota. These successive modifications result in their transformation to C-6–C-5 phenylvalerolactones and phenylvaleric acids, followed by their conversion into C-6–C-1 phenolic and aromatic acids, which are absorbed by the colon, enter the bloodstream, and are excreted in urine. The total amount that finally exits the body through urine is approximately a third of the ingested flavan-3-ols [21]. Moreover, it is believed that these transformations that occur in the colon might have important bioactive effects, and that these effects might vary between individuals because of differences in the microbiota composition. Even so, further studies are needed to make such assumptions [25].

It has been found, comparing two acute green tea feeding studies, one with volunteers subjected to an ileostomy [26] and the other with healthy individuals [5], that there were almost no differences in the plasmatic flavan-3-ol pharmacokinetics. These results indicated that flavan-3-ol monomers are principally absorbed in the upper part of the gastrointestinal tract [6]. Even so, it was also reported in the study with human subjects with an ileostomy that the ileal fluid contained 70% of the initially supplemented green tea flavan-3-ols [26]. Therefore, it can be stated that, in healthy subjects, the major part of favan-3-ols consumed will pass from the small to large intestines [6].

2. Muscle in Obesity: The Problem of Inflammation

Obesity is a term defined by the World Health Organization (WHO) that involves an abnormal or excessive amount of body fat accumulation that presents a risk to health [27]. Nowadays, obesity is becoming a global public health issue because affected individuals are at a major risk of developing a big range of comorbidities such as cardiovascular disease, type 2 diabetes (T2D) and respiratory disorders, among others [28,29].

Recent insights in obesity indicate that the adipose tissue exerts an inflammatory influence on the body. The metabolic effects of inflammation include insulin insensitivity, hyperlipidemia, muscle protein loss and oxidant stress [30]. Activation of the immune system increases the production of oxidant molecules. Moreover, oxidants could take part in the inflammatory response activating the nuclear factor kappa-B (NF-κB) which is linked to many of the genes related to the inflammatory response [31]. White adipose tissue derivatives, either fatty acids (FA) or inflammatory cytokines, in obesity have many adverse and synergistic effects on the skeletal metabolism [32]. High levels of interleukin-6 (IL-6), an inflammatory cytokine, are associated with insulin resistance (IR) and T2D [33–35] likely due to greater white adipose tissue IL-6 secretion [36,37].

In obesity and T2D subjects, the IL-6 signaling pathway in muscle cells has an abnormal function because there is a reduction in the expression of IL-6 receptor and also an abnormal STAT3/suppressor of cytokine signaling 3 (SOCS3) in adipose tissue [35,38]. SOCS3 is involved in the inhibition of leptin and insulin signaling, and has been found to be elevated in the skeletal muscle of mice fed with a high fat diet [39] and in insulin resistant states [40]. Overexpression of SOCS3 impairs leptin-stimulated AMPK activation, reduces tyrosine phosphorylation of IRS-1, PI-3-kinase activity, and AKT phosphorylation [39]. Thus, the reduction of SOCS3 expression in most cases could improve leptin and insulin resistance [41].

In addition, the lipid excess observed in obesity damages the muscle, causing cellular dysfunctions. Indeed, lipid excess in skeletal muscle activates endoplasmic reticulum (ER) stress and, consequently, the accumulation of unfolded or misfolded proteins in the ER lumen. Furthermore, it has been shown that the muscles of obese insulin-resistant individuals contain almost 30% less mitochondria than normal individuals [42], which suggests that muscles have less capacity to oxidize fatty acids, and thus contribute to insulin resistance.

Currently, there are many studies focusing on the treatment of the systemic inflammation induced by obesity and T2D, and particularly, through the use of natural bioactive compounds [43,44], which are usually harmless and more secure than synthetic drugs [45]. Moreover, targeting obesity-induced inflammation would be useful for the treatment of obesity and related diseases, since this state is linked to many illnesses or problematics, such as an overall activation of the immune system [46], cancer [47] or metabolic diseases [48].

3. EGCG on Energy Metabolism: Animal Models and Human Studies

In recent years, the interest in the health benefits of dietary components for preventing obesity and T2D has increased [49]. Specifically, polyphenol compounds such as a green tea extract rich in

EGCG exert anti-obesogenic properties [50,51]. Preclinical studies on animals and some studies on humans have confirmed the beneficial effects of EGCG [29] on obesity-related parameters including decreased body weight [52–54], decreased adipose mass [52], reduction of food intake [55], decreased total lipids, cholesterol and triglyceride in the liver and plasma, and an improvement in glucose homeostasis [52,53,56]. Various mechanisms have been proposed to produce these responses, including suppression of dietary fat absorption [52,57,58], enhancement of fat oxidation in adipose tissue and skeletal muscle [53,59], increase of glucose utilization [52,60,61], and decrease of de novo lipogenesis [59,62,63].

Moreover, data also provide evidence that green tea extracts have beneficial effects improving body composition and weight [53,64,65], reducing body fat [53,60,61], improving glucose and lipid metabolism [53,61,65], and protecting against ER stress, oxidative stress and protein degradation induced by high fat diet in skeletal muscle [66].

Treatment of C57b1/6J mice with 0.32% dietary EGCG for 16 weeks has been shown to reduce body weight gain and markers of T2D [52] induced by a high fat diet. In obese KK-ay mice, EGCG reduces ROS content, decreases glucose levels and increases glucose tolerance in animals [67]. Some of these effects are mediated by epigenetic mechanisms because, one of the mechanisms of EGCG appears to be the direct inhibition of DNA methyltransferases (DNMT) [68,69].

Laboratory studies with animal models have generally demonstrated that green tea and EGCG play a role in the prevention of obesity and have beneficial effects on glucose homeostasis, oxidative stress and lipid metabolism [49]. However, the effects on humans have been less studied. Epidemiological studies have suggested some of the possible effects of EGCG on humans, but there are few controlled intervention studies and many of these have different methodological designs. Therefore, more studies are needed to elucidate the action mechanisms [70]. A few studies have been carried out on humans with the aim of determining whether EGCG and/or green tea extract mediates the effects of lipid metabolism or energy expenditure in skeletal muscle. A study [71] researched the effect of 3-day supplementation of 282 mg/day EGCG on overweight subjects and found a non-significant effect on skeletal muscle lipolysis. It also found decreased lactate concentration, which suggests a shift towards a more oxidative muscle phenotype and also indicates that a longer period is necessary for the prevention of obesity [71,72]. Additionally, a systematic review on the effects on metabolic parameters such as respiratory quotient and energy expenditure concluded that EGCG could have a positive effect on both parameters, however, the authors conclude that further and larger prospective trials are needed [73].

The findings on humans suggest that EGCG alone also has a potential effect on fat oxidation. A randomized, double-blind, placebo-controlled, crossover pilot study showed that the administration of 300 mg EGCG/day for two days decreased the respiratory quotient during the first postprandial phase, suggesting an increase in fat oxidation and a potential anti-obesity effect [74]. Another study conducted with human subjects reported a decrease in body weight and body fat as well as an increase in fat oxidation and thermogenesis; these findings were confirmed in cell culture systems and animal models of obesity [63]. Other studies and designed experiments with green tea consumption combined with resistance training aimed to determine whether the observed beneficial effects were increased with exercise. Results demonstrated that there was a decrease in body fat, waist circumference and triglyceride levels, and an increase in body mass and muscle strength [75]. In contrast, in a randomized controlled trial study, overweight or obese male subjects randomly took 400 mg capsules of EGCG twice a day over 8 weeks. The results conclude that EGCG had no effect on insulin sensitivity, insulin secretion or glucose tolerance measured in blood extractions [50]. Therefore, well-designed and controlled clinical studies are necessary to validate the results of these human studies. Moreover, it must be stated that the concentrations used in many animal studies or the extrapolation of the doses from cell culture experiment into those equivalents in humans, greatly surpass what would be considered a physiological dose in humans. This might explain the differences in observed results between the different models and should be taken into account in future studies.

4. Metabolic Effects of EGCG in the Muscle and Muscle Cell Lines

4.1. Mitochondria and Oxidative Stress

The main role of mitochondria is energy production. For this reason, an impairment of their function could be implicated in insulin resistance and obesity [76]. The oxygen available for the respiratory chain activity may undergo incomplete reduction giving rise to ROS that is scavenged by the antioxidant defenses of the organelle. Likewise, there are several other ROS producers that have been identified in muscle cells that are activated by different stimuli including nicotinamide adenine dinucleotide phosphate (NADPH), oxidases (NOXs), phospholipase A2 (PLA2), xanthine oxidase (XO) and lipoxygenases [77]. Moreover, ROS can also be produced from non-muscle sources, such as immune cells, in response to muscle injures from exercise [78]. Furthermore, it has also been proposed that ROS activates ERK and/or JNK and induces autophagy in skeletal muscle [79]. The overproduction of ROS could lead to oxidative stress. To protect against this oxidative stress, enzymatic and non-enzymatic antioxidant systems could regulate ROS. The enzymatic systems, which include superoxide dismutase, glutathione peroxidase and catalase, have the capacity to convert ROS into less active molecules and prevent the transformation of these less active species into a more deleterious form. However, non-enzymatic antioxidants, such as EGCG, can protect against this undesirable effect and prevent pathological states that involve oxidative cell damage [80]. Indeed, the intake of EGCG by Wistar rats also reveals a decrease in plasma markers of oxidative stress, and an increase in antioxidant enzymes. Thus modulating and protecting from the effects of oxidant species by increasing antioxidant enzymatic systems and also due to their antioxidant capacity [81].

In skeletal muscle, the oral gavage of 100 mg EGCG/kg/day for 3 months in diabetic rats significantly reduced the expression levels of Beclin1 and dynamin-related protein 1 (DRP1) [79]. This implies that EGCG regulated mitochondrial-involved autophagy and ameliorated excessive muscle autophagy through down regulation of the ROS/ERK/JNK-p53 pathway [79]. Muscle is a major site of ATP production and energy consumption where the uptake and oxidation of glucose and fatty acids are key molecular events [64]. Moreover, EGCG has also been reported to inhibit mitochondrial oxidative phosphorylation to decrease ATP levels [82]. All these actions would result in an increase in the ADP/ATP ratio to activate AMPK, although these possibilities are still being researched.

4.2. Endoplasmic Reticulum

It has been shown that a high fat and sucrose diet, apart from dysregulation of lipid homeostasis, can also activate endoplasmic reticulum (ER) in skeletal muscle [83,84]. ER is an organelle that regulates a variety of post-transcriptional protein modifications, so its disruption leads to the accumulation of unfolded or misfolded proteins in the ER that affects a variety of cellular signaling processes, including energy production, inflammation and apoptosis. Several studies suggest that altered redox homeostasis in the ER causes ER stress and induces ROS production in ER and mitochondria [85,86]. If the ER stress is prolonged and cannot be restored, the functional homeostasis of the ER is impaired, which can induce an inflammatory state, protein degradation and cell death [85,87]. In mice fed with a high fat diet and receiving green tea extract rich in EGCG for 20 weeks, Rodriguez [66] found that there was a protective effect in muscle against oxidative stress and ER stress due to the repression of the increase in Binding immunoglobulin protein (BiP), Activating transcription factor 4 (ATF4), X-box binding protein 1s (XBP1s) and X-box binding protein 1u (XBP1u) in skeletal muscle protecting the cell from apoptosis and cell death.

4.3. Lipids

Other studies have also shown that EGCG may modulate muscle lipid metabolism by increasing lipid use, suggesting that thermogenesis and fat oxidation are increased [60] and, thus, that EGCG has lipid lowering properties [88]. Human and animal studies have revealed that excessive lipid accumulation in addition to obesity could also lead to insulin resistance or heart failure. Therefore, this lipid accumulation deteriorates cell signaling pathways and causes cellular dysfunctions [66,89]. It has been shown that chronic feeding of green tea extract could be implicated in fatty acid oxidation; elevating gene expression factors involved in lipid transport and oxidation such as fatty acid translocase (FAT)/CD36, medium-chain acyl-CoA dehydrogenase (MCAD) and uncoupling protein 3 (UCP3) [49,60]. Another study demonstrated that the treatment of 1% dietary EGCG for 4 weeks in mice reduced high fat diet-induced increase in body weight and body fat mass as well as increased mRNA expression of UCP2 and UCP3 in liver and skeletal muscle. These two genes are related to fatty acid oxidation, explaining the effects of EGCG on body weight gain. EGCG in this experiment also downregulates genes related to fatty acid synthesis and storage in the liver and white adipose tissue [54,90]. Moreover, β-oxidation in the gastrocnemius muscle of lean mice, fed with green tea, was elevated and exercise capacity was increased, as well as the expression of FAT/CD36 mRNA in skeletal muscle [60]. Friedrich [91] studied the acute effect of EGCG on oxidation and fat depots, and showed that in male C57BL/6 mice fed with different high fat diets, and an EGCG supplement, there was an increase of postprandial dietary fat oxidation and a decrease of dietary fat incorporation in skeletal muscle. These results were correlated with the downregulation of lipogenesis genes (ACC, FAS, SCD1) and lipid synthesis in liver and skeletal muscle in the postprandial state after 2 and 4 days of treatment.

4.4. Glucose

The role of EGCG in the modulation of glucose uptake and disposition has also been studied. Skeletal muscle is a key regulator of glucose homeostasis and contributes to postprandial blood glucose levels [92]. Skeletal muscle accounts for about 75% of insulin-stimulated whole-body glucose uptake [93]. To stimulate glucose uptake in the muscle cells, insulin promotes the translocation of GLUT4 from intracellular storage vesicles to the plasma membrane [94]. Many studies have focused on the regulation of the expression of genes involved in glucose uptake and insulin signaling to determine the mechanism behind the antidiabetic activities of green tea [57]. An experiment with mice fed with a high fat diet and treated with 0.32% EGCG for 16 weeks found a reduction in body weight and insulin resistance and an increase in the mRNA levels of the nuclear respiratory factor (Nrf1), medium chain acyl coA decarboxylase (Mcad), UCP3 and peroxisome proliferator α (PPAR-α) related to lipid metabolism [49]. Serisier et al. [95] carried out an experiment with dogs and showed that green tea can affect insulin sensitivity. Obese, insulin-resistant dogs were treated orally with green tea extract (80 mg/kg bw per day) over 12 weeks. The results showed that insulin resistance was decreased by 20% and in skeletal muscle the expression of PPARα and LPL mRNA increased; however, GLUT4 mRNA did not increase. In contrast, an experiment on Wistar rats with 0.1–0.2% dietary green tea treatment over 6 weeks concomitant with a high fructose diet showed that mRNA GLUT4 and IRS1 levels increased in muscle [96]. Similar results were found in an experiment carried out with male C57BL/6J mice fed with a high-fat diet and green and black tea supplements, where body weight gain and fat deposition in white adipose tissue were suppressed due to the stimulation of glucose uptake and the upregulation of the GLUT4 expression in the plasma membrane of muscle cells [97]. Experiments on Wistar rats revealed that EGCG attenuated free fatty-induced insulin resistance by activating the AMPK pathway [81]. Enhanced GLUT4 translocation and activation of AMPK in skeletal muscle have also been observed in lean mice treated with oolong, black or Pu-erh tea (2% extract as drinking fluid) for 7 days [98]. AMPK is a phosphorylating enzyme that regulates metabolic homeostasis of fatty acid and glucose metabolism in skeletal muscle and the inhibition of adipocyte lipolysis and the modulation of insulin secretion by pancreatic β-cells [99]. For this reason, there is interest in developing AMPK activators as a potential therapy for diabetes and obesity [94,100,101]. This AMPK activation would decrease gluconeogenesis and fatty acid synthesis while increasing catabolism, leading to a reduction in body weight [64]. Therefore, the effects of green tea rich in EGCG on glucose metabolism associated with T2D seems to be mediated in various ways, including glucose production, increased insulin secretion and insulin sensitivity, and increased uptake of glucose into skeletal muscle [102]. Various authors have discussed these mechanisms and their beneficial effects [103,104]. Indeed, experiments carried out on rodents have detected several other mechanisms attributed to the decrease on body weight. EGCG may modulate energy expenditure by inhibiting catechol-o-methyltransferase (COMT), which would lead to increased fat oxidation [105,106]. Another mechanism is the involvement of EGCG in sirtuins activation, especially Sirtuin 1 (SIRT1), which deacetylates histones and non-histone proteins including transcription factors [107]. The activation of SIRT1 in various types of polyphenols, such as EGCG, is beneficial for reducing energy absorption and increasing fat oxidation in diet-induced obesity in mice [54]. Moreover, SIRT1 is associated with the transcriptional co-factor peroxisome proliferator-activated receptor-y-coactivator 1 α (PGC1 α) activation, thereby also improving the mitochondrial function and protecting against metabolic diseases [107,108].

In experiments with isolated myocytes, it was found that EGCG stimulates GLUT4 translocation and results in an increased glucose uptake [56,61,97]. A study in male Wistar rats with an intake of EGCG during 3 weeks, also ameliorated glucose homeostasis [92]. EGCG acts as a potent antioxidant and protects against oxidant agents such as docosahexaenoic acid (DHA) in in vitro experiments by decreasing ROS levels and restring changes in mitochondrial morphology induced by DHA [109]. Moreover, other experiments with mouse C2C12 muscle cells treated with EGCG have shown a reduction in ROS levels [110,111], and a beneficial effect on fatty acid-induced peripheral insulin resistance [112]. There are many mechanisms involved in such response including: inhibition of PKC activation enhanced by the AMPK cascade, IRS1 serine phosphorylation and other kinases such as ERK1/2 and p38 MAPK, essential for maximal stimulation of glucose uptake in response to insulin [113,114]; and finally, the suppression of lipid accumulation via the AMPK/ACC signaling pathway [112,115]. In mouse C2C12 myotubes, the inhibition of AMPK following glutamate dehydrogenase (GDH) activation was reversed by EGCG. GDH senses mitochondrial energy supply, and its stimulation in primary human myotubes caused lowering of insulin-induced 2-deoxy-glucose uptake, which was partially counteracted by EGCG. Thus, mitochondrial energy provision, through anaplerotic input via GDH, influences the activity of the cytosolic energy sensor AMPK [116]. In addition, an in vitro experiment with L6 cells with insulin resistance and treated with 20 μM EGCG, demonstrated an improvement in glucose uptake by GLUT 4 translocation to the plasma membrane [94,117], which depended on the key regulator AMPK [118] and PI3-K/Akt activation [56,117,119]. Other studies on EGCG reported that it stimulates the MAPK pathway and the Nrf2 transcription factor leading to the transcription activation of the ARE-mediated Phase II genes induction [120].

Some of EGCG effects are mediated by epigenetic mechanisms because EGCG inhibits directly DNMT by interacting with the catalytic site of the DNMT molecule [121]. Studies with structural analogues of EGCG suggest the importance of D and B ring structures in the inhibitory activity. Molecular modelling studies also support the direct inhibitory effect of EGCG on DNMT; EGCG forms hydrogen bonds with Pro(1223), Glu(1265), Cys(1225), Ser(1229) and Arg(1309) in the catalytic pocket of DNMT [68]. EGCG also acts by inhibiting histone acetyl transferase activity and NF-κB activation [122].

5. Future Approaches

As exposed in this review, there are numerous studies focusing on EGCG and its effects on the many metabolic disturbances that affect the skeletal muscle in obesity and T2D, however, more research must be done to identify the specific metabolic pathways implicated on its response or the appropriate treatment for human patients. Moreover, the low systemic bioavailability of EGCG raises doubts about the feasibility of this molecule for the treatment or prevention of particular diseases.

In order to overcome the problem of EGCG instability and low bioavailability, several studies have tried the use of nanocarriers, such as liposomes and gold nanoparticles, which have shown to greatly increase the effects of EGCG in particular diseases [123]. On the other hand, scientists are studying the possibility of combining different bioactive ingredients with known beneficial activities on the causes of obesity or the inflammatory state. In this sense, there are studies focusing on the combination of these ingredients in order to obtain additive or synergic effects that could increase the overall effect of the individual ingredients [124,125]. Specifically for EGCG, it has been shown that combining EGCG with other bioactive ingredients with similar activities, and its supplementation to obese individuals, improved many of the obesity related parameters [126,127].

6. Conclusions

In conclusion, EGCG may be useful to treat obesity by re-sensitizing insulin-resistant muscle, increasing muscle lipid oxidation and stimulating the glucose uptake of muscle cells. Likewise, EGCG may revert the increase of ROS production, ER stress and protein degradation in skeletal muscle in obesity by regulating mitochondrial-involved autophagy and ameliorating excessive muscle autophagy (Figure 2). Despite being a potent antioxidant, EGCG does not seem to act in vivo as conventional hydrogen-donating antioxidants due to its low bioavailability. The circulating EGCG concentration is in the nanoM interval, similar to hormones. Thus, rather than acting as a chemical antioxidant, in vivo EGCG generates signals for inducing protective enzymes and may exert modulatory actions in cells acting as signaling molecules and/or regulating gene expression. In this sense, EGCG, among other mechanisms, up-regulates genes encoding for phase II enzymes with antioxidant response elements (AREs) in the promoter region; has insulin-mimetic actions via the PI3K/Akt signaling pathway; activates AMPK, an energy-responsive and redox sensing enzyme; and inhibits DNA methyltransferases and histone acetyl transferases, thus mediating epigenetic mechanisms.

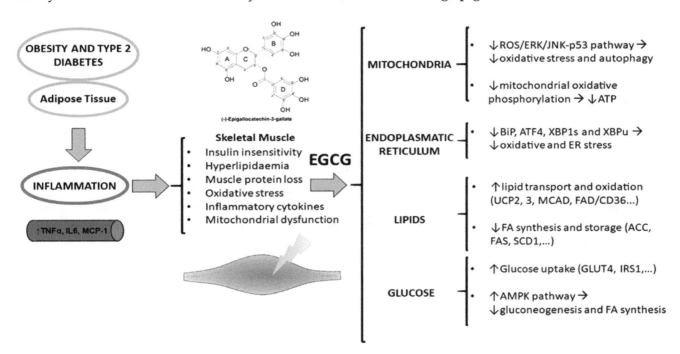

Figure 2. Summary of the effects of (−)-Epigallocatechin-3-gallate on the modulation of muscle homeostasis in obesity and type 2 diabetes. Arrows indicate an increase (↑) or decrease (↓) of that particular molecule or the pathway's activity.

It would be interesting to apply these results to counteract obesity, where EGCG could be used as a complement to sport programmes and good eating habits to obtain better responses against obesity.

References

1. Bhagwat, S.; Haytowitz, D.B.; Holden, J.M. *USDA Database for the Flavonoid Content of Selected Foods Release 3*; U.S. Department of Argiculture: Washington, DC, USA, 2011; pp. 1–156.

2. Del Rio, D.; Stewart, A.J.; Mullen, W.; Burns, J.; Lean, M.E.J.; Brighenti, F.; Crozier, A. HPLC-MS[n] Analysis of Phenolic Compounds and Purine Alkaloids in Green and Black Tea. *J. Agric. Food Chem.* **2004**, *52*, 2807–2815. [CrossRef]

3. Kanwar, J.; Taskeen, M.; Mohammad, I.; Huo, C.; Chan, T.H.; Dou, Q.P. Recent advances on tea polyphenols. *Front. Biosci.* **2012**, *4*, 111–131. [CrossRef]

4. Renaud, J.; Nabavi, S.M.; Daglia, M.; Nabavi, S.F.; Martinoli, M.-G. Epigallocatechin-3-gallate, a promising molecule for Parkinson's disease? *Rejuvenation Res.* **2015**, *18*, 257–269. [CrossRef] [PubMed]

5. Stalmach, A.; Troufflard, S.; Serafini, M.; Crozier, A. Absorption, metabolism and excretion of Choladi green tea flavan-3-ols by humans. *Mol. Nutr. Food Res.* **2009**, *53*, 44–53. [CrossRef] [PubMed]

6. Del Rio, D.; Rodriguez-Mateos, A.; Spencer, J.P.E.; Tognolini, M.; Borges, G.; Crozier, A. Dietary (Poly)phenolics in Human Health: Structures, Bioavailability, and Evidence of Protective Effects Against Chronic Diseases. *Antioxid. Redox Signal.* **2013**, *18*, 1818–1892. [CrossRef] [PubMed]

7. Shahrzad, S.; Bitsch, I. Determination of gallic acid and its metabolites in human plasma and urine by high-performance liquid chromatography. *J. Chromatogr. B. Biomed. Sci. Appl.* **1998**, *705*, 87–95. [CrossRef]

8. Shahrzad, S.; Aoyagi, K.; Winter, A.; Koyama, A.; Bitsch, I. Pharmacokinetics of gallic acid and its relative bioavailability from tea in healthy humans. *J. Nutr.* **2001**, *131*, 1207–1210. [CrossRef] [PubMed]

9. Chow, H.H.; Cai, Y.; Alberts, D.S.; Hakim, I.; Dorr, R.; Shahi, F.; Crowell, J.A.; Yang, C.S.; Hara, Y. Phase I pharmacokinetic study of tea polyphenols following single-dose administration of epigallocatechin gallate and polyphenon E. *Cancer Epidemiol. Biomar. Prev.* **2001**, *10*, 53–58.

10. Lee, M.-J.; Maliakal, P.; Chen, L.; Meng, X.; Bondoc, F.Y.; Prabhu, S.; Lambert, G.; Mohr, S.; Yang, C.S. Pharmacokinetics of tea catechins after ingestion of green tea and (-)-epigallocatechin-3-gallate by humans: Formation of different metabolites and individual variability. *Cancer Epidemiol. Biomark. Prev.* **2002**, *11*, 1025–1032.

11. Meng, X.; Sang, S.; Zhu, N.; Lu, H.; Sheng, S.; Lee, M.-J.; Ho, C.-T.; Yang, C.S. Identification and characterization of methylated and ring-fission metabolites of tea catechins formed in humans, mice, and rats. *Chem. Res. Toxicol.* **2002**, *15*, 1042–1050. [CrossRef]

12. Ullmann, U.; Haller, J.; Decourt, J.D.; Girault, J.; Spitzer, V.; Weber, P. Plasma-kinetic characteristics of purified and isolated green tea catechin epigallocatechin gallate (EGCG) after 10 days repeated dosing in healthy volunteers. *Int. J. Vitam. Nutr. Res.* **2004**, *74*, 269–278. [CrossRef] [PubMed]

13. Okushio, K.; Suzuki, M.; Matsumoto, N.; Nanjo, F.; Hara, Y. Identification of (−)-Epicatechin Metabolites and Their Metabolic Fate in the Rat. *Drug Metab. Dispos.* **1999**, *27*, 309–316. [PubMed]

14. Eaton, J.D.; Williamson, M.P. Multi-site binding of epigallocatechin gallate to human serum albumin measured by NMR and isothermal titration calorimetry. *Biosci. Rep.* **2017**, *37*, BSR20170209. [CrossRef] [PubMed]

15. Kim, S.; Lee, M.J.; Hong, J.; Li, C.; Smith, T.J.; Yang, G.Y.; Seril, D.N.; Yang, C.S. Plasma and tissue levels of tea catechins in rats and mice during chronic consumption of green tea polyphenols. *Nutr. Cancer* **2000**, *37*, 41–48. [CrossRef] [PubMed]

16. Lin, L.-C.; Wang, M.-N.; Tseng, T.-Y.; Sung, J.-S.; Tsai, T.-H. Pharmacokinetics of (-)-epigallocatechin-3-gallate in conscious and freely moving rats and its brain regional distribution. *J. Agric. Food Chem.* **2007**, *55*, 1517–1524. [CrossRef] [PubMed]

17. Suganuma, M.; Okabe, S.; Oniyama, M.; Tada, Y.; Ito, H.; Fujiki, H. Wide distribution of [3H](-)-epigallocatechin gallate, a cancer preventive tea polyphenol, in mouse tissue. *Carcinogenesis* **1998**, *19*, 1771–1776. [CrossRef] [PubMed]

18. Kohri, T.; Matsumoto, N.; Yamakawa, M.; Suzuki, M.; Nanjo, F.; Hara, Y.; Oku, N. Metabolic fate of (-)-[4-(3)H]epigallocatechin gallate in rats after oral administration. *J. Agric. Food Chem.* **2001**, *49*, 4102–4112. [CrossRef]

19. Unno, T.; Kondo, K.; Itakura, H.; Takeo, T. Analysis of (-)-epigallocatechin gallate in human serum obtained after ingesting green tea. *Biosci. Biotechnol. Biochem.* **1996**, *60*, 2066–2068. [CrossRef]

20. Henning, S.M.; Niu, Y.; Liu, Y.; Lee, N.H.; Hara, Y.; Thames, G.D.; Minutti, R.R.; Carpenter, C.L.; Wang, H.; Heber, D. Bioavailability and antioxidant effect of epigallocatechin gallate administered in purified form versus as green tea extract in healthy individuals. *J. Nutr. Biochem.* **2005**, *16*, 610–616. [CrossRef]

21. Clifford, M.; van der Hooft, J.; Crozier, A. Human studies on the absorption, distribution, metabolism, and excretion of tea polyphenols. *Am. J. Clin. Nutr.* **2013**, *98*, 1619S–1630S. [CrossRef]

22. Auger, C.; Mullen, W.; Hara, Y.; Crozier, A. Bioavailability of polyphenon E flavan-3-ols in humans with an ileostomy. *J. Nutr.* **2008**, *138*, 1535S–1542S. [CrossRef] [PubMed]

23. Kida, K.; Suzuki, M.; Matsumoto, N.; Nanjo, F.; Hara, Y. Identification of biliary metabolites of (-)-epigallocatechin gallate in rats. *J. Agric. Food Chem.* **2000**, *48*, 4151–4155. [CrossRef] [PubMed]

24. Kohri, T.; Nanjo, F.; Suzuki, M.; Seto, R.; Matsumoto, N.; Yamakawa, M.; Hojo, H.; Hara, Y.; Desai, D.; Amin, S.; et al. Synthesis of (-)-[4-3H]epigallocatechin gallate and its metabolic fate in rats after intravenous administration. *J. Agric. Food Chem.* **2001**, *49*, 1042–1048. [CrossRef] [PubMed]

25. Del Rio, D.; Calani, L.; Cordero, C.; Salvatore, S.; Pellegrini, N.; Brighenti, F. Bioavailability and catabolism of green tea flavan-3-ols in humans. *Nutrition* **2010**, *26*, 1110–1116. [CrossRef] [PubMed]

26. Stalmach, A.; Mullen, W.; Steiling, H.; Williamson, G.; Lean, M.E.J.; Crozier, A. Absorption, metabolism, and excretion of green tea flavan-3-ols in humans with an ileostomy. *Mol. Nutr. Food Res.* **2010**, *54*, 323–334. [CrossRef] [PubMed]

27. World Health Organization (WHO) Obesity and Overweight, Factsheet No. 311. Available online: http://www.who.int/mediacentre/factsheets/fs311/en/ (accessed on 13 February 2018).

28. Fruh, S.M. Obesity: Risk factors, complications, and strategies for sustainable long-term weight management. *J. Am. Assoc. Nurse Pract.* **2017**, *29*, S3–S14. [CrossRef] [PubMed]

29. Wang, S.; Moustaid-Moussa, N.; Chen, L.; Mo, H.; Shastri, A.; Su, R.; Bapat, P.; Kwun, I.S.; Shen, C.L. Novel insights of dietary polyphenols and obesity. *J. Nutr. Biochem.* **2014**, *25*, 1–18. [CrossRef] [PubMed]

30. Grimble, R.F. Gene Polymorphisms, Nutrition, and the Inflammatory Response. In *Nutritional Genomics: Impact on Health and Disease*; Brigelius-Flohé, R., Joost, H.G., Eds.; Wiley-Blackwell: Hoboken, NJ, USA, 2006; pp. 1–442, ISBN 9783527312948.

31. Liu, T.; Zhang, L.; Joo, D.; Sun, S.-C. NF-κB signaling in inflammation. *Signal Transduct. Target. Ther.* **2017**, *2*, 17023. [CrossRef] [PubMed]

32. McArdle, M.A.; Finucane, O.M.; Connaughton, R.M.; McMorrow, A.M.; Roche, H.M. Mechanisms of obesity-induced inflammation and insulin resistance: Insights into the emerging role of nutritional strategies. *Front. Endocrinol.* **2013**, *4*, 52. [CrossRef] [PubMed]

33. Spranger, J.; Kroke, A.; Möhlig, M.; Hoffmann, K.; Bergmann, M.M.; Ristow, M.; Boeing, H.; Pfeiffer, A.F.H. Inflammatory cytokines and the risk to develop type 2 diabetes: Results of the prospective population-based European Prospective Investigation into Cancer and Nutrition (EPIC)-Potsdam Study. *Diabetes* **2003**, *52*, 812–817. [CrossRef] [PubMed]

34. Pedersen, B.K.; Febbraio, M.A. Muscle as an endocrine organ: Focus on muscle-derived interleukin-6. *Physiol. Rev.* **2008**, *88*, 1379–1406. [CrossRef] [PubMed]

35. Rehman, K.; Akash, M.S.H.; Liaqat, A.; Kamal, S.; Qadir, M.I.; Rasul, A. Role of Interleukin-6 in Development of Insulin Resistance and Type 2 Diabetes Mellitus. *Crit. Rev. Eukaryot. Gene Expr.* **2017**, *27*, 229–236. [CrossRef] [PubMed]

36. Hoene, M.; Weigert, C. The role of interleukin-6 in insulin resistance, body fat distribution and energy balance. *Obes. Rev.* **2008**, *9*, 20–29. [CrossRef] [PubMed]

37. Sindhu, S.; Thomas, R.; Shihab, P.; Sriraman, D.; Behbehani, K.; Ahmad, R. Obesity Is a Positive Modulator of IL-6R and IL-6 Expression in the Subcutaneous Adipose Tissue: Significance for Metabolic Inflammation. *PLoS ONE* **2015**, *10*, e0133494. [CrossRef] [PubMed]

38. Palanivel, R.; Fullerton, M.D.; Galic, S.; Honeyman, J.; Hewitt, K.A.; Jorgensen, S.B.; Steinberg, G.R. Reduced Socs3 expression in adipose tissue protects female mice against obesity-induced insulin resistance. *Diabetologia* **2012**, *55*, 3083–3093. [CrossRef] [PubMed]

39. Yang, Z.; Hulver, M.; McMillan, R.P.; Cai, L.; Kershaw, E.E.; Yu, L.; Xue, B.; Shi, H. Regulation of Insulin and Leptin Signaling by Muscle Suppressor of Cytokine Signaling 3 (SOCS3). *PLoS ONE* **2012**, *7*, e47493. [CrossRef] [PubMed]

40. Boucher, J.; Kleinridders, A.; Kahn, C.R. Insulin Receptor Signaling in Normal and Insulin-Resistant States. *Cold Spring Harb. Perspect. Biol.* **2014**, *6*, a009191. [CrossRef]

41. Pedroso, J.A.B.; Ramos-Lobo, A.M.; Donato, J. SOCS3 as a future target to treat metabolic disorders. *Hormones* **2018**. [CrossRef] [PubMed]

42. Karimfar, M.H.; Haghani, K.; Babakhani, A.; Bakhtiyari, S. Rosiglitazone, but Not Epigallocatechin-3-Gallate, Attenuates the Decrease in PGC-1α Protein Levels in Palmitate-Induced Insulin-Resistant C2C12 Cells. *Lipids* **2015**, *50*, 521–528. [CrossRef] [PubMed]

43. Aggarwal, B.B. Targeting inflammation-induced obesity and metabolic diseases by curcumin and other nutraceuticals. *Annu. Rev. Nutr.* **2010**, *30*, 173–199. [CrossRef] [PubMed]

44. Lee, Y.-M.; Yoon, Y.; Yoon, H.; Park, H.-M.; Song, S.; Yeum, K.-J. Dietary Anthocyanins against Obesity and Inflammation. *Nutrients* **2017**, *9*, 1049. [CrossRef] [PubMed]

45. Torres-Fuentes, C.; Schellekens, H.; Dinan, T.G.; Cryan, J.F. A natural solution for obesity: Bioactives for the prevention and treatment of weight gain. A review. *Am. J. Clin. Nutr.* **2015**, *18*, 49–65. [CrossRef] [PubMed]

46. Asghar, A.; Sheikh, N. Role of immune cells in obesity induced low grade inflammation and insulin resistance. *Cell. Immunol.* **2017**, *315*, 18–26. [CrossRef] [PubMed]

47. Deng, T.; Lyon, C.J.; Bergin, S.; Caligiuri, M.A.; Hsueh, W.A. Obesity, Inflammation, and Cancer. *Annu. Rev. Pathol. Mech. Dis.* **2016**, *11*, 421–449. [CrossRef] [PubMed]

48. Saltiel, A.R.; Olefsky, J.M. Inflammatory mechanisms linking obesity and metabolic disease. *J. Clin. Investig.* **2017**, *127*, 1–4. [CrossRef] [PubMed]

49. Sae-tan, S.; Grove, K.A.; Kennett, M.J.; Lambert, J.D. (-)-Epigallocatechin-3-gallate increases the expression of genes related to fat oxidation in the skeletal muscle of high fat-fed mice. *Food Funct.* **2011**, *2*, 111–116. [CrossRef] [PubMed]

50. Brown, A.L.; Lane, J.; Coverly, J.; Stocks, J.; Jackson, S.; Stephen, A.; Bluck, L.; Coward, A.; Hendrickx, H. Effects of dietary supplementation with the green tea polyphenol epigallocatechin-3-gallate on insulin resistance and associated metabolic risk factors: Randomized controlled trial. *Br. J. Nutr.* **2009**, *101*, 886–894. [CrossRef] [PubMed]

51. Santamarina, A.B.; Oliveira, J.L.; Silva, F.P.; Carnier, J.; Mennitti, L.V.; Santana, A.A.; de Souza, G.H.I.; Ribeiro, E.B.; Oller do Nascimento, C.M.; Lira, F.S.; et al. Green Tea Extract Rich in Epigallocatechin-3-Gallate Prevents Fatty Liver by AMPK Activation via LKB1 in Mice Fed a High-Fat Diet. *PLoS ONE* **2015**, *10*, e0141227. [CrossRef] [PubMed]

52. Bose, M.; Lambert, J.D.; Ju, J.; Reuhl, K.R.; Shapses, S.A.; Yang, C.S. The Major Green Tea Polyphenol, (-)-Epigallocatechin-3-Gallate, Inhibits Obesity, Metabolic Syndrome, and Fatty Liver Disease in High-Fat–Fed Mice. *J. Nutr.* **2008**, *138*, 1677–1683. [CrossRef] [PubMed]

53. Chen, N.; Bezzina, R.; Hinch, E.; Lewandowski, P.A.; Cameron-Smith, D.; Mathai, M.L.; Jois, M.; Sinclair, A.J.; Begg, D.P.; Wark, J.D.; et al. Green tea, black tea, and epigallocatechin modify body composition, improve glucose tolerance, and differentially alter metabolic gene expression in rats fed a high-fat diet. *Nutr. Res.* **2009**, *29*, 784–793. [CrossRef] [PubMed]

54. Klaus, S.; Pultz, S.; Thone-Reineke, C.; Wolfram, S. Epigallocatechin gallate attenuates diet-induced obesity in mice by decreasing energy absorption and increasing fat oxidation. *Int. J. Obes. Relat. Metab. Disord.* **2005**, *29*, 615–623. [CrossRef] [PubMed]

55. Li, H.; Kek, H.C.; Lim, J.; Gelling, R.W.; Han, W. Green tea (-)-epigallocatechin-3-gallate counteracts daytime overeating induced by high-fat diet in mice. *Mol. Nutr. Food Res.* **2016**, *60*, 2565–2575. [CrossRef] [PubMed]

56. Ueda, M.; Nishiumi, S.; Nagayasu, H.; Fukuda, I.; Yoshida, K.; Ashida, H. Epigallocatechin gallate promotes GLUT4 translocation in skeletal muscle. *Biochem. Biophys. Res. Commun.* **2008**, *377*, 286–290. [CrossRef] [PubMed]

57. Sae-tan, S.; Grove, K.A.; Lambert, J.D. Weight control and prevention of metabolic syndrome by green tea. *Pharmacol. Res.* **2011**, *64*, 146–154. [CrossRef] [PubMed]

58. Yu, C.; Chen, Y.; Cline, G.W.; Zhang, D.; Zong, H.; Wang, Y.; Bergeron, R.; Kim, J.K.; Cushman, S.W.; Cooney, G.J.; et al. Mechanism by which fatty acids inhibit insulin activation of insulin receptor substrate-1 (IRS-1)-associated phosphatidylinositol 3-kinase activity in muscle. *J. Biol. Chem.* **2002**, *277*, 50230–50236. [CrossRef] [PubMed]

59. Lu, C.; Zhu, W.; Shen, C.-L.; Gao, W. Green Tea Polyphenols Reduce Body Weight in Rats by Modulating Obesity-Related Genes. *PLoS ONE* **2012**, *7*, e0038332. [CrossRef] [PubMed]

60. Murase, T.; Haramizu, S.; Shimotoyodome, A.; Nagasawa, A.; Tokimitsu, I. Green tea extract improves endurance capacity and increases muscle lipid oxidation in mice. *Am. J. Physiol. Regul. Integr. Comp. Physiol.* **2005**, *288*, R708–R715. [CrossRef] [PubMed]

61. Ashida, H.; Furuyashiki, T.; Nagayasu, H.; Bessho, H.; Sakakibara, H.; Hashimoto, T.; Kanazawa, K. Anti-obesity actions of green tea: Possible involvements in modulation of the glucose uptake system and suppression of the adipogenesis-related transcription factors. *BioFactors* **2004**, *22*, 135–140. [CrossRef]

62. Kim, H.-J.; Jeon, S.-M.; Lee, M.-K.; Jung, U.J.; Shin, S.-K.; Choi, M.-S. Antilipogenic effect of green tea extract in C57BL/6J-Lepob/ob mice. *Phyther. Res.* **2009**, *23*, 467–471. [CrossRef]

63. Wolfram, S.; Wang, Y.; Thielecke, F. Anti-obesity effects of green tea: From bedside to bench. *Mol. Nutr. Food Res.* **2006**, *50*, 176–187. [CrossRef]

64. Yang, C.S.; Zhang, J.; Zhang, L.; Huang, J.; Wang, Y. Mechanisms of Body Weight Reduction and Metabolic Syndrome Alleviation by Tea. *Mol. Nutr. Food Res.* **2016**, *60*, 160–174. [CrossRef] [PubMed]

65. Ramadan, G.; El-Beih, N.M.; Abd El-Ghffar, E.A. Modulatory effects of black v. green tea aqueous extract on hyperglycaemia, hyperlipidaemia and liver dysfunction in diabetic and obese rat models. *Br. J. Nutr.* **2009**, *102*, 1611–1619. [CrossRef] [PubMed]

66. Rodriguez, J.; Gilson, H.; Jamart, C.; Naslain, D.; Pierre, N.; Deldicque, L.; Francaux, M. Pomegranate and green tea extracts protect against ER stress induced by a high-fat diet in skeletal muscle of mice. *Eur. J. Nutr.* **2015**, *54*, 377–389. [CrossRef] [PubMed]

67. Yan, J.; Zhao, Y.; Suo, S.; Liu, Y.; Zhao, B. Green tea catechins ameliorate adipose insulin resistance by improving oxidative stress. *Free Radic. Biol. Med.* **2012**, *52*, 1648–1657. [CrossRef] [PubMed]

68. Fang, M.Z.; Wang, Y.; Ai, N.; Hou, Z.; Sun, Y.; Lu, H.; Welsh, W.; Yang, C.S. Tea polyphenol (-)-epigallocatechin-3-gallate inhibits DNA methyltransferase and reactivates methylation-silenced genes in cancer cell lines. *Cancer Res.* **2003**, *63*, 7563–7570.

69. Li, Y.; Tollefsbol, T.O. Impact on DNA methylation in cancer prevention and therapy by bioactive dietary components. *Curr. Med. Chem.* **2010**, *17*, 2141–2151. [CrossRef]

70. Grove, K.A.; Lambert, J.D. Laboratory, Epidemiological, and Human Intervention Studies Show That Tea (Camellia sinensis) May Be Useful in the Prevention of Obesity. *J. Nutr.* **2010**, *140*, 446–453. [CrossRef] [PubMed]

71. Most, J.; van Can, J.G.P.; van Dijk, J.-W.; Goossens, G.H.; Jocken, J.; Hospers, J.J.; Bendik, I.; Blaak, E.E. A 3-day EGCG-supplementation reduces interstitial lactate concentration in skeletal muscle of overweight subjects. *Sci. Rep.* **2016**, *5*, 17896. [CrossRef] [PubMed]

72. Corpeleijn, E.; Saris, W.H.M.; Blaak, E.E. Metabolic flexibility in the development of insulin resistance and type 2 diabetes: Effects of lifestyle. *Obes. Rev.* **2009**, *10*, 178–193. [CrossRef] [PubMed]

73. Kapoor, M.P.; Sugita, M.; Fukuzawa, Y.; Okubo, T. Physiological effects of epigallocatechin-3-gallate (EGCG) on energy expenditure for prospective fat oxidation in humans: A systematic review and meta-analysis. *J. Nutr. Biochem.* **2017**, *43*, 1–10. [CrossRef]

74. Boschmann, M.; Thielecke, F. The effects of epigallocatechin-3-gallate on thermogenesis and fat oxidation in obese men: A pilot study. *J. Am. Coll. Nutr.* **2007**, *26*, 389S–395S. [CrossRef] [PubMed]

75. Cardoso, G.A.; Salgado, J.M.; de Castro Cesar, C.; Donado-Pestana, C.M. The effects of green tea consumption and resistance training on body composition and resting metabolic rate in overweight or obese women. *J. Med. Food* **2013**, *16*, 120–127. [CrossRef] [PubMed]

76. Porter, C.; Wall, B.T. Skeletal muscle mitochondrial function: Is it quality or quantity that makes the difference in insulin resistance? *J. Physiol.* **2012**, *590*, 5935–5936. [CrossRef] [PubMed]

77. Steinbacher, P.; Eckl, P. Impact of Oxidative Stress on Exercising Skeletal Muscle. *Biomolecules* **2015**, *5*, 356–377. [CrossRef] [PubMed]

78. Powers, S.K.; Jackson, M.J. Exercise-Induced Oxidative Stress: Cellular Mechanisms and Impact on Muscle Force Production. *Physiol. Rev.* **2010**, *88*, 1243–1276. [CrossRef] [PubMed]

79. Yan, J.; Feng, Z.; Liu, J.; Shen, W.; Wang, Y.; Wertz, K.; Weber, P.; Long, J.; Liu, J. Enhanced autophagy plays a cardinal role in mitochondrial dysfunction in type 2 diabetic Goto-Kakizaki (GK) rats: Ameliorating effects of (-)-epigallocatechin-3-gallate. *J. Nutr. Biochem.* **2012**, *23*, 716–724. [CrossRef] [PubMed]

80. Dorta, D.J.; Pigoso, A.A.; Mingatto, F.E.; Rodrigues, T.; Pestana, C.R.; Uyemura, S.A.; Santos, A.C.; Curti, C. Antioxidant activity of flavonoids in isolated mitochondria. *Phyther. Res.* **2008**, *22*, 1213–1218. [CrossRef]

81. Li, Y.; Zhao, S.; Zhang, W.; Zhao, P.; He, B.; Wu, N.; Han, P. Epigallocatechin-3-O-gallate (EGCG) attenuates FFAs-induced peripheral insulin resistance through AMPK pathway and insulin signaling pathway in vivo. *Diabetes Res. Clin. Pract.* **2011**, *93*, 205–214. [CrossRef]

82. Valenti, D.; de Bari, L.; Manente, G.A.; Rossi, L.; Mutti, L.; Moro, L.; Vacca, R.A. Negative modulation of mitochondrial oxidative phosphorylation by epigallocatechin-3 gallate leads to growth arrest and apoptosis in human malignant pleural mesothelioma cells. *Biochim. Biophys. Acta* **2013**, *1832*, 2085–2096. [CrossRef]

83. Deldicque, L.; Cani, P.D.; Philp, A.; Raymackers, J.-M.; Meakin, P.J.; Ashford, M.L.J.; Delzenne, N.M.; Francaux, M.; Baar, K. The unfolded protein response is activated in skeletal muscle by high-fat feeding: Potential role in the downregulation of protein synthesis. *Am. J. Physiol. Endocrinol. Metab.* **2010**, *299*, E695–E705. [CrossRef]

84. Pierre, N.; Deldicque, L.; Barbé, C.; Naslain, D.; Cani, P.D.; Francaux, M. Toll-Like Receptor 4 Knockout Mice Are Protected against Endoplasmic Reticulum Stress Induced by a High-Fat Diet. *PLoS ONE* **2013**, *8*, e65061. [CrossRef] [PubMed]

85. Zhang, K.; Kaufman, R.J. From endoplasmic-reticulum stress to the inflammatory response. *Nature* **2008**, *454*, 455–462. [CrossRef] [PubMed]

86. Cao, S.S.; Kaufman, R.J. Endoplasmic Reticulum Stress and Oxidative Stress in Cell Fate Decision and Human Disease. *Antioxid. Redox Signal.* **2014**, *21*, 396–413. [CrossRef] [PubMed]

87. Gandeboeuf, D.; Dupre, C.; Roeckel-Drevet, P.; Nicolas, P.; Chevalier, G. Typing Tuber ectomycorrhizae by polymerase chain amplification of the internal transcribed spacer of rDNA and the sequence characterized amplified region markers. *Can. J. Microbiol.* **1997**, *43*, 723–728. [CrossRef]

88. Pajuelo, D.; Diaz, S.; Quesada, H.; Fernandez-Iglesias, A.; Mulero, M.; Arola-Arnal, A.; Salvado, M.J.; Blade, C.; Arola, L. Acute administration of grape seed proanthocyanidin extract modulates energetic metabolism in skeletal muscle and BAT mitochondria. *J. Agric. Food Chem.* **2011**, *59*, 4279–4287. [CrossRef] [PubMed]

89. Tsiotra, P.C.; Tsigos, C. Stress, the endoplasmic reticulum, and insulin resistance. *Ann. N. Y. Acad. Sci.* **2006**, *1083*, 63–76. [CrossRef]

90. Wolfram, S.; Raederstorff, D.; Wang, Y.; Teixeira, S.R.; Elste, V.; Weber, P. TEAVIGO™ (Epigallocatechin Gallate) Supplementation Prevents Obesity in Rodents by Reducing Adipose Tissue Mass. *Ann. Nutr. Metab.* **2005**, *49*, 54–63. [CrossRef]

91. Friedrich, M.; Petzke, K.J.; Raederstorff, D.; Wolfram, S.; Klaus, S. Acute effects of epigallocatechin gallate from green tea on oxidation and tissue incorporation of dietary lipids in mice fed a high-fat diet. *Int. J. Obes.* **2012**, *36*, 735–743. [CrossRef]

92. Keske, M.A.; Ng, H.L.H.; Premilovac, D.; Rattigan, S.; Kim, J.; Munir, K.; Yang, P.; Quon, M.J. Vascular and Metabolic Actions of the Green Tea Polyphenol Epigallocatechin Gallate. *Curr. Med. Chem.* **2015**, *22*, 59–69. [CrossRef] [PubMed]

93. Kumar, N.; Kaushik, N.K.; Park, G.; Choi, E.H.; Uhm, H.S. Enhancement of glucose uptake in skeletal muscle L6 cells and insulin secretion in pancreatic hamster-insulinoma-transfected cells by application of non-thermal plasma jet. *Appl. Phys. Lett.* **2013**, *103*, 203701. [CrossRef]

94. Yamashita, Y.; Wang, L.; Nanba, F.; Ito, C.; Toda, T.; Ashida, H. Procyanidin Promotes Translocation of Glucose Transporter 4 in Muscle of Mice through Activation of Insulin and AMPK Signaling Pathways. *PLoS ONE* **2016**, *11*, e0161704. [CrossRef] [PubMed]

95. Serisier, S.; Leray, V.; Poudroux, W.; Magot, T.; Ouguerram, K.; Nguyen, P. Effects of green tea on insulin sensitivity, lipid profile and expression of PPARalpha and PPARgamma and their target genes in obese dogs. *Br. J. Nutr.* **2008**, *99*, 1208–1216. [CrossRef] [PubMed]

96. Cao, H.; Hininger-Favier, I.; Kelly, M.A.; Benaraba, R.; Dawson, H.D.; Coves, S.; Roussel, A.M.; Anderson, R.A. Green Tea Polyphenol Extract Regulates the Expression of Genes Involved in Glucose Uptake and Insulin Signaling in Rats Fed a High Fructose Diet. *J. Agric. Food Chem.* **2007**, *55*, 6372–6378. [CrossRef] [PubMed]

97. Nishiumi, S.; Bessyo, H.; Kubo, M.; Aoki, Y.; Tanaka, A.; Yoshida, K.; Ashida, H. Green and black tea suppress hyperglycemia and insulin resistance by retaining the expression of glucose transporter 4 in muscle of high-fat diet-fed C57BL/6J mice. *J. Agric. Food Chem.* **2010**, *58*, 12916–12923. [CrossRef] [PubMed]

98. Yamashita, Y.; Wang, L.; Tinshun, Z.; Nakamura, T.; Ashida, H. Fermented tea improves glucose intolerance in mice by enhancing translocation of glucose transporter 4 in skeletal muscle. *J. Agric. Food Chem.* **2012**, *60*, 11366–11371. [CrossRef]

99.   Yuliana, N.D.; Korthout, H.; Wijaya, C.H.; Kim, H.K.; Verpoorte, R. Plant-derived food ingredients for stimulation of energy expenditure. *Crit. Rev. Food Sci. Nutr.* **2014**, *54*, 373–388. [CrossRef] [PubMed]

100. Carling, D.; Thornton, C.; Woods, A.; Sanders, M.J. AMP-activated protein kinase: New regulation, new roles? *Biochem. J.* **2012**, *445*, 11–27. [CrossRef] [PubMed]

101. O'Neill, H.M.; Holloway, G.P.; Steinberg, G.R. AMPK regulation of fatty acid metabolism and mitochondrial biogenesis: Implications for obesity. *Mol. Cell. Endocrinol.* **2013**, *366*, 135–151. [CrossRef]

102. Thielecke, F.; Boschmann, M. The potential role of green tea catechins in the prevention of the metabolic syndrome—A review. *Phytochemistry* **2009**, *70*, 11–24. [CrossRef]

103. Crespy, V.; Williamson, G. A review of the health effects of green tea catechins in in vivo animal models. *J. Nutr.* **2004**, *134*, 3431S–3440S. [CrossRef]

104. Kao, Y.-H.; Chang, H.-H.; Lee, M.-J.; Chen, C.-L. Tea, obesity, and diabetes. *Mol. Nutr. Food Res.* **2006**, *50*, 188–210. [CrossRef]

105. Dulloo, A.G.; Duret, C.; Rohrer, D.; Girardier, L.; Mensi, N.; Fathi, M.; Chantre, P.; Vandermander, J. Efficacy of a green tea extract rich in catechin polyphenols and caffeine in increasing 24-h energy expenditure and fat oxidation in humans. *Am. J. Clin. Nutr.* **1999**, *70*, 1040–1045. [CrossRef] [PubMed]

106. Hursel, R.; Janssens, P.L.H.R.; Bouwman, F.G.; Mariman, E.C.; Westerterp-Plantenga, M.S. The Role of Catechol-O-Methyl Transferase Val(108/158)Met Polymorphism (rs4680) in the Effect of Green Tea on Resting Energy Expenditure and Fat Oxidation: A Pilot Study. *PLoS ONE* **2014**, *9*, e106220. [CrossRef] [PubMed]

107. Chung, S.; Yao, H.; Caito, S.; Hwang, J.; Arunachalam, G.; Rahman, I. Regulation of SIRT1 in cellular functions: Role of polyphenols. *Arch. Biochem. Biophys.* **2010**, *501*, 79–90. [CrossRef] [PubMed]

108. Lagouge, M.; Argmann, C.; Gerhart-Hines, Z.; Meziane, H.; Lerin, C.; Daussin, F.; Messadeq, N.; Milne, J.; Lambert, P.; Elliott, P.; et al. Resveratrol improves mitochondrial function and protects against metabolic disease by activating SIRT1 and PGC-1alpha. *Cell* **2006**, *127*, 1109–1122. [CrossRef] [PubMed]

109. Casanova, E.; Baselga-Escudero, L.; Ribas-Latre, A.; Arola-Arnal, A.; Bladé, C.; Arola, L.; Salvadó, M.J. Epigallocatechin gallate counteracts oxidative stress in docosahexaenoxic acid-treated myocytes. *Biochim. Biophys. Acta Bioenerg.* **2014**, *1837*, 783–791. [CrossRef] [PubMed]

110. Wang, L.; Wang, Z.; Yang, K.; Shu, G.; Wang, S.; Gao, P.; Zhu, X.; Xi, Q.; Zhang, Y.; Jiang, Q. Epigallocatechin Gallate Reduces Slow-Twitch Muscle Fiber Formation and Mitochondrial Biosynthesis in C2C12 Cells by Repressing AMPK Activity and PGC-1α Expression. *J. Agric. Food Chem.* **2016**, *64*, 6517–6523. [CrossRef]

111. Wei, H.; Meng, Z. Protective effects of epigallocatechin-3-gallate against lead-induced oxidative damage. *Hum. Exp. Toxicol.* **2011**, *30*, 1521–1528. [CrossRef]

112. Deng, Y.-T.; Chang, T.-W.; Lee, M.-S.; Lin, J.-K. Suppression of free fatty acid-induced insulin resistance by phytopolyphenols in C2C12 mouse skeletal muscle cells. *J. Agric. Food Chem.* **2012**, *60*, 1059–1066. [CrossRef]

113. Babu, P.V.A.; Liu, D.; Gilbert, E.R. Recent advances in understanding the anti-diabetic actions of dietary flavonoids. *J. Nutr. Biochem.* **2013**, *24*, 1777–1789. [CrossRef]

114. Green, C.J.; Macrae, K.; Fogarty, S.; Hardie, D.G.; Sakamoto, K.; Hundal, H.S. Counter-modulation of fatty acid-induced pro-inflammatory nuclear factor kappaB signalling in rat skeletal muscle cells by AMP-activated protein kinase. *Biochem. J.* **2011**, *435*, 463–474. [CrossRef] [PubMed]

115. Dong, Z. Effects of food factors on signal transduction pathways. *Biofactors* **2000**, *12*, 17–28. [CrossRef] [PubMed]

116. Pournourmohammadi, S.; Grimaldi, M.; Stridh, M.H.; Lavallard, V.; Waagepetersen, H.S.; Wollheim, C.B.; Maechler, P. Epigallocatechin-3-gallate (EGCG) activates AMPK through the inhibition of glutamate dehydrogenase in muscle and pancreatic ß-cells: A potential beneficial effect in the pre-diabetic state? *Int. J. Biochem. Cell Biol.* **2017**, *88*, 220–225. [CrossRef] [PubMed]

117. Zhang, Z.F.; Li, Q.; Liang, J.; Dai, X.Q.; Ding, Y.; Wang, J.B.; Li, Y. Epigallocatechin-3-O-gallate (EGCG) protects the insulin sensitivity in rat L6 muscle cells exposed to dexamethasone condition. *Phytomedicine* **2010**, *17*, 14–18. [CrossRef] [PubMed]

118. Sheena, A.; Mohan, S.S.; Haridas, N.P.A.; Anilkumar, G. Elucidation of the Glucose Transport Pathway in Glucose Transporter 4 via Steered Molecular Dynamics Simulations. *PLoS ONE* **2011**, *6*, e25747. [CrossRef]

119. Jung, K.H.; Choi, H.S.; Kim, D.H.; Han, M.Y.; Chang, U.J.; Yim, S.-V.; Song, B.C.; Kim, C.-H.; Kang, S.A. Epigallocatechin gallate stimulates glucose uptake through the phosphatidylinositol 3-kinase-mediated pathway in L6 rat skeletal muscle cells. *J. Med. Food* **2008**, *11*, 429–434. [CrossRef]

120. Kong, A.-N.T.; Owuor, E.; Yu, R.; Hebbar, V.; Chen, C.; Hu, R.; Mandlekar, S. Induction of xenobiotic enzymes by the map kinase pathway and the antioxidant or electrophile response element (ARE/EpRE)[†,‡]. *Drug Metab. Rev.* **2001**, *33*, 255–271. [CrossRef]

121. Lee, W.J.; Shim, J.-Y.; Zhu, B.T. Mechanisms for the Inhibition of DNA Methyltransferases by Tea Catechins and Bioflavonoids. *Mol. Pharmacol.* **2005**, *68*, 1018–1030. [CrossRef]

122. Choi, K.-C.; Jung, M.G.; Lee, Y.-H.; Yoon, J.C.; Kwon, S.H.; Kang, H.-B.; Kim, M.-J.; Cha, J.-H.; Kim, Y.J.; Jun, W.J.; et al. Epigallocatechin-3-gallate, a histone acetyltransferase inhibitor, inhibits EBV-induced B lymphocyte transformation via suppression of RelA acetylation. *Cancer Res.* **2009**, *69*, 583–592. [CrossRef]

123. Granja, A.; Frias, I.; Neves, A.R.; Pinheiro, M.; Reis, S. Therapeutic Potential of Epigallocatechin Gallate Nanodelivery Systems. *Biomed. Res. Int.* **2017**, *2017*. [CrossRef]

124. Liu, R.H. Potential Synergy of Phytochemicals in Cancer Prevention: Mechanism of Action. *J. Nutr.* **2004**, *134*, 3479S–3485S. [CrossRef] [PubMed]

125. de Kok, T.M.; van Breda, S.G.; Manson, M.M. Mechanisms of combined action of different chemopreventive dietary compounds. *Eur. J. Nutr.* **2008**, *47*, 51–59. [CrossRef] [PubMed]

126. Rondanelli, M.; Opizzi, A.; Perna, S.; Faliva, M.; Solerte, S.B.; Fioravanti, M.; Klersy, C.; Edda, C.; Maddalena, P.; Luciano, S.; et al. Improvement in insulin resistance and favourable changes in plasma inflammatory adipokines after weight loss associated with two months' consumption of a combination of bioactive food ingredients in overweight subjects. *Endocrine* **2013**, *44*, 391–401. [CrossRef]

127. Belza, A.; Frandsen, E.; Kondrup, J. Body fat loss achieved by stimulation of thermogenesis by a combination of bioactive food ingredients: A placebo-controlled, double-blind 8-week intervention in obese subjects. *Int. J. Obes.* **2007**, *31*, 121–130. [CrossRef] [PubMed]

2

Adipose Tissue-Derived Stromal Cells in Matrigel Impact the Regeneration of Severely Damaged Skeletal Muscles

Iwona Grabowska, Malgorzata Zimowska, Karolina Maciejewska, Zuzanna Jablonska⑩,
Anna Bazga, Michal Ozieblo, Wladyslawa Streminska, Joanna Bem, Edyta Brzoska⑩
and Maria A. Ciemerych *⑩

Department of Cytology, Faculty of Biology, University of Warsaw, Miecznikowa 1, 02-096 Warsaw, Poland
* Correspondence: ciemerych@biol.uw.edu.pl

Abstract: In case of large injuries of skeletal muscles the pool of endogenous stem cells, i.e., satellite cells, might be not sufficient to secure proper regeneration. Such failure in reconstruction is often associated with loss of muscle mass and excessive formation of connective tissue. Therapies aiming to improve skeletal muscle regeneration and prevent fibrosis may rely on the transplantation of different types of stem cell. Among such cells are adipose tissue-derived stromal cells (ADSCs) which are relatively easy to isolate, culture, and manipulate. Our study aimed to verify applicability of ADSCs in the therapies of severely injured skeletal muscles. We tested whether 3D structures obtained from Matrigel populated with ADSCs and transplanted to regenerating mouse gastrocnemius muscles could improve the regeneration. In addition, ADSCs used in this study were pretreated with myoblasts-conditioned medium or anti-TGFβ antibody, i.e., the factors modifying their ability to proliferate, migrate, or differentiate. Analyses performed one week after injury allowed us to show the impact of 3D cultured control and pretreated ADSCs at muscle mass and structure, as well as fibrosis development immune response of the injured muscle.

Keywords: skeletal muscle; Matrigel; ADSCs; regeneration; TGFβ

---

1. Introduction

Skeletal muscles are built of the tissue which is characterized by the prominent ability to regenerate after injury. On daily basis many muscles groups are subjected to the damage caused by exercise or accidental mechanical injuries. Next, all of the muscles are affected during aging or in case of degenerative diseases, such as muscular dystrophies. Under physiological conditions skeletal muscle regeneration depends on the muscle specific unipotent stem cells, i.e., satellite cells that remain quiescent residing between sarcolemma and basal lamina surrounding muscle fiber. Injury which destroys muscle fibers, causing the release and/or activation various factors, leads to the satellite cell activation [1]. As a result, these cells start to proliferate, differentiate, and fuse to reconstruct functional muscle fibers. Each time satellite cells become activated to differentiate they also undergo self-renewal, allowing them to sustain their population. Importantly, with aging or disease progression the reservoir of satellite cells might be drained what could lead to the failure in proper skeletal muscle regeneration. Therapeutic approaches to treat such pathologies take into consideration various strategies. Among them is the support of muscle regeneration which could be achieved by the transplantation of cells able to undergo myogenic differentiation. Such cells should be readily available for clinicians, relatively easy to expand in vitro, and able to populate damaged and regenerating tissue. Satellite cells and myoblasts derived from them were among the "obvious" candidates for such cell-based therapies, however, not the perfect ones. The usefulness of these cells was limited by the fact that after transplantation they underwent necrosis, apoptosis, or anoikis [2–5]; failed to proliferate and colonize either the injured or dystrophic muscle [4,6]; or were eliminated by the host immune system [4,7]. Counteracting these phenomena relied on various experimental interventions, such as manipulating certain signaling pathways enhancing cell survival or migration [8–15] or using various scaffolds and gels to improve cell survival or colonization of injured or dystrophic muscles of mdx mice [16–18]. Obstacles preventing the application of satellite cells were among the impulses stimulating the studies on other stem cell types. Importantly, other subpopulations of cells residing within the muscle were shown to be able to undergo myogenic differentiation in vitro and in some cases to participate in and improve muscle regeneration [1]. Among such cells are mesoangioblasts [19–21], pericytes [22,23], muscle-resident interstitial cells that do not express paired box protein 7 (Pax7) but synthesize cell stress mediator PW1 [24], muscle side population cells [25], or so-called muscle-derived stem cells (MDSCs) [26]. Interestingly, tissue regeneration could be improved by enhancing the colonization of regenerating area by transplanting bio-scaffolds, such as muscle acellular scaffolds [27]. In such cases, transplantation of such extracellular matrix reach biomaterial was shown to attract the resident cells specific for the adjacent tissue.

Except the muscle-residing cells also those ones isolated form other tissues are extensively tested as the ones able to improve skeletal muscle regeneration. Various studies focus at the bone marrow and adipose tissue as the source of so-called mesenchymal stem or stromal cells (MSCs). Bone marrow-derived mesenchymal stromal cells (BM-MSCs) and adipose tissue-derived stromal cells (ADSCs) are characterized by fibroblast-like morphology, ability to adhere and grow in plastic culture dishes, expression of CD73, CD90, CD105 and lack of CD45, CD34, CD14 or CD11b, CD79a, or CD19, and HLA-DR antigens, as well as the ability to undergo at least osteo- and adipogenesis [28–31]. The fact that ADSC isolation is relatively simple and involves minimally invasive methods causes that these cells are extensively studied. As far as myogenic differentiation of BM-MSCs is concerned they do not possess the ability to undergo this process without additional stimulation. Many lines of evidence prove that MSCs can differentiate into myoblasts and form myotubes either in vitro or in vivo. For example, in vitro cultured BM-MSCs exposed to DNA demethylating agent 5-azacitidine were able to form myoblast-like structures [32]. In vivo, these cells were also shown to be able to incorporate into regenerating injured [33,34] or dystrophic muscles [35,36]. Unfortunately, proportion of myofibers formed with the participation of BM-MSCs was very low, thus, such transplantation did not present sufficient therapeutic potential [37].

As mentioned above, ADSCs could be differentiated, both in vitro and in vivo, to tissues other than adipose one. Multiple lines of evidence document that they could serve as a source for bone cells [38] or even neuronal cells. Santos et al showed that treatment of human ADSCs with cyclic ketamine compounds triggers processes resulting in the changes in the molecular patterns characteristic for neuronal cells [39]. Neuronal differentiation of ADSCs can be also achieved by such different interventions, as manipulation of the level of miRNA-124 [40], overexpression of BNDF [41], or overexpression of Sox2 [42].

In case of ADSCs myogenic potential it was documented both in vitro and in vivo [43]. In fact, some studies suggest that ADSC are more prone to undergo myogenic differentiation than BM-MSCs [44–47]. Importantly, it is widely accepted that transplantation of these cells, i.e., BM-MSCs and ADSCs, into regenerating muscles often improves regeneration via their immunomodulatory properties [48]. Moreover, such cells could be used in the combination with other factors impacting at various aspects of tissue repair. For example, combination of ADSCs with losartan—transforming growth factor beta (TGFβ) inhibitor—prevented fibrosis and improved repair of regenerating skeletal muscles of mdx mice [49]. TGFβ negatively regulates myoblast proliferation and differentiation [50]. Importantly, it stimulates extracellular matrix (ECM) production, modulates the expression of ECM-degrading enzymes and proteinase inhibitors, resulting in the development of fibrosis in regenerating muscle [51]. Thus, reduction of TGFβ signaling was previously shown by us [52] and others [49,53] to be beneficial for the skeletal muscle regeneration [54].

Next, the cell-based therapy could benefit from the application of various biomaterials or scaffolds mimicking cell niche, securing safe delivery or being a medium to deliver and release beneficial factor. It is also important in case of large, volumetric injures of skeletal muscles, which regeneration might not proceed properly, leading to the excessive connective tissue development. Many lines of evidence document that support of stem cells with materials substituting for extracellular matrix could improve the function and action of transplanted stem cells. For example, as we previously shown, in vitro culture of mouse myoblasts in Matrigel increase the level of adhesion proteins crucial for cell fusion [55]. Moreover, the delivery of cells seeded onto various scaffolds could be the only possible method to deliver stem cells into the site of massive skeletal muscle injury. BM-MSCs transplanted within the Matrigel [56], fibrin [57], or alginate cryogel improved skeletal muscle regeneration [58]. In addition, the latter study involved the application of recombinant growth factors, i.e., IGF-1 and VEGF, to enhance paracrine effect of BM-MSCs [58]. Except the application of selected growth factors the use of the whole secretome present within media conditioned by differentiating myoblasts was also tested as a "tool" to improve regeneration. As previously shown the secretome of differentiating myoblasts contains among other proteins at least 35 growth factors and 40 cytokines [59]. Another study revealed that human differentiating myoblasts secrete at least 253 conventionally, including 43 previously implicated in myogenesis [60]. Importantly, many of these factors were released in extracellular vesicles [60]. Thus, contact with myoblasts or exposure to the myoblast conditioned medium could significantly impact the function of other cells. For example, ADSCs cultured in such conditioned medium proliferated normally, expressed myogenic markers, and presented increased myogenic potential [47]. Moreover, other studies showed that use of media conditioned by differentiating muscles and myofibers had positive impact at regeneration and revascularization of ischemic skeletal muscle [61].

In the current study, using mouse model, we decided to combine various approaches aiming at the improvement of skeletal muscle regeneration—simultaneous application of cells, biomaterial, and growth factors. We choose ADSCs, as cells that could be easily isolated and expanded in combination with Matrigel infused with either anti-TGFβ antibody or myoblast-conditioned medium. We tested if such cell-based approach could positively impact repair of the skeletal muscle large injuries. Thus, as a model we choose mouse skeletal muscles which were induced to regenerate after the volumetric damage.

2. Results

The aim of our study was to investigate the impact of mouse ADSCs embedded either in Matrigel infused with medium conditioned by in vitro differentiating C2C12 myoblasts or Matrigel infused with anti-TGFβ antibody. As a control we used Matrigel subjected to control medium or to medium containing TGFβ. We hypothesized that transplantation of Matrigel containing ADSCs and infused with additional factors could be beneficial for the regeneration of muscle which underwent volumetric injury. Matrigel could fill the damaged space and support ADSCs that could impose their immunomodulatory action supported either by growth factors present in conditioned medium or by silencing of TGFβ signaling.

2.1. ADSC Reaction to Myoblast-Conditioned Medium or Manipulation of TGFβ Signaling

First, we analyzed ADSCs that were cultured in vitro under four different experimental conditions: (1) in control medium, (2) in medium conditioned by differentiating C2C12 myoblasts (at 7th day of culture), (3) medium containing TGFβ, and (4) medium containing antibody against TGFβ. We decided to use TGFβ as a control for the treatment in which signaling dependent on this factor was silenced. ADSC morphology (Figure 1A), expression of mesenchymal cell markers and mesoderm marker (Figure 1B), cell proliferation (Figure 1C), and migration (Figure 1D) was analyzed at day 1, 3, and 7 of culture. Analysis of all types of cultures suggested that conditioned medium influenced the ADSC morphology—cells became more elongated, resembling myoblasts. TGFβ treatment resulted in flattened, outstretched morphology of ADSCs, and significant reduction in their number (Figure 1A). Inhibiting TGFβ signaling with specific antibody did not impacted at cell morphology. Analysis of the expression of mRNAs encoding CD90 (Thy-1) and CD73 (ecto-5'-nukleotydase), which are considered the major markers of MSCs [30], showed their mRNAs were detectable in all types of cell culture at all analyzed stages of cell culture, except the one involving TGFβ. Analysis of mRNA encoding PDGFRα, i.e., the marker of paraxial mesoderm which during embryonic development gives rise to myogenic precursor cells [62], revealed that again its level was the lowest in TGFβ treated cells (Figure 1B). Each of the culture conditions tested decreased the proliferation of ADSCs, however to a different extend (Figure 1C). Thus, TGFβ completely abolished and conditioned medium significantly prevented cell proliferation. Antibody against TGFβ decreased number of cells, as compared to those one cultured in control medium and analyzed at day 7. However, this drop in proliferation was not as profound as in case of conditioned medium. Since TGFβ, used by as a control treatment, completely blocked proliferation of ADSCs it was excluded from subsequent experiments. The influence of culture conditions tested at the migration of ADSCs was assessed using in vitro scratch wound healing assay. The surface of the culture dish from which the cells were removed by scratch (0 h) was calculated. Next, the area which was not invaded by migrating cells was presented. Comparison between control cultures and the other ones showed that at 6 h it was the conditioned medium had a most profound impact at cell migration. At 24 h, however, anti-TGFβ antibody treatment caused the best effects, i.e., the resulted in the biggest area covered by migrating ADSCs (Figure 1D). Thus, the most profound effect at migration could be attributed to anti-TGFβ antibody treatment.

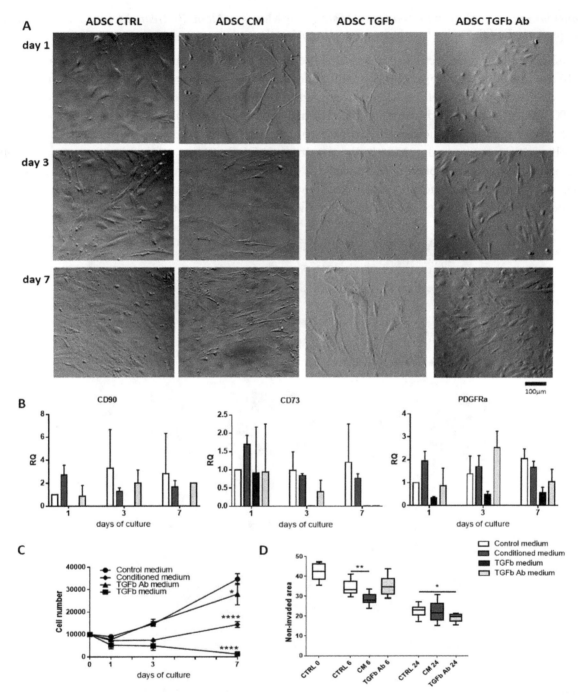

Figure 1. Impact of myoblast-conditioned medium or TGFβ signaling at mouse tissue-derived stromal cells (ADSCs). (**A**) ADSC morphology at 1 (24 h), 3, and 7 day of culture in control (CTRL), myoblast-conditioned (CM), and supplemented either with TGFβ (TGFb) or antibody against TGFβ (TGFb Ab) medium. (**B**) Expression of mRNAs encoding CD90, CD73, and PDGFRα. Expression was related to the levels observed in cells cultured in control medium at day 1, and normalized to the level of mRNA encoding β-actin. RQ: relative quantity. (**C**) ADSC growth curve at 1 (24 h), 3, and 7 day of culture in control, or myoblasts-conditioned, supplemented either with TGFβ or antibody against TGFβ medium. (**D**) In vitro scratch wound healing assay—cells were scratched from culture dish and the area which was not invaded by migrating cells was presented (at 6 h and 24 h). For each time point or experimental group $n \geq 3$. Data are presented as mean ± SD. *represent results of Student's t-test: * $p \leq 0.05$; ** $p \leq 0.01$, **** $p \leq 0.0001$.

2.2. Transplantation of ADSCs Embedded in Matrigel or Matrigel Alone Pretreated with Myoblast-Conditioned Medium or Anti-TGFβ Antibody into Regenerating Muscle

We showed that ADSC culture in myoblast-conditioned medium or in the presence of anti-TGFβ antibody decreased but not prevented proliferation and have an impact at the migration of these cells. Thus, we decided to test whether ADSCs, supported by Matrigel pretreated with conditioned medium or anti-TGFβ antibody, could improve skeletal muscle regeneration. ADSCs used in this study were labeled by BacMam Transduction Control vector coding GFP what allowed us to visualize position of the cells within the muscle. Matrigel containing ADSCs (7.5×10^5/mL) was preconditioned by incubation with myoblast-conditioned medium or medium containing anti-TGFβ antibody for 48 h. Analysis performed after such pretreatment revealed that cells "suspended" in Matrigel remained round and their morphology was similar regardless of the treatment (Figure 2).

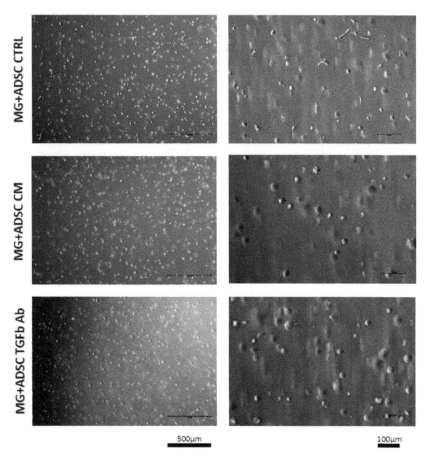

Figure 2. Morphology of ADSCs embedded in Matrigel. ADSC morphology at 48 h of treatment with control (CTRL), myoblast-conditioned (CM), or supplemented with antibody against TGFβ (TGFb Ab) medium.

Matrigel containing ADSCs was then transplanted to gastrocnemius muscle which was injured by deep incision. Transplantation of Matrigel alone or Matrigel containing ADSCs was performed just after injury. Injured muscles or muscles that received Matrigel only served as control. Seven days after transplantation muscles were dissected, weighted (Figure 3A), and processed for further analyzes. Transplantation of ADSCs within the Matrigel which was pretreated with either the myoblast-conditioned medium or anti-TGFβ antibody resulted in higher muscle mass, as compared to muscles that received only Matrigel (Figure 3A). Next, we localized transplanted Matrigel and ADSCs on the basis of GFP fluorescence within the muscle sections in that we also immunolocalized laminin to visualize muscle fiber borders (Figure 3B). Such analysis documented the presence of ADSCs within the muscle tissue. They did not participate in the formation of new myofibers, but were localized between them (Figure 3B). We did not see any substantial differences in ADSC localization between the muscles that received cells within Matrigel treated with control medium, conditioned medium, or medium supplemented with anti-TGFβ antibody. We did, however, notice the differences in the muscle structure. These aspects we analyzed using histological sections (Figure 4A).

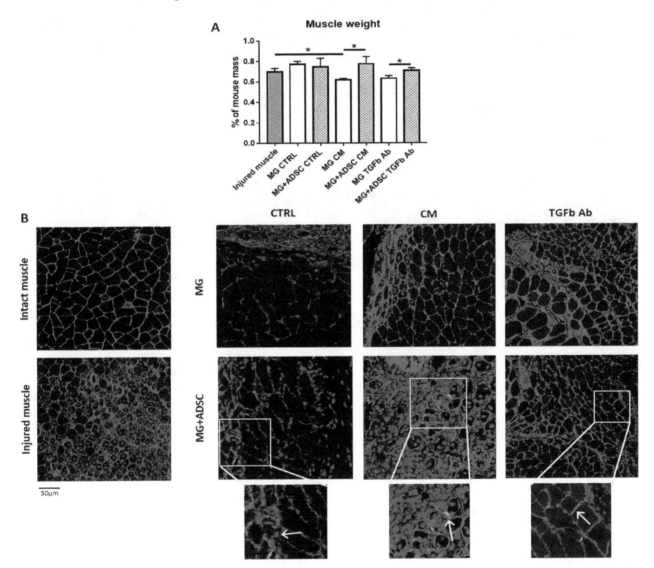

Figure 3. Analysis of skeletal muscles to which ADSCs embedded in Matrigel were transplanted. (**A**) Muscle weight (7 day of regeneration) of injured muscles and muscles that received Matrigel or Matrigel with ADSC pretreated in control (CTRL), myoblast-conditioned (CM), or supplemented with antibody against TGFβ (TGFb Ab) medium. For each experimental group $n \geq 3$. Data are presented as mean ± SD. * represent results of Student's t-test: * $p \leq 0.05$. (**B**) Localization of ADSCs in muscles which received Matrigel or Matrigel with ADSC pretreated in control (CTRL), myoblast-conditioned (CM), or supplemented with antibody against TGFβ (TGFb Ab) medium. Inserts: magnification of selected area of muscle cross-sections. Arrows indicates localization of GFP-expressing ADSCs. Green—ADSC-expressing GFP; red—laminin; blue—nuclei. Bar: 50 μm.

We compared histology of intact muscle, and injured muscles at day 7 of regeneration. The transplantation of control or conditioned medium treated Matrigel did not improve muscle regeneration—its structure was comparable to control injured muscles. Thus, the degeneration of injured tissue and accumulation of inflammatory cells was clearly visible. However, the introduction of Matrigel preincubated with anti-TGFβ antibody was beneficial for regenerating tissue—regenerated myofibers were more abundant (Figure 4A). Even better results were achieved when such Matrigel contained ADSCs. In such case improvement of regeneration was noticed in muscles that received Matrigel and ADSCs either conditioned medium treated or exposed to anti-TGFβ antibody (Figure 4A).

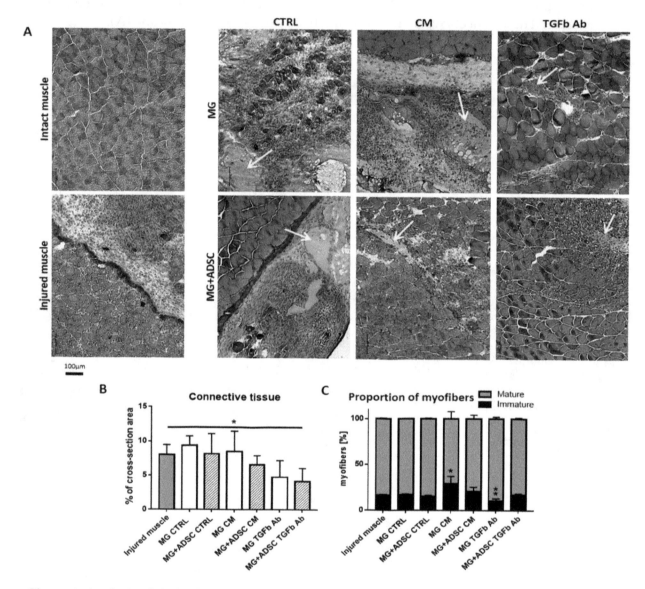

Figure 4. Analysis of skeletal muscle and connective tissue morphology. (**A**) Morphology of skeletal muscles (blue) stained with Harris hematoxylin and Gomori Trichrome dye, at 7 day of regeneration. Intact muscles, injured muscles, and muscles which received Matrigel or Matrigel with ADSC pretreated with control (CTRL), myoblast-conditioned (CM), or supplemented with antibody against TGFβ (TGFb Ab) medium. Arrows indicates localization of Matrigel. (**B**) Area occupied by connective tissue analyzed on cross-sections of injured muscles and muscles which received Matrigel or Matrigel with ADSC pretreated with control (CTRL), myoblast-conditioned (CM) or supplemented with antibody against TGFβ (TGFb Ab) medium. (**C**) Analysis of the proportion of mature and immature muscle fibers present in regenerating skeletal muscles of all analyzed groups. For each experimental group $n \geq 3$. Data are presented as mean ± SD. * represent results of Student's t-test: * $p \leq 0.05$, ** $p \leq 0.01$. Bar - 100 μm.

Skeletal muscle regeneration is often accompanied with the excessive production of connective tissue fibers. Such adversary effect might hamper proper function of regenerated muscle. Treatments that result in the decrease of connective tissue development and deposition of excessive amounts of extracellular matrix components are beneficial for regeneration [52,63]. Proportion of connective tissue was assessed within regenerating muscles of all group studied, i.e., control ones, transplanted with Matrigel treated with conditioned medium with or without ADSCs, treated with anti-TGFβ antibody containing medium with or without ASCs. Significant reduction of the amount of connective tissue was detected in muscles that received anti-TGFβ antibody pretreated Matrigel-containing ADSCs (Figure 4B).

Analysis of the differences in proportion between mature and immature myofibers, i.e., those ones undergoing reconstruction, showed that the presence of myoblast-conditioned medium treated Matrigel delayed the regeneration, as compared to control injured muscle. In such muscles proportion of myofibers with centrally positioned nuclei was significantly higher, while it was similar in other groups of analyzed muscles (Figure 4B). Interestingly, Matrigel delivering anti-TGFβ antibody significantly accelerated the maturation of muscle fibers, while when it contained ADSCs proportion of immature fibers was again comparable to control, suggesting that cells produced some factors ameliorating the inhibition of TGFβ signaling.

2.3. Inflammation-Related Response of Regenerating Muscles

The successful regeneration of skeletal muscles is a result of properly executed degeneration and regeneration phase. First one is associated with the removal of damaged muscle fibers, infiltration with immune cells and activation of satellite cells. Second one covers the differentiation of satellite cells derived myoblasts into myotubes maturing into myofibers and reconstruction of extracellular matrix. The success of both of the phases depends not only of satellite cells function but to great extent on proper timing of action of immune cells infiltrating the site of injury [64–66]. Thus, we analyzed the proportion of lymphocytes characterized by the expression of CD45, proinflammatory M1-macrophages expressing CD68, and anti-inflammatory M2 macrophages expressing CD163 [66,67]. At day 7 after injury the proportion of CD45+ cells was significantly increased in all muscles that received Matrigel with ADSCs, regardless of additional treatments, and also Matrigel pretreated with myoblast-conditioned medium (Figure 5A,B). Next, the influx of proinflammatory M1 macrophages was higher in regenerating muscle implanted with Matrigel pretreated with myoblast-conditioned medium and that one pretreated with anti-TGFβ antibody and containing ADSCs. Importantly, only in latter case, i.e., Matrigel pretreated with anti-TGFβ with ADSCs we noticed significant increase in the proportion of anti-inflammatory M2 macrophages (Figure 5A,B).

Next, we analyzed the levels of mRNAs encoding selected cytokines playing important role during skeletal muscle regeneration. We have chosen to analyze CCL2 (C-C Motif Chemokine Ligand 2)—a macrophage-produced cytokine responsible for attracting neutrophils, which is necessary to remove cellular debris [68]; IL-1b, IL-6, and TNFα mediate the inflammatory response and are proinflammatory cytokines produced, e.g., by infiltrated monocytes/macrophages [69–71] and IL-10—an anti-inflammatory cytokine that regulates changes in macrophage phenotype [72] and improves skeletal muscle regeneration [73,74]. At day 7 after injury the levels of proinflammatory cytokines were increased, as compared to control intact muscle. The level of mRNA encoding anti-inflammatory IL-10 remained low (Figure 6A). Transplantation of Matrigel alone or Matrigel containing ADSCs, control or treated either with myoblast-conditioned medium or anti-TGFβ antibody did not have substantial beneficial effect at inflammation (Figure 6B). In general proinflammatory cytokines were increased in every analyzed group of muscle, as compared to control injured muscle. Interestingly, muscles that received ADSCs embedded in Matrigel pretreated with anti-TGFβ antibody were characterized by levels of CCL2, IL-1b, IL-6, and TNFα similar to that observed in control injured muscle (Figure 6B). IL-1b and IL-6 mRNA levels were increased in muscle transplanted with ADSC containing Matrigel which was pretreated with myoblast-conditioned medium. The mRNA encoding anti-inflammatory IL-10 was upregulated in all analyzed samples, as compared to injured control. Importantly, the presence of ADSCs lowered the expression of these interleukin (Figure 6B).

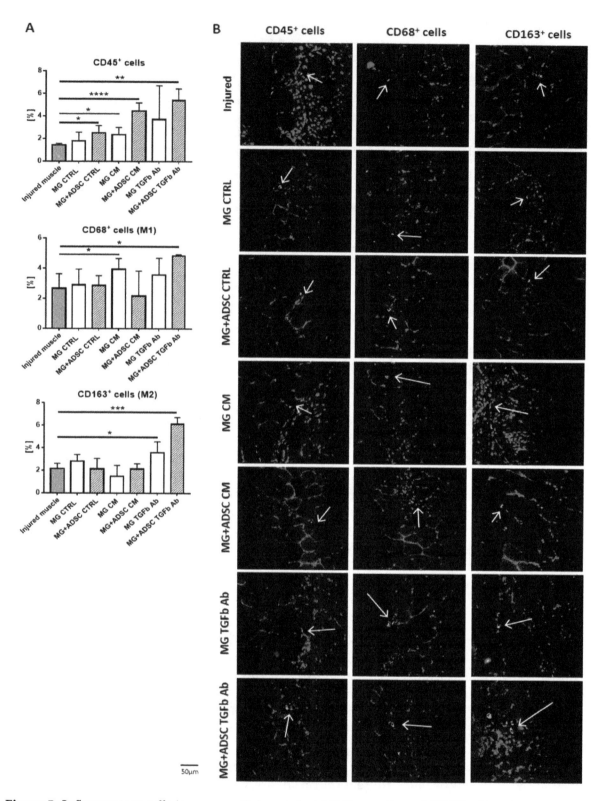

Figure 5. Inflammatory cells in regenerating muscles. (**A**) Proportion of CD45$^+$, CD68$^+$, and CD163$^+$ cells, presented as percentage of all nuclei, present in regenerating skeletal muscles of all analyzed groups. (**B**) Localization of CD45$^+$, CD68$^+$, and CD163$^+$ cells in regenerating skeletal muscles of all analyzed groups. Green - CD45$^+$, CD68$^+$ or CD163$^+$ cells, red - nuclei. Arrows indicates localization of analyzed cells. For each experimental group $n \geq 3$. Data are presented as mean ± SD. *represent results of Student's *t*-test: * $p \leq 0.05$; ** $p \leq 0.01$, *** $p \leq 0.001$, **** $p \leq 0.0001$. Bar: 500 μm.

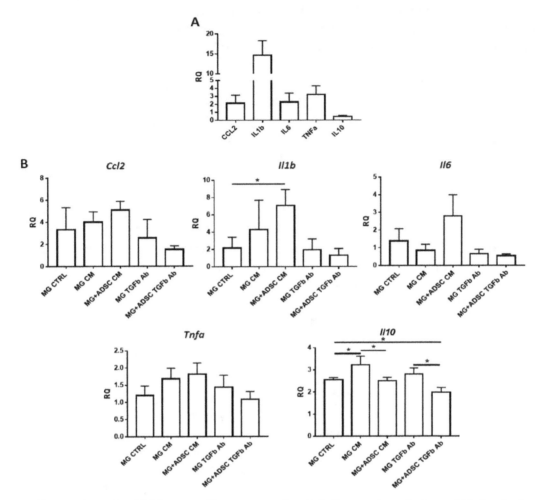

Figure 6. Expression of mRNAs encoding pro- and anti-inflammatory factors. (**A**) Analysis of the level of mRNAs encoding CCL2, IL1b, IL6, TNFα, and IL10 in control injured muscles. (**B**) Expression of cytokines studied in muscles which received Matrigel only or Matrigel with ADSC pretreated in control (CTRL), myoblast-conditioned (CM), or supplemented with antibody against TGFβ (TGFb Ab) medium. Expression was related to the levels observed in injured muscles, and normalized to mRNA encoding β-actin. RQ - relative quantity. For each experimental group $n \geq 3$. Data are presented as mean ± SD. * represent results of Student's t-test: * $p \leq 0.05$.

Thus, an increased proportion of M2 macrophages and level of anti-inflammatory factors in muscles, to which Matrigel pretreated with anti-TGFβ antibody and containing ADSCs was transplanted, significantly improved skeletal muscle regeneration.

3. Discussion

Various types of cells are widely tested as a "material" that can be used in therapies supporting tissues and organs repair or function. In such context, the "ideal cell" should present the ability to differentiate into required cell or tissue type and/or support regeneration by other means, e.g., by releasing growth or anti-inflammatory factors. Unfortunately, such ideal stem cell was not identified so far. The best ability to differentiate is attributed to pluripotent stem cells, i.e., embryonic stem cells (ESCs) or induced pluripotent stem cells (iPSCs). They were shown to be extremely easy to propagate and able to differentiate into any given tissue [75–77]. In addition, iPSCs could be produced from patient somatic cells what would allow the derivation of syngeneic cells for transplantation. Unfortunately, the methods of pluripotent stem cells differentiation are still not perfect, and some of the cell types, such as skeletal muscle myoblasts, are not easy to derive [37,78]. Moreover, there are also well-founded worries that if not properly prepared these cells can differentiate chaotically within the recipient tissue, forming so-called teratomas, what might pose serious health risk [79]. For these reason multipotent stem cells, such as MSCs and among them ADSCs, attract increasing attention. Their characteristic is quite different from that of ESCs or iPSCs. MSCs could be isolated from various sources, such as bone marrow or adipose tissue, present limited ability to differentiate and for this reason do not form teratomas. However, when appropriately treated they do undergo chondro-, osteo-, and adipogenesis [80,81]. Many lines of evidence indicate that under certain experimental conditions they can also differentiate into such cell types as myoblasts [32] or even those ones of other than mesodermal origin, e.g., neurons [82,83]. However, the efficiency of such differentiation is still not the highest. In vitro analyzes showed that MSCs, isolated from umbilical cord connective tissue are able, for example, to form hybrid myotubes with C2C12 cells [84]. Moreover, MSCs were shown to be able to colonize regenerating muscle and participate in the formation of new myofibers, however, with very low frequency [34–36,84]. ADSCs were also documented to be able to undergo myogenic differentiation in vitro or in vivo, i.e., when transplanted to the muscles of *mdx* mice [43]. These and other lines of evidence documented that they are able to colonize the tissue and participate in its regeneration. In our study we introduced Matrigel embedded ADSCs into severely damaged mouse gastrocnemius muscle. Our in vitro study showed that such cells are able to proliferate and migrate under culture conditions applied by us, i.e., either in control, myoblast-conditioned medium, or in the presence of anti-TGFβ antibody. Based on previous reports we also hoped that they will be able to participate in the formation of new myofibers. Unfortunately, ADSCs introduced by us were not able to participate in myofiber regeneration; however, they were detectable within the muscle at day 7 after injury. Such results are in agreement with our previous study during which we were able to detect other MSCs within the regenerating muscle [84,85]. This inconsistency between our findings and those ones of Zhang et al. [43] could be a result of different experimental settings used in these two studies. First of all, we analyzed regeneration of massively injured muscles transplanted with Matrigel containing ADSC which were pretreated either with conditioned medium or anti-TGFβ antibody. Zhang et al studied mdx mouse muscles transplanted with ADSCs that were treated with BIO, bFGF, and forskolin for as long as 7 days, followed by their exposition to ADSC culture supernatant. Such experimental conditions resulted in the participation of these cells in the muscle regeneration. Apparently, the treatment proposed by us is not as efficient. However, despite that ADSCs transplanted within Matrigel did not participate in the skeletal muscle regeneration they were able to impact at this process. Thus, the differentiation into required cell or tissue type is not the action which makes MSCs, such as ADSCs, useful as a tool to improve regeneration. The major impact of MSCs at the regenerating tissue relies at their ability to immunomodulate the function of other cells present within the site of the injury [86–88]

We showed that introduction of Matrigel and ADSCs increased the number of CD45+ and CD68+ cells, increasing the local inflammation. However, the most important phenotype we observed in case of CD163+ cells, i.e., anti-inflammatory macrophages which were dramatically increased in skeletal muscles which received anti-TGFβ antibody pretreated Matrigel containing ADSCs. TGFβ modifies activation and proliferation of lymphocytes, induces maturation of monocytes to macrophages, and also acts as macrophage chemoattractant. Thus, the modification of TGFβ level may modulate inflammation and result in the improvement of muscle repair. The development of inflammatory response and its effective silencing are crucial for skeletal muscle regeneration. M2 macrophages play an important role in improving skeletal muscle regeneration. They do not phagocytose degenerating skeletal muscle fibers but rather produce growth factors, such as fibroblast growth factor (FGF) and insulin-like growth factor (IGF-1), and as a result of myoblast proliferation. [73,89,90]. The action of M2 macrophages relies at their secretory activity. Many studies have shown that they secrete various soluble factors as well as release exosomes and by such action may impact at other cell function [91]. Moreover, pretreatment of ADSCs with various growth factors or cytokines may modulate their function [92–95]. Our current result showed that presence of ADSCs within the transplanted Matrigel significantly improved the structure of regenerating muscle. For example, transplantation of Matrigel treated with myoblast-preconditioned medium resulted in the higher number of immature muscle fibers, as compared to control, i.e., injured muscle. Presence of ADSCs in such Matrigel increased the number of mature fibers, i.e., with peripherally positioned nuclei. Moreover, ADSCs modulated the outcome of anti-TGFβ antibody treatment—in the presence of cells development of connective tissue was significantly limited. Analyzing the level of mRNAs encoding proinflammatory cytokines we noticed that combination of anti-TGFβ antibody infused Matrigel and ADSCs resulted in the level of mRNAs comparable to nontreated, injured muscle. This is especially important since we showed that transplantation of Matrigel increases the level of inflammation, as judged by the expression of CCL2, IL-1b, or IL-6. Thus, the presence of biomaterial might not necessarily be beneficial for the skeletal muscle regeneration and if such is used to improve the regeneration of volumetric injuries it might be of important combine it with certain regeneration-supporting factors or MSCs. In fact, many lines of evidence document that 3D cultures of cells in Matrigel could be beneficial for proliferation and/or differentiation. For example, differentiation of myoblasts cultured in Matrigel was shown to be improved [96]. As far as MSCs are concerned those ones isolated from bone marrow and transplanted within Matrigel was shown to improve soleus muscle regeneration. This was manifested by fewer immature myofibers, however, no impact at fibrosis development was noticed and immune status of such muscles was not analyzed [56].

Combining Matrigel as a stem cell scaffold with additional factors might be another approach to improve tissue repair. The benefits of silencing of TGFβ signaling during skeletal muscle regeneration have been previously shown by us for slow-twitch Soleus muscles, which regeneration is affected by the excessive ECM deposition. Blocking TGFβ action with specific antibodies decreased fibrosis and significantly improved regeneration [52]. Decrease in ECM deposition was also characteristic for muscles treated with such factors inhibiting TGFβ activity as suramin [97], angiotensin receptor blocker [98] or as a result of blocking of TGFβ receptor—TβRI [99]. Importantly, TGFβ was also shown to inhibit proliferation and differentiation of myoblasts [50,100]. Thus, our results documenting complete abolishment of ADSC proliferation by TGFβ and improvement of the regeneration of muscles to which Matrigel pretreated with anti-TGFβ antibody containing ADSCs was transplanted are in agreement with abovementioned findings. The use of myoblast-conditioned medium tested in our study did not appear as beneficial as expected. Transplantation of Matrigel pretreated with such medium resulted with lower muscle mass and affected muscle regeneration, what was documented by increased number of immature myofibers. This effect was counteracted by the addition of ADSCs to such Matrigel. In other experimental setting, however, such medium was shown to improve tissue regeneration impacting revascularization of damaged skeletal muscle tissue [61] or preventing intramuscular adipose tissue differentiation and lipid accumulation [101].

4. Materials and Methods

All procedures involving animals were approved by Local Ethics Committee No. 1 in Warsaw, Poland, permissions number 626/2014 (6 December 2014) and 493/2017 (4 January 2018).

4.1. Cell Culture

Adipose tissue was isolated from C57BL/6J male mice (aged 6–8 weeks) and transferred to betadine solution (8μL/mL, EGIS Polska sp. z o.o.) and then washed with Phospate Buffered Saline. ADSC were isolated by digestion of fragmented adipose tissue with 0.2% type I collagenase solution (Sigma-Aldrich, Saint Louis, MI, USA) for 90 min at 37 °C. Cells were cultured in Dulbecco's Modified Eagle's Medium (DMEM, Invitrogen, Carlsbad, CA, USA) (4.5 g glucose/L) supplemented with 50% FBS (Invitrogen), and gentamycin (Sigma-Aldrich). Cells were cultured at 37 °C in the atmosphere of 5% CO_2 and analyzed at day 1 (24 h), day 3 and day 7 of culture.

Control ADSCs were cultured under the standard conditions. ADSC were additionally pretreated for 48 h either with 10 μL/mL anti-TGFβ antibody (Santa Cruz Biotechnology, Dallas, TX, USA) or 0.25 ng/mL Recombinant Mouse TGF-β1 (carrier-free) (BioLegend, San Diego, CA, USA) dissolved in 1% Bovine Serum Albumin or conditioned by myoblast medium. Conditioned medium was obtained from confluent culture of fusing/differentiating C2C12 mouse myoblasts cell line. Twenty-four hours before application to ADSC culture, the medium (DMEM 4.5 g glucose/L, supplemented with 15% FBS, and gentamycin was changed in the culture of C2C12 cells. After 24 h the medium was filtered using a 40 μm pore filter. The filtered medium was used for ADSC cell culture. Optimal concentration of reagents and necessary frequency of cell treatments were determined experimentally.

The morphology of cultured cells was analyzed using Nikon Eclipse, TE200 microscope with Hoffman contrast. Cell proliferation was assessed by counting the total number of cells at day 1 (24 h), day 3 and day 7 of culture after their detachment from 10 mm culture dishes using 0.05% trypsin (Invitrogen).

4.2. Migration Assay

Migration of ADSC was analyzed using scratch wound healing assay [102]. Briefly, cells were plated in the 8 cm^2 culture dish and cultured until they reached 90% of confluency. Next, the cells were scratched from the plate using plastic automatic pipette tip to create the "wound." The wound healing manifested by the ability of the cells to refill the created gap was monitored after 6 and 24 h of culture. Three independent experiments were performed.

4.3. qPCR

RNA isolation was performed with the High Pure RNA Isolation Kit (ADSC) or mirVana miRNA Isolation Kit (muscles) according to the manufacturer's (Roche or Thermo Fisher Scientific, respectively) recommendation. Reverse transcription was performed using 0.5 μg total RNA and RevertAid First Strand cDNA Synthesis Kit (Thermo Fisher Scientific, Waltham, MA, USA), according to the manufacturer's instruction. qPCR was performed using the following specific TaqMan® probes; mm00493682_g1 (Thy1-CD90), mm00440701_m1 (Pdgfra), mm00501910_m1 (Nt5e-CD73), Mm00441242 (CCL2), Mm00434228 (IL1b), Mm00446190 (IL6), Mm00443258 (TNF-α), and Mm01288386 (IL10), using the TaqMan Gene Expression Master Mix (Thermo Fisher Scientific) and Light Cycler 96 instrument (Roche, Basel, Switzerland). Data was collected and analyzed with Light Cycler 96 SW1.1 software (Roche). Analysis of relative gene expression using quantitative PCR and the 2(T) (-Delta Delta Ct) method was performed according to Livak and Schmittgen [103].

4.4. ADSC Labeling Using BacMam GFP Transduction Control

BacMam GFP Transduction Control (Invitrogen) was added to ADSC culture medium (150 μL/12 mL culture medium, i.e., approximately 1.5×10^6 cells). Incubated for 10 min at room temperature and then left overnight in ADSC culture. After this time the BacMam GFP medium was removed and the culture was supplemented with a fresh medium. The procedure was carried out as recommended, based on the manufacturer's protocol.

4.5. Three-Dimensional ADSC Culture in Matrigel and Pretreatment with TGFβ Antibody or Conditioned Medium

ADSC was cultured under standard conditions (monolayer culture) until the desired number of cells was obtained and then cells were labeled with BacMam GFP Transduction Control. Cells marked with GFP marker were washed three times with PBS. Cells were removed from the dish by adding trypsin and a few minutes incubation (~5–7 min) at 37 °C. Suspended cells were transferred to a centrifuge tube and centrifuged at 1300 rpm for 8 min. After centrifugation the supernatant was discarded and the sediment was suspended in ADSC culture medium to obtain solution of 250,000 in 10 μL of the medium. The next steps in the procedure were carried out on ice, i.e., 290 μL of Matrigel was collected and then 10 μL of cell suspension was added (250,000 ADSC). The cells in Matrigel were distributed by pipetting several times and the suspension was transferred to the 1 cm^2 well of the 4-well dish. In variants without cells 300 μL of Matrigel was collected and transferred to the dish. The procedure was repeated until all the necessary variants were prepared. The Matrigel was maintained at a temperature of about 4 °C all the time in order to keep it in the liquid form. Then the

Matrigel seeded with cells or Matrigel itself was incubated for 30 min at 37 °C to form a gel, after which 300 μL of medium (control, or containing 10 μL/mL anti-TGFβ antibody, or 0.25 ng/mL Recombinant Mouse TGF-β1, or conditioned by myoblasts medium) was added to each well. Matrigel with cells was photographed (Nikon TE200 microscope using NIS Elements program, Minato, Tokyo, Japan). The 3D structures were left in the incubator (37 °C, 5% CO_2) for 48 h. After this time the medium was discarded and the gel transplanted into the muscles.

4.6. Skeletal Muscle Injury and Transplantation of Matrigel

After the animals (6–8-week-old male C57BL/6J) were anesthetized with isoflurane the surgical field, was cleared from fur and this area was topically anaesthetized with 4% Lidocain. Next, right gastrocnemius muscle was exposed (from the Achilles tendon to the knee) by cutting the skin and making 3-mm-long and 3-mm-deep incision within the middle part of the muscle belly. Then Matrigel with/without ADSC cells was introduced to such site of muscle injury and the skin was sutured. Each variant of the experiment was performed in three biological repeats. After the procedure mice were kept under standard conditions with free access to food and water. Additional control was provided by (1) muscles not subjected to any procedures (intact) and (2) muscles injured (without ADSC transplantation in Matrigel)—three biological repeats for each variant. After 7 days mice were killed by spinal cord dislocation. Muscles and mouse from which the muscle was taken were weighed. The isolated muscles were frozen in isopentane cooled in liquid nitrogen and stored at −80 °C.

4.7. Histological Analyzes—Myofibers Number and Connective Tissue Area

The frozen muscles were cut into sections of 10 μm thickness using cryostat (Microm HM505N). Cross-sections were placed on slides and after drying were stored at 4 °C. Sections were hydrated in PBS (10 min), and then stained in Harris hematoxylin solution for 40 min, washed gently under tap water (about 5 min), and stained in Gomori trichrome solution (30 min). After staining, sections were rinsed again under tap water (~5 min). Dehydrated in 96% ethanol (2 × 3 min) and then in 100% ethanol (2 × 3 min). Dehydrated preparations were immersed twice in Neoclear xylene equivalent (2 × 8 min), and closed with Entalan. The samples were analyzed using Nikon TE200 microscope and NIS Elements program. The number of newly formed myofibers (immature) was determined in relation to the number of undamaged myofibers (mature) at the day 7 of regeneration. The photos of sections from each of the 3 replicates for each variant were analyzed and the results were presented as a proportion of the number of mature and immature myofibers on the sections. The area occupied by the connective tissue in relation to the area of the entire section was calculated using ImageJ software. The sections of each of the 3 repetitions for each variant were analyzed. The obtained data were averaged and presented on a graph.

4.8. Immunolocalization

In the first stage muscle cross-sections were rehydrated for 10 min. in PBS, and then fixed for 10 min in 3% paraformaldehyde (Sigma-Aldrich) in PBS. Next, cells or muscle sections were permeabilized with 0.1% Triton X-100/PBS (Sigma-Aldrich) and incubated with 0.25% glycine for 15 min (Sigma-Aldrich). Nonspecific binding of antibodies was blocked with 3% bovine serum albumin (BSA, Sigma-Aldrich) in PBS, at room temperature, for 30 min. Next, sections were incubated for with primary antibodies: rabbit against Laminin (Sigma-Aldrich), rat against CD45 (Abcam), rat anti-CD68 (Abcam), and rabbit anti-CD163 (Abcam) diluted 1:100 in 3% BSA in PBS overnight, washed with PBS, and incubated at room temperature with secondary donkey antibodies with Alexa Fluor 594, (Life Technologies, Carlsbad, CA, USA) diluted 1:200 in 3% BSA in PBS. After washing with PBS, cell nuclei were visualized by incubation with DRAQ5 (Biostatus Limited, Shepshed, Loughborough, Great Britain) diluted 1:1000 in PBS for 10 min. Specimens were mounted with Fluorescent Mounting Medium (Dako Cytomation, Glostrup, Denmark). After the procedure was completed samples were analyzed using Axio Observer Z1 scanning confocal microscope (Zeiss, Oberkochen, Germany) equipped with LSM 700 software (Zeiss). For the analysis of leukocytes and macrophages presence the photos of sections from each of the 3 independent replicates for each variant were analyzed and the results were presented as a proportion of the number of $CD45^+$, $CD68^+$, or $CD163^+$ cells and all nuclei on the 3 pictures of each of three sections were analyzed. The obtained data were averaged and presented on a graph.

4.9. Statistical Analysis

Results were analyzed using GraphPad Software (San Diego, CaliphCA, USA) and nonpaired *t*-test was performed to compare treated with the control cells/muscles. The differences were considered statistically significant when $p < 0.05$. Each analysis was repeated three times. Data are expressed as mean ± standard deviation. Statistical significance was determined using a Student's *t*-test - * $p < 0.05$; ** $p < 0.01$; *** $p < 0.005$.

5. Conclusions

ADSCs can be considered as a suitable material for replacement therapies. Results of our study document that transplantation of preconditioned ADSCs in Matrigel 3D structures in combination with silencing of TGFβ signaling could improve skeletal muscle regeneration as judged by muscle mass and structure, proportion of mature myofibers, decreased level of fibrosis, and an increase in the number of anti-inflammatory macrophages and appropriate levels of inflammation-regulating factors. Thus, by silencing this signaling pathway the regeneration could be improved. However, the molecular basis of this phenomenon is still unclear. Elucidation of molecular changes triggered by silencing TGFβ signaling would uncover more precise targets which could be "used" as a tool to improve skeletal muscle regeneration. Also other preconditioning treatments, such as application of selected cytokines, in combination with 3D scaffolds should be investigated.

Author Contributions: Conceptualization: I.G. and M.A.C.; methodology: I.G., M.Z., and E.B.; formal analysis: I.G.; investigation: I.G., M.Z., K.M., Z.J., A.B., M.O., W.S., J.B., and E.B.; data curation: I.G., M.Z., J.B., and E.B.; writing—original draft preparation, M.A.C. and IG; writing—review and editing, I.G., M.Z., E.B., and M.A.C.; visualization: I.G.; supervision: I.G. and M.A.C.; project administration: I.G. and M.A.C.; funding acquisition: M.A.C.

Acknowledgments: The authors thank Katarzyna Janczyk-Ilach for her excellent technical support.

Abbreviations

ADSC	adipose tissue-derived stromal cell
BM-MSC	bone marrow-derived mesenchymal stromal cell
CM	myoblast-conditioned medium
CTRL	control medium
ECM	extracellular matrix
ESC	embryonic stem cell
FBS	fetal bovine serum
iPSC	induced pluripotent stem cell
MDSC	muscle-derived stem cell
MG	Matrigel
MSC	mesenchymal stem/stromal cell
TGFβ	transforming growth factor beta
TGFb	medium supplemented with TGFβ
TGFb Ab	medium supplemented with antibody against TGFβ

References

1.   Schmidt, M.; Schuler, S.C.; Huttner, S.S.; von Eyss, B.; von Maltzahn, J. Adult stem cells at work: Regenerating skeletal muscle. *Cell Mol. Life Sci.* **2019**. [CrossRef] [PubMed]

2. Bouchentouf, M.; Benabdallah, B.F.; Rousseau, J.; Schwartz, L.M.; Tremblay, J.P. Induction of Anoikis following myoblast transplantation into SCID mouse muscles requires the Bit1 and FADD pathways. *Am. J. Transplant.* **2007**, *7*, 1491–1505. [CrossRef] [PubMed]

3. Skuk, D.; Caron, N.J.; Goulet, M.; Roy, B.; Tremblay, J.P. Resetting the problem of cell death following muscle-derived cell transplantation: Detection, dynamics and mechanisms. *J. Neuropathol. Exp. Neurol.* **2003**, *62*, 951–967. [CrossRef] [PubMed]

4. Fan, Y.; Maley, M.; Beilharz, M.; Grounds, M. Rapid death of injected myoblasts in myoblast transfer therapy. *Muscle Nerve* **1996**, *19*, 853–860. [CrossRef]

5. Skuk, D.; Tremblay, J.P. Cell Therapy in Myology: Dynamics of Muscle Precursor Cell Death after Intramuscular Administration in Non-human Primates. *Mol. Ther Methods Clin. Dev.* **2017**, *5*, 232–240. [CrossRef] [PubMed]

6. Rando, T.A.; Blau, H.M. Primary mouse myoblast purification, characterization, and transplantation for cell-mediated gene therapy. *J. Cell Biol.* **1994**, *125*, 1275–1287. [CrossRef] [PubMed]

7. Rando, T.A.; Pavlath, G.K.; Blau, H.M. The fate of myoblasts following transplantation into mature muscle. *Exp. Cell Res.* **1995**, *220*, 383–389. [CrossRef]

8. Ito, H.; Hallauer, P.L.; Hastings, K.E.; Tremblay, J.P. Prior culture with concanavalin A increases intramuscular migration of transplanted myoblast. *Muscle Nerve* **1998**, *21*, 291–297. [CrossRef]

9. Morgan, J.; Rouche, A.; Bausero, P.; Houssaini, A.; Gross, J.; Fiszman, M.Y.; Alameddine, H.S. MMP-9 overexpression improves myogenic cell migration and engraftment. *Muscle Nerve* **2011**, *42*, 584–595. [CrossRef]

10. Lafreniere, J.F.; Mills, P.; Tremblay, J.P.; El Fahime, E. Growth factors improve the in vivo migration of human skeletal myoblasts by modulating their endogenous proteolytic activity. *Transplantation* **2004**, *77*, 1741–1747. [CrossRef]

11. Torrente, Y.; El Fahime, E.; Caron, N.J.; Bresolin, N.; Tremblay, J.P. Intramuscular migration of myoblasts transplanted after muscle pretreatment with metalloproteinases. *Cell Transplant.* **2000**, *9*, 539–549. [CrossRef] [PubMed]

12. Bouchentouf, M.; Benabdallah, B.F.; Tremblay, J.P. Myoblast survival enhancement and transplantation success improvement by heat-shock treatment in mdx mice. *Transplantation* **2004**, *77*, 1349–1356. [CrossRef] [PubMed]

13. El Fahime, E.; Bouchentouf, M.; Benabdallah, B.F.; Skuk, D.; Lafreniere, J.F.; Chang, Y.T.; Tremblay, J.P. Tubulyzine, a novel tri-substituted triazine, prevents the early cell death of transplanted myogenic cells and improves transplantation success. *Biochem. Cell Biol.* **2003**, *81*, 81–90. [CrossRef] [PubMed]

14. Fakhfakh, R.; Lamarre, Y.; Skuk, D.; Tremblay, J.P. Losartan enhances the success of myoblast transplantation. *Cell Transplant.* **2011**. [CrossRef] [PubMed]

15. Benabdallah, B.F.; Bouchentouf, M.; Rousseau, J.; Bigey, P.; Michaud, A.; Chapdelaine, P.; Scherman, D.; Tremblay, J.P. Inhibiting myostatin with follistatin improves the success of myoblast transplantation in dystrophic mice. *Cell Transplant.* **2008**, *17*, 337–350. [CrossRef] [PubMed]

16. Boldrin, L.; Malerba, A.; Vitiello, L.; Cimetta, E.; Piccoli, M.; Messina, C.; Gamba, P.G.; Elvassore, N.; De Coppi, P. Efficient delivery of human single fiber-derived muscle precursor cells via biocompatible scaffold. *Cell Transplant.* **2008**, *17*, 577–584. [CrossRef]

17. Gerard, C.; Forest, M.A.; Beauregard, G.; Skuk, D.; Tremblay, J.P. Fibrin gel improves the survival of transplanted myoblasts. *Cell Transplant.* **2011**. [CrossRef]

18. Cezar, C.A.; Mooney, D.J. Biomaterial-based delivery for skeletal muscle repair. *Adv. Drug Deliv Rev.* **2015**, *84*, 188–197. [CrossRef]

19. Morosetti, R.; Gidaro, T.; Broccolini, A.; Gliubizzi, C.; Sancricca, C.; Tonali, P.A.; Ricci, E.; Mirabella, M. Mesoangioblasts from facioscapulohumeral muscular dystrophy display in vivo a variable myogenic ability predictable by their in vitro behavior. *Cell Transplant.* **2011**, *20*, 1299–1313. [CrossRef]

20. Rotini, A.; Martinez-Sarra, E.; Duelen, R.; Costamagna, D.; Di Filippo, E.S.; Giacomazzi, G.; Grosemans, H.; Fulle, S.; Sampaolesi, M. Aging affects the in vivo regenerative potential of human mesoangioblasts. *Aging Cell* **2018**, *17*. [CrossRef]

21. Quattrocelli, M.; Costamagna, D.; Giacomazzi, G.; Camps, J.; Sampaolesi, M. Notch signaling regulates myogenic regenerative capacity of murine and human mesoangioblasts. *Cell Death Dis.* **2014**, *5*, e1448. [CrossRef] [PubMed]

22. Dellavalle, A.; Maroli, G.; Covarello, D.; Azzoni, E.; Innocenzi, A.; Perani, L.; Antonini, S.; Sambasivan, R.; Brunelli, S.; Tajbakhsh, S.; et al. Pericytes resident in postnatal skeletal muscle differentiate into muscle fibres and generate satellite cells. *Nat. Commun.* **2011**, *2*, 499. [CrossRef] [PubMed]

23. Dellavalle, A.; Sampaolesi, M.; Tonlorenzi, R.; Tagliafico, E.; Sacchetti, B.; Perani, L.; Innocenzi, A.; Galvez, B.G.; Messina, G.; Morosetti, R.; et al. Pericytes of human skeletal muscle are myogenic precursors distinct from satellite cells. *Nat. Cell Biol.* **2007**, *9*, 255–267. [CrossRef] [PubMed]

24. Mitchell, K.J.; Pannerec, A.; Cadot, B.; Parlakian, A.; Besson, V.; Gomes, E.R.; Marazzi, G.; Sassoon, D.A. Identification and characterization of a non-satellite cell muscle resident progenitor during postnatal development. *Nat. Cell Biol.* **2010**, *12*, 257–266. [CrossRef] [PubMed]

25. Tanaka, K.K.; Hall, J.K.; Troy, A.A.; Cornelison, D.D.; Majka, S.M.; Olwin, B.B. Syndecan-4-expressing muscle progenitor cells in the SP engraft as satellite cells during muscle regeneration. *Cell Stem Cell* **2009**, *4*, 217–225. [CrossRef] [PubMed]

26. Lee, J.Y.; Qu-Petersen, Z.; Cao, B.; Kimura, S.; Jankowski, R.; Cummins, J.; Usas, A.; Gates, C.; Robbins, P.; Wernig, A.; et al. Clonal isolation of muscle-derived cells capable of enhancing muscle regeneration and bone healing. *J. Cell Biol.* **2000**, *150*, 1085–1100. [CrossRef] [PubMed]

27. Aulino, P.; Costa, A.; Chiaravalloti, E.; Perniconi, B.; Adamo, S.; Coletti, D.; Marrelli, M.; Tatullo, M.; Teodori, L. Muscle Extracellular Matrix Scaffold Is a Multipotent Environment. *Int. J. Med. Sci.* **2015**, *12*, 336–340. [CrossRef]

28. Zuk, P.A.; Zhu, M.; Ashjian, P.; De Ugarte, D.A.; Huang, J.I.; Mizuno, H.; Alfonso, Z.C.; Fraser, J.K.; Benhaim, P.; Hedrick, M.H. Human adipose tissue is a source of multipotent stem cells. *Mol. Biol. Cell* **2002**, *13*, 4279–4295. [CrossRef]

29. Lv, F.J.; Tuan, R.S.; Cheung, K.M.; Leung, V.Y. Concise review: The surface markers and identity of human mesenchymal stem cells. *Stem Cells* **2014**, *32*, 1408–1419. [CrossRef]

30. Dominici, M.; Le Blanc, K.; Mueller, I.; Slaper-Cortenbach, I.; Marini, F.; Krause, D.; Deans, R.; Keating, A.; Prockop, D.; Horwitz, E. Minimal criteria for defining multipotent mesenchymal stromal cells. The International Society for Cellular Therapy position statement. *Cytotherapy* **2006**, *8*, 315–317. [CrossRef]

31. Buhring, H.J.; Battula, V.L.; Treml, S.; Schewe, B.; Kanz, L.; Vogel, W. Novel markers for the prospective isolation of human MSC. *Ann. N Y Acad Sci.* **2007**, *1106*, 262–271. [CrossRef] [PubMed]

32. Wakitani, S.; Saito, T.; Caplan, A.I. Myogenic cells derived from rat bone marrow mesenchymal stem cells exposed to 5-azacytidine. *Muscle Nerve* **1995**, *18*, 1417–1426. [CrossRef] [PubMed]

33. LaBarge, M.A.; Blau, H.M. Biological progression from adult bone marrow to mononucleate muscle stem cell to multinucleate muscle fiber in response to injury. *Cell* **2002**, *111*, 589–601. [CrossRef]

34. Brazelton, T.R.; Nystrom, M.; Blau, H.M. Significant differences among skeletal muscles in the incorporation of bone marrow-derived cells. *Dev. Biol.* **2003**, *262*, 64–74. [CrossRef]

35. Gussoni, E.; Soneoka, Y.; Strickland, C.D.; Buzney, E.A.; Khan, M.K.; Flint, A.F.; Kunkel, L.M.; Mulligan, R.C. Dystrophin expression in the mdx mouse restored by stem cell transplantation. *Nature* **1999**, *401*, 390–394. [CrossRef] [PubMed]

36. Fukada, S.; Miyagoe-Suzuki, Y.; Tsukihara, H.; Yuasa, K.; Higuchi, S.; Ono, S.; Tsujikawa, K.; Takeda, S.; Yamamoto, H. Muscle regeneration by reconstitution with bone marrow or fetal liver cells from green fluorescent protein-gene transgenic mice. *J. Cell Sci.* **2002**, *115*, 1285–1293.

37. Archacka, K.; Brzoska, E.; Ciemerych, M.A.; Czerwinska, A.M.; Grabowska, I.; Kowalski, K.K.; Zimowska, M. Pluripotent and Mesenchymal Stem Cells—Challenging Sources for Derivation of Myoblast. In *Cardiac Cell Culture Technologies*; Brzozka, Z., Jastrzebska, E., Eds.; Springer International Publishing: Berlin/Heidelberg, Germany, 2018; pp. 109–154.

38. Paduano, F.; Marrelli, M.; Amantea, M.; Rengo, C.; Rengo, S.; Goldberg, M.; Spagnuolo, G.; Tatullo, M. Adipose Tissue as a Strategic Source of Mesenchymal Stem Cells in Bone Regeneration: A Topical Review on the Most Promising Craniomaxillofacial Applications. *Int. J. Mol. Sci.* **2017**, *18*. [CrossRef]

39. Santos, J.; Milthorpe, B.K.; Padula, M.P. Proteomic Analysis of Cyclic Ketamine Compounds Ability to Induce Neural Differentiation in Human Adult Mesenchymal Stem Cells. *Int. J. Mol. Sci.* **2019**, *20*. [CrossRef]

40. Shi, F.S.; Yang, Y.; Wang, T.C.; Kouadir, M.; Zhao, D.M.; Hu, S.H. Cellular Prion Protein Promotes Neuronal Differentiation of Adipose-Derived Stem Cells by Upregulating miRNA-124 (vol 59, pg 48, 2016). *J. Mol. Neurosci.* **2016**, *59*, 56–57. [CrossRef]

41. Ji, W.; Zhang, X.; Ji, L.; Wang, K.; Qiu, Y. Effects of brainderived neurotrophic factor and neurotrophin3 on the neuronal differentiation of rat adiposederived stem cells. *Mol. Med. Rep.* **2015**, *12*, 4981–4988. [CrossRef]

42. Qin, Y.; Zhou, C.; Wang, N.; Yang, H.; Gao, W.Q. Conversion of Adipose Tissue-Derived Mesenchymal Stem Cells to Neural Stem Cell-Like Cells by a Single Transcription Factor, Sox2. *Cell Reprogram* **2015**, *17*, 221–226. [CrossRef] [PubMed]

43. Zhang, Y.; Zhu, Y.; Li, Y.; Cao, J.; Zhang, H.; Chen, M.; Wang, L.; Zhang, C. Long-term engraftment of myogenic progenitors from adipose-derived stem cells and muscle regeneration in dystrophic mice. *Hum. Mol. Genet.* **2015**, *24*, 6029–6040. [CrossRef] [PubMed]

44. de la Garza-Rodea, A.S.; van der Velde, I.; Boersma, H.; Goncalves, M.A.; van Bekkum, D.W.; de Vries, A.A.; Knaan-Shanzer, S. Long-Term Contribution of Human Bone Marrow Mesenchymal Stromal Cells to Skeletal Muscle Regeneration in Mice. *Cell Transplant.* **2010**. [CrossRef] [PubMed]

45. Mizuno, H.; Hyakusoku, H. Mesengenic potential and future clinical perspective of human processed lipoaspirate cells. *J. Nippon Med. Sch* **2003**, *70*, 300–306. [CrossRef] [PubMed]

46. Mizuno, H.; Zuk, P.A.; Zhu, M.; Lorenz, H.P.; Benhaim, P.; Hedrick, M.H. Myogenic differentiation by human processed lipoaspirate cells. *Plast. Reconstr. Surg.* **2002**, *109*, 199–209; discussion 191–210. [CrossRef] [PubMed]

47. Stern-Straeter, J.; Bonaterra, G.A.; Juritz, S.; Birk, R.; Goessler, U.R.; Bieback, K.; Bugert, P.; Schultz, J.; Hormann, K.; Kinscherf, R.; et al. Evaluation of the effects of different culture media on the myogenic differentiation potential of adipose tissue- or bone marrow-derived human mesenchymal stem cells. *Int. J. Mol. Med.* **2014**, *33*, 160–170. [CrossRef] [PubMed]

48. Pinheiro, C.H.; de Queiroz, J.C.; Guimaraes-Ferreira, L.; Vitzel, K.F.; Nachbar, R.T.; de Sousa, L.G.; de Souza, A.L., Jr.; Nunes, M.T.; Curi, R. Local injections of adipose-derived mesenchymal stem cells modulate inflammation and increase angiogenesis ameliorating the dystrophic phenotype in dystrophin-deficient skeletal muscle. *Stem Cell Rev.* **2012**, *8*, 363–374. [CrossRef] [PubMed]

49. Lee, E.M.; Kim, A.Y.; Lee, E.J.; Park, J.K.; Lee, M.M.; Hwang, M.; Kim, C.Y.; Kim, S.Y.; Jeong, K.S. Therapeutic effects of mouse adipose-derived stem cells and losartan in the skeletal muscle of injured mdx mice. *Cell Transplant.* **2015**, *24*, 939–953. [CrossRef]

50. Massague, J.; Cheifetz, S.; Endo, T.; Nadal-Ginard, B. Type beta transforming growth factor is an inhibitor of myogenic differentiation. *Proc. Natl. Acad. Sci. USA* **1986**, *83*, 8206–8210. [CrossRef]

51. Mauviel, A. Transforming growth factor-beta: A key mediator of fibrosis. *Methods Mol. Med.* **2005**, *117*, 69–80. [CrossRef]

52. Zimowska, M.; Duchesnay, A.; Dragun, P.; Oberbek, A.; Moraczewski, J.; Martelly, I. Immunoneutralization of TGFbeta1 Improves Skeletal Muscle Regeneration: Effects on Myoblast Differentiation and Glycosaminoglycan Content. *Int. J. Cell Biol.* **2009**, *2009*, 659372. [CrossRef] [PubMed]

53. Lefaucheur, J.P.; Sebille, A. Muscle regeneration following injury can be modified in vivo by immune neutralization of basic fibroblast growth factor, transforming growth factor beta 1 or insulin-like growth factor I. *J. Neuroimmunol.* **1995**, *57*, 85–91. [CrossRef]

54. Delaney, K.; Kasprzycka, P.; Ciemerych, M.A.; Zimowska, M. The role of TGF-beta1 during skeletal muscle regeneration. *Cell Biol. Int.* **2017**, *41*, 706–715. [CrossRef] [PubMed]

55. Grabowska, I.; Szeliga, A.; Moraczewski, J.; Czaplicka, I.; Brzoska, E. Comparison of satellite cell-derived myoblasts and C2C12 differentiation in two- and three-dimensional cultures: Changes in adhesion protein expression. *Cell Biol. Int.* **2011**, *35*, 125–133. [CrossRef] [PubMed]

56. Andrade, B.M.; Baldanza, M.R.; Ribeiro, K.C.; Porto, A.; Pecanha, R.; Fortes, F.S.; Zapata-Sudo, G.; Campos-de-Carvalho, A.C.; Goldenberg, R.C.; Werneck-de-Castro, J.P. Bone marrow mesenchymal cells improve muscle function in a skeletal muscle re-injury model. *PLoS ONE* **2015**, *10*, e0127561. [CrossRef] [PubMed]

57. Natsu, K.; Ochi, M.; Mochizuki, Y.; Hachisuka, H.; Yanada, S.; Yasunaga, Y. Allogeneic bone marrow-derived mesenchymal stromal cells promote the regeneration of injured skeletal muscle without differentiation into myofibers. *Tissue Eng.* **2004**, *10*, 1093–1112. [CrossRef] [PubMed]

58. Pumberger, M.; Qazi, T.H.; Ehrentraut, M.C.; Textor, M.; Kueper, J.; Stoltenburg-Didinger, G.; Winkler, T.; von Roth, P.; Reinke, S.; Borselli, C.; et al. Synthetic niche to modulate regenerative potential of MSCs and enhance skeletal muscle regeneration. *Biomaterials* **2016**, *99*, 95–108. [CrossRef] [PubMed]

59. Henningsen, J.; Rigbolt, K.T.; Blagoev, B.; Pedersen, B.K.; Kratchmarova, I. Dynamics of the skeletal muscle secretome during myoblast differentiation. *Mol. Cell Proteom.* **2010**, *9*, 2482–2496. [CrossRef] [PubMed]

60. Le Bihan, M.C.; Bigot, A.; Jensen, S.S.; Dennis, J.L.; Rogowska-Wrzesinska, A.; Laine, J.; Gache, V.; Furling, D.; Jensen, O.N.; Voit, T.; et al. In-depth analysis of the secretome identifies three major independent secretory pathways in differentiating human myoblasts. *J. Proteom.* **2012**, *77*, 344–356. [CrossRef]

61. Kozakowska, M.; Kotlinowski, J.; Grochot-Przeczek, A.; Ciesla, M.; Pilecki, B.; Derlacz, R.; Dulak, J.; Jozkowicz, A. Myoblast-conditioned media improve regeneration and revascularization of ischemic muscles in diabetic mice. *Stem Cell Res. Ther.* **2015**, *6*, 61. [CrossRef]

62. Kataoka, H.; Takakura, N.; Nishikawa, S.; Tsuchida, K.; Kodama, H.; Kunisada, T.; Risau, W.; Kita, T.; Nishikawa, S.I. Expressions of PDGF receptor alpha, c-Kit and Flk1 genes clustering in mouse chromosome 5 define distinct subsets of nascent mesodermal cells. *Dev. Growth Differ.* **1997**, *39*, 729–740. [CrossRef] [PubMed]

63. Zimowska, M.; Olszynski, K.H.; Swierczynska, M.; Streminska, W.; Ciemerych, M.A. Decrease of MMP-9 Activity Improves Soleus Muscle Regeneration. *Tissue Eng. Part. A* **2012**, *18*, 1183–1192. [CrossRef] [PubMed]

64. Zimowska, M.; Kasprzycka, P.; Bocian, K.; Delaney, K.; Jung, P.; Kuchcinska, K.; Kaczmarska, K.; Gladysz, D.; Streminska, W.; Ciemerych, M.A. Inflammatory response during slow- and fast-twitch muscle regeneration. *Muscle Nerve* **2017**, *55*, 400–409. [CrossRef] [PubMed]

65. Brzoska, E.; Ciemerych, M.A.; Przewozniak, M.; Zimowska, M. Regulation of muscle stem cells activation: The role of growth factors and extracellular matrix. *Vitam. Horm.* **2011**, *87*, 239–276.

66. Juban, G.; Chazaud, B. Metabolic regulation of macrophages during tissue repair: Insights from skeletal muscle regeneration. *FEBS Lett.* **2017**, *591*, 3007–3021. [CrossRef]

67. Chazaud, B. Macrophages: Supportive cells for tissue repair and regeneration. *Immunobiology* **2014**, *219*, 172–178. [CrossRef]

68. Tidball, J.G. Regulation of muscle growth and regeneration by the immune system. *Nat. Rev. Immunol.* **2017**, *17*, 165–178. [CrossRef]

69. Cohen, T.V.; Many, G.M.; Fleming, B.D.; Gnocchi, V.F.; Ghimbovschi, S.; Mosser, D.M.; Hoffman, E.P.; Partridge, T.A. Upregulated IL-1beta in dysferlin-deficient muscle attenuates regeneration by blunting the response to pro-inflammatory macrophages. *Skelet Muscle* **2015**, *5*, 24. [CrossRef]

70. Zhang, C.; Li, Y.; Wu, Y.; Wang, L.; Wang, X.; Du, J. Interleukin-6/signal transducer and activator of transcription 3 (STAT3) pathway is essential for macrophage infiltration and myoblast proliferation during muscle regeneration. *J. Biol. Chem.* **2013**, *288*, 1489–1499. [CrossRef]

71. Warren, G.L.; Hulderman, T.; Jensen, N.; McKinstry, M.; Mishra, M.; Luster, M.I.; Simeonova, P.P. Physiological role of tumor necrosis factor alpha in traumatic muscle injury. *FASEB J.* **2002**, *16*, 1630–1632. [CrossRef]

72. Akdis, M.; Aab, A.; Altunbulakli, C.; Azkur, K.; Costa, R.A.; Crameri, R.; Duan, S.; Eiwegger, T.; Eljaszewicz, A.; Ferstl, R.; et al. Interleukins (from IL-1 to IL-38), interferons, transforming growth factor beta, and TNF-alpha: Receptors, functions, and roles in diseases. *J. Allergy Clin. Immunol.* **2016**, *138*, 984–1010. [CrossRef] [PubMed]

73. Liu, X.; Liu, Y.; Zhao, L.; Zeng, Z.; Xiao, W.; Chen, P. Macrophage depletion impairs skeletal muscle regeneration: The roles of regulatory factors for muscle regeneration. *Cell Biol. Int.* **2017**, *41*, 228–238. [CrossRef] [PubMed]

74. Deng, B.; Wehling-Henricks, M.; Villalta, S.A.; Wang, Y.; Tidball, J.G. IL-10 triggers changes in macrophage phenotype that promote muscle growth and regeneration. *J. Immunol.* **2012**, *189*, 3669–3680. [CrossRef] [PubMed]

75. Evans, M. Discovering pluripotency: 30 years of mouse embryonic stem cells. *Nat. Rev. Mol. Cell Biol.* **2011**, *12*, 680–686. [CrossRef] [PubMed]

76. Takahashi, K.; Yamanaka, S. Induction of pluripotent stem cells from mouse embryonic and adult fibroblast cultures by defined factors. *Cell* **2006**, *126*, 663–676. [CrossRef] [PubMed]

77. Takahashi, K.; Tanabe, K.; Ohnuki, M.; Narita, M.; Ichisaka, T.; Tomoda, K.; Yamanaka, S. Induction of pluripotent stem cells from adult human fibroblasts by defined factors. *Cell* **2007**, *131*, 861–872. [CrossRef]

78. Swierczek, B.; Ciemerych, M.A.; Archacka, K. From pluripotency to myogenesis: A multistep process in the dish. *J. Muscle Res. Cell Motil.* **2015**, *36*, 363–375. [CrossRef]

79. Cao, F.; van der Bogt, K.E.; Sadrzadeh, A.; Xie, X.; Sheikh, A.Y.; Wang, H.; Connolly, A.J.; Robbins, R.C.; Wu, J.C. Spatial and temporal kinetics of teratoma formation from murine embryonic stem cell transplantation. *Stem Cells Dev.* **2007**, *16*, 883–891. [CrossRef]

80. Pittenger, M.F.; Mackay, A.M.; Beck, S.C.; Jaiswal, R.K.; Douglas, R.; Mosca, J.D.; Moorman, M.A.; Simonetti, D.W.; Craig, S.; Marshak, D.R. Multilineage potential of adult human mesenchymal stem cells. *Science* **1999**, *284*, 143–147. [CrossRef]

81. Chamberlain, G.; Fox, J.; Ashton, B.; Middleton, J. Concise review: Mesenchymal stem cells: Their phenotype, differentiation capacity, immunological features, and potential for homing. *Stem Cells* **2007**, *25*, 2739–2749. [CrossRef]

82. Woodbury, D.; Schwarz, E.J.; Prockop, D.J.; Black, I.B. Adult rat and human bone marrow stromal cells differentiate into neurons. *J. Neurosci Res.* **2000**, *61*, 364–370. [CrossRef]

83. Buzanska, L.; Jurga, M.; Stachowiak, E.K.; Stachowiak, M.K.; Domanska-Janik, K. Neural stem-like cell line derived from a nonhematopoietic population of human umbilical cord blood. *Stem Cells Dev.* **2006**, *15*, 391–406. [CrossRef] [PubMed]

84. Grabowska, I.; Brzoska, E.; Gawrysiak, A.; Streminska, W.; Moraczewski, J.; Polanski, Z.; Hoser, G.; Kawiak, J.; Machaj, E.K.; Pojda, Z.; et al. Restricted Myogenic Potential of Mesenchymal Stromal Cells Isolated From Umbilical Cord. *Cell Transplant.* **2012**, *21*, 1711–1726. [CrossRef] [PubMed]

85. Brzoska, E.; Grabowska, I.; Hoser, G.; Streminska, W.; Wasilewska, D.; Machaj, E.K.; Pojda, Z.; Moraczewski, J.; Kawiak, J. Participation of stem cells from human cord blood in skeletal muscle regeneration of SCID mice. *Exp. Hematol* **2006**, *34*, 1262–1270. [CrossRef] [PubMed]

86. Abarbanell, A.M.; Coffey, A.C.; Fehrenbacher, J.W.; Beckman, D.J.; Herrmann, J.L.; Weil, B.; Meldrum, D.R. Proinflammatory cytokine effects on mesenchymal stem cell therapy for the ischemic heart. *Ann. Thorac. Surg.* **2009**, *88*, 1036–1043. [CrossRef] [PubMed]

87. Shohara, R.; Yamamoto, A.; Takikawa, S.; Iwase, A.; Hibi, H.; Kikkawa, F.; Ueda, M. Mesenchymal stromal cells of human umbilical cord Wharton's jelly accelerate wound healing by paracrine mechanisms. *Cytotherapy* **2012**, *14*, 1171–1181. [CrossRef] [PubMed]

88. Heo, S.C.; Jeon, E.S.; Lee, I.H.; Kim, H.S.; Kim, M.B.; Kim, J.H. Tumor necrosis factor-alpha-activated human adipose tissue-derived mesenchymal stem cells accelerate cutaneous wound healing through paracrine mechanisms. *J. Invest. Dermatol* **2011**, *131*, 1559–1567. [CrossRef] [PubMed]

89. Tidball, J.G. Inflammatory processes in muscle injury and repair. *Am. J. Physiol Regul Integr Comp. Physiol* **2005**, *288*, R345–R353. [CrossRef] [PubMed]

90. Kharraz, Y.; Guerra, J.; Mann, C.J.; Serrano, A.L.; Munoz-Canoves, P. Macrophage plasticity and the role of inflammation in skeletal muscle repair. *Mediators Inflamm.* **2013**, *2013*, 491497. [CrossRef] [PubMed]

91. Zimmerlin, L.; Park, T.S.; Zambidis, E.T.; Donnenberg, V.S.; Donnenberg, A.D. Mesenchymal stem cell secretome and regenerative therapy after cancer. *Biochimie* **2013**, *95*, 2235–2245. [CrossRef] [PubMed]

92. de Witte, S.F.H.; Merino, A.M.; Franquesa, M.; Strini, T.; van Zoggel, J.A.A.; Korevaar, S.S.; Luk, F.; Gargesha, M.; O'Flynn, L.; Roy, D.; et al. Cytokine treatment optimises the immunotherapeutic effects of umbilical cord-derived MSC for treatment of inflammatory liver disease. *Stem Cell Res. Ther.* **2017**, *8*, 140. [CrossRef] [PubMed]

93. Fukuyo, S.; Yamaoka, K.; Sonomoto, K.; Oshita, K.; Okada, Y.; Saito, K.; Yoshida, Y.; Kanazawa, T.; Minami, Y.; Tanaka, Y. IL-6-accelerated calcification by induction of ROR2 in human adipose tissue-derived mesenchymal stem cells is STAT3 dependent. *Rheumatology (Oxford).* **2014**, *53*, 1282–1290. [CrossRef] [PubMed]

94. Sonomoto, K.; Yamaoka, K.; Oshita, K.; Fukuyo, S.; Zhang, X.; Nakano, K.; Okada, Y.; Tanaka, Y. Interleukin-1beta induces differentiation of human mesenchymal stem cells into osteoblasts via the Wnt-5a/receptor tyrosine kinase-like orphan receptor 2 pathway. *Arthritis Rheum.* **2012**, *64*, 3355–3363. [CrossRef] [PubMed]

95. Cho, J.W.; Kang, M.C.; Lee, K.S. TGF-beta1-treated ADSCs-CM promotes expression of type I collagen and MMP-1, migration of human skin fibroblasts, and wound healing in vitro and in vivo. *Int. J. Mol. Med.* **2010**, *26*, 901–906. [PubMed]

96. Grefte, S.; Vullinghs, S.; Kuijpers-Jagtman, A.M.; Torensma, R.; Von den Hoff, J.W. Matrigel, but not collagen I, maintains the differentiation capacity of muscle derived cells in vitro. *Biomed. Mater.* **2012**, *7*, 055004. [CrossRef] [PubMed]

97. Chan, Y.S.; Li, Y.; Foster, W.; Horaguchi, T.; Somogyi, G.; Fu, F.H.; Huard, J. Antifibrotic effects of suramin in injured skeletal muscle after laceration. *J. Appl. Physiol.* **2003**, *95*, 771–780. [CrossRef] [PubMed]

98. Bedair, H.S.; Karthikeyan, T.; Quintero, A.; Li, Y.; Huard, J. Angiotensin II receptor blockade administered after injury improves muscle regeneration and decreases fibrosis in normal skeletal muscle. *Am. J. Sports Med.* **2008**, *36*, 1548–1554. [CrossRef] [PubMed]

99. Yousef, H.; Conboy, M.J.; Morgenthaler, A.; Schlesinger, C.; Bugaj, L.; Paliwal, P.; Greer, C.; Conboy, I.M.; Schaffer, D. Systemic attenuation of the TGF-beta pathway by a single drug simultaneously rejuvenates hippocampal neurogenesis and myogenesis in the same old mammal. *Oncotarget* **2015**, *6*, 11959–11978. [CrossRef]

100. Brennan, T.J.; Edmondson, D.G.; Li, L.; Olson, E.N. Transforming growth factor beta represses the actions of myogenin through a mechanism independent of DNA binding. *Proc. Natl. Acad. Sci. USA* **1991**, *88*, 3822–3826. [CrossRef]

101. Han, H.; Wei, W.; Chu, W.; Liu, K.; Tian, Y.; Jiang, Z.; Chen, J. Muscle Conditional Medium Reduces Intramuscular Adipocyte Differentiation and Lipid Accumulation through Regulating Insulin Signaling. *Int. J. Mol. Sci.* **2017**, *18*. [CrossRef]

102. Kowalski, K.; Kolodziejczyk, A.; Sikorska, M.H.; Placzkiewicz, J.; Cichosz, P.; Kowalewska, M.; Streminska, W.; Janczyk-Ilach, K.; Koblowska, M.; Fogtman, A.; et al. Stem cells migration during skeletal muscle regeneration—the role of Sdf-1/Cxcr4 and Sdf-1/Cxcr7 axis. *Cell Adh. Migr.* **2016**. [CrossRef]

103. Livak, K.J.; Schmittgen, T.D. Analysis of relative gene expression data using real-time quantitative PCR and the 2(T)(-Delta Delta C) method. *Methods* **2001**, *25*, 402–408. [CrossRef] [PubMed]

3

Key Components of Human Myofibre Denervation and Neuromuscular Junction Stability are Modulated by Age and Exercise

Casper Soendenbroe [1,2], Cecilie J. L. Bechshøft [1,3], Mette F. Heisterberg [1], Simon M. Jensen [1], Emma Bomme [1], Peter Schjerling [1,3], Anders Karlsen [1,3], Michael Kjaer [1,3], Jesper L. Andersen [1,3] and Abigail L. Mackey [1,2,3,*]

[1] Institute of Sports Medicine Copenhagen, Department of Orthopedic Surgery M, Bispebjerg Hospital, Building 8, Nielsine Nielsens vej 11, 2400 Copenhagen NV, Denmark; caspersoendenbroe@outlook.dk (C.S.); cjleidersdorff@gmail.com (C.J.L.B.); metteflindt@hotmail.com (M.F.H.); simonmarqvard@gmail.com (S.M.J.); emmabomme@gmail.com (E.B.); Peter@mRNA.dk (P.S.); ak@anderskarlsen.dk (A.K.); michaelkjaer@sund.ku.dk (M.K.); Jesper.Loevind.Andersen@regionh.dk (J.L.A.)

[2] Xlab, Department of Biomedical Sciences, Faculty of Health and Medical Sciences, University of Copenhagen, Blegdamsvej 3, 2200 Copenhagen N, Denmark

[3] Center for Healthy Aging, Faculty of Health and Medical Sciences, University of Copenhagen, Blegdamsvej 3, 2200 Copenhagen N, Denmark

* Correspondence: abigailmac@sund.ku.dk;

Abstract: The decline in muscle mass and function with age is partly caused by a loss of muscle fibres through denervation. The purpose of this study was to investigate the potential of exercise to influence molecular targets involved in neuromuscular junction (NMJ) stability in healthy elderly individuals. Participants from two studies (one group of 12 young and 12 elderly females and another group of 25 elderly males) performed a unilateral bout of resistance exercise. Muscle biopsies were collected at 4.5 h and up to 7 days post exercise for tissue analysis and cell culture. Molecular targets related to denervation and NMJ stability were analysed by immunohistochemistry and real-time reverse transcription polymerase chain reaction. In addition to a greater presence of denervated fibres, the muscle samples and cultured myotubes from the elderly individuals displayed altered gene expression levels of acetylcholine receptor (AChR) subunits. A single bout of exercise induced general changes in AChR subunit gene expression within the biopsy sampling timeframe, suggesting a sustained plasticity of the NMJ in elderly individuals. These data support the role of exercise in maintaining NMJ stability, even in elderly inactive individuals. Furthermore, the cell culture findings suggest that the transcriptional capacity of satellite cells for AChR subunit genes is negatively affected by ageing.

Keywords: sarcopenia; denervation; neuromuscular junction; heavy resistance exercise; acetylcholine receptor; cell culture; myogenesis; neonatal myosin; neural cell adhesion molecule

1. Introduction

The rate of loss of muscle mass increases with advancing age [1], and ultimately leads to impaired physical function in elderly individuals [2–4]. This age-dependent decline in muscle mass is partly due to a loss of individual muscle fibres [5] as a result of muscle fibre denervation [6–8]. While physical exercise is recognized as a strong countermeasure against the loss of muscle mass and has consistently been shown to maintain physical function and health in the last ten years of life [9,10], it is currently unclear whether denervation can be ameliorated or reversed by exercise.

It has been shown in animals that exercise causes positive adaptations to the neuromuscular junction (NMJ) that to some extent can attenuate the age-related degeneration of the NMJ [11]. Changes in expression of acetylcholine receptors (AChRs) with acute exercise have been suggested to indicate NMJ remodelling in animals [12,13] and represent a potential target for studying this in humans [14]. AChR are present in abundance at the NMJ [15] and are almost non-existent in the extra-synaptic region of the muscle fibre [16]. Upon experimental denervation, however, the $\alpha 1$, $\beta 1$, γ, and δ subunits increase extra synaptically [16–19], raising the possibility that these AChR subunits can be used as indicators of denervation associated with ageing. We recently observed a correlation between age and gene expression levels of the foetal γ AChR subunit in a large group ($n = 70$) of healthy elderly men ranging in age from 65 to 94 years, in conjunction with tissue markers of muscle fibre denervation, neural cell adhesion molecule (NCAM) and neonatal myosin (MHCn), at the protein level [20]. Direct comparisons with a younger cohort as well as the potential for exercise to influence AChR expression patterns are however lacking.

One of the challenges for ageing skeletal muscle is related to the decline in satellite cell function with age. Not only is satellite cell function important for tissue repair and maintenance, but it also has potential implications for maintenance of the NMJ, where myonuclei at this site must be capable of carrying out the specialization necessary to complete the formation of the NMJ. This includes producing a high concentration of AChRs at the membrane and a clustering of myonuclei, which become transcriptionally specialized and distinct from adjacent extra-synaptic myonuclei [21,22]. Whether this capacity declines with age is currently unknown. Satellite cells have been shown to play a vital role in maintaining the post-synaptic region in mice, both in terms of myonuclear clusters of AChRs and re-innervation of the regenerating NMJ [23,24]. In this context it is interesting that we have recently observed a poorer fusion capacity of satellite cells derived from old women compared to young women, accompanied by a distinctly different molecular profile throughout the myogenic program [25]. It remains unknown, however, to what extent this dysfunction in human satellite cells has implications for NMJ maintenance with increasing age.

Based on the above, the main purpose of this study was to investigate the influence of age and exercise on molecular markers of NMJ stability and muscle fibre denervation in healthy elderly individuals. An additional focus was to determine how ageing would alter the capacity of myonuclei in cell culture to produce key transcriptional elements for NMJ formation.

2. Materials and Methods

2.1. Experimental Design

This study is based on muscle biopsies collected from two studies, on 12 young and 12 elderly women [25], and on 25 elderly men [26], respectively. Both studies were approved by The Committees on Health Research Ethics for The Capital Region of Denmark (Ref: H-15017223, H-3-2012-081). All procedures conformed to the Declaration of Helsinki of 1975, revised in 2013, and the subjects gave written informed consent before participation. All participants were healthy, non-smokers, non-obese, and did not perform strenuous physical exercise on a regular basis. The men were part of a randomized controlled trial investigating the effect of the blood pressure-lowering medication losartan on the muscle response to exercise, where half of the participants received losartan and the other half placebo. Given the general lack of drug effect, the two groups were merged in the present study (separate group data are also provided for reference in online Supplementary Figure S1).

All participants performed a maximal strength test in a Leg Extension machine (M52, TechnoGym, Cesena, Italy) to determine the one-repetition maximum (1 RM), which was used to determine the load lifted during the subsequent bout of heavy resistance exercise. The Leg Extension exercise protocols consisted of both concentric and eccentric contractions. First, 4–5 sets of 12 concentric contractions at 70% of 1 RM were performed, followed by four sets of 4–6 eccentric contractions at 110% of 1 RM, as previously described [25,26]. The exercise was performed with one leg only, leaving the contralateral leg as a control. No other exercise was allowed during the study period.

2.2. Muscle Biopsies

For all participants, muscle biopsies were obtained from the vastus lateralis muscle, under local anaesthetic (1% lidocaine), using the percutaneous needle biopsy technique of Bergström [27], with five 6-mm needles and manual suction. Pieces of muscle tissue were aligned, embedded in Tissue-Tek, and then frozen in isopentane, pre-cooled in liquid nitrogen, and stored at −80 °C. The men had six muscle biopsies taken over 17 days, at the following time points: −10 and −3 days before exercise from the control, non-exercised leg, and from the exercised leg at +4.5 h and on days +1, +4, and +7 post exercise. The day −3 sample was excluded from the current study since its purpose was to investigate a potential effect of losartan in the rested state and is therefore superfluous in the current context. The young and elderly women had muscle biopsies collected from each leg five days after exercise, from which a part was embedded as described above and a part was used for cell culture, where myoblasts were plated in 12-well plates for three days of proliferation (12,000 cells per well), or three days of proliferation followed by four days of differentiation (20,000 cells per well), as previously described in detail [25].

2.3. RNA Extraction

100 cryo sections, 10 μm thick, from the embedded muscle tissue were homogenized in 1 mL of TriReagent (Molecular Research Center, Cincinnati, OH, USA) containing five stainless steel balls of 2.3 mm in diameter (BioSpec Products, Bartlesville, OK, USA), and one silicon-carbide sharp particle of 1 mm (BioSpec Products), by shaking in a FastPrep®-24 instrument (MP Biomedicals, Illkirch, France) at speed level four for 15 s. Cell culture cells were dissolved directly in the Trireagent. Bromo-chloropropane was added in order to separate the samples into an aqueous and an organic phase. Following isolation of the aqueous phase, RNA was precipitated using isopropanol. The RNA pellet was then washed in ethanol and subsequently dissolved in 20 μL RNAse-free water. Total RNA concentrations and purity were determined by spectroscopy at 260, 280, and 240 nm. Good RNA integrity was ensured by gel electrophoresis.

2.4. Real-Time RT-PCR

mRNA targets related to innervation were analysed for the current study. The specific primers are given in Table 1. Total RNA (500 ng for muscle and 150 ng for cell culture) was converted into cDNA in 20 μL using OmniScript reverse transcriptase (Qiagen, Redwood City, CA, USA) and 1 μM poly-dT (Invitrogen, Naerum, Denmark) according to the manufacturer's protocol (Qiagen). The same pool of cDNA used previously for the cells in culture [25] and the male muscle tissue [26] was used here. For each target mRNA, 0.25 μL cDNA were amplified in a 25-μL SYBR Green polymerase chain reaction (PCR) containing 1 × Quantitect SYBR Green Master Mix (Qiagen) and 100 nM of each primer (Table 1). The amplification was monitored real time using the MX3005P Real-time PCR machine (Stratagene, San Diego, CA, USA). The Ct values were related to a standard curve made with known concentrations of cloned PCR products or DNA oligonucleotides (Ultramer™ oligos, Integrated DNA Technologies, Inc., Leuven, Belgium) with a DNA sequence corresponding to the sequence of the expected PCR product. The specificity of the PCR products was confirmed by melting curve analysis after amplification. Ribosomal Protein Lateral Stalk Subunit P0 (RPLP0) mRNA was chosen as internal control. To validate this use, another unrelated "constitutive" mRNA, Glyceraldehyde-3-Phosphate Dehydrogenase (GAPDH), was measured and normalized with RPLP0. In the cell culture experiment GAPDH mRNA normalized to RPLP0 mRNA was constant, indicating that RPLP0 (and GAPDH) was indeed constant and suitable for normalization. However, in tissue the GAPDH/RPLP0 ratio was lower in the elderly female subjects and one and four days after exercise in the males, showing either a GAPDH decrease or a RPLP0 increase. However, the decrease in GAPDH was not reflected in the general pattern of the other mRNA when normalized to RPLP0, arguing against a general normalization error. We therefore chose to use retain RPLP0 for normalization. The GAPDH mRNA data from cell culture of the females and tissue of the males have been used as internal control in already published papers [25,26].

Table 1. Primers used for PCR. RPLP0: Ribosomal Protein Lateral Stalk Subunit P0; GAPDH: Glyceraldehyde-3-Phosphate Dehydrogenase; AChR: acetylcholine receptor; MuSK: muscle-specific-kinase; MHCn: neonatal myosin; MHCe: embryonic myosin heavy chain.

mRNA	Genbank	Sense	Antisense
RPLP0	NM_053275.3	GGAAACTCTGCATTCTCGCTTCCT	CCAGGACTCGTTTGTACCCGTTG
AchRα1	NM_000079.3	GCAGAGACCATGAAGTCAGACCAGGAG	CCGATGATGCAAACAAGCATGAA
AchRβ1	NM_000747.2	TTCATCCGGAAGCCGCCAAG	CCGCAGATCAGGGGCAGACA
AchRδ	NM_000751.2	CAGCTGTGGATGGGGCAAAC	GCCACTCGGTTCCAGCTGTCTT
AchRε	NM_000080.4	TGGCAGAACTGTTCGCTTATTTTCC	TTGATGGTCTTGCCGTCGTTGT
AchRγ	NM_005199.4	GCCTGCAACCTCATTGCCTGT	ACTCGGCCCACCAGGAACCAC
MuSK	NM_005592.3	TCATGGCAGAATTTGACAACCCTAAC	GGCTTCCCGACAGCACACAC
MHCe	NM_002470.3	CGGATATCGCAGAATCTCAAGTCAA	CTCCAGAAGGGCTGGCTCACTC
MHCn	NM_002472.2	CGGAAACATGAGCGACGAGTAAAA	CAGCCTGAGAACATTCTTGCGATCTT
GAPDH	NM_002046.6	GAGGGGCCATCCACAGTCTTCT	GACATGCCCAAGACCCAGAAGGA

2.5. Immunohistochemistry

For the female participants, cross sections (10 μm) from the biopsies of the exercised and control legs were cut at −20 °C in a cryostat. Sections from both legs of one individual were placed on the same glass slide (Thermo Scientific, Waltham, MA, USA) and stored at −80 °C until staining. For staining, two primary antibodies were diluted in 1% bovine serum albumin (BSA) in Tris-buffered saline (TBS) and applied to the sections (see Table 2), and then incubated in the refrigerator overnight. Afterwards two secondary antibodies (see Table 2) diluted in 1% BSA in TBS were applied for 45 min. At this point, the sections were fixed in 5% formaldehyde (Histofix, Histolab, Gothenburg, Sweden) for 12 min and then mounted with Prolong-Gold-Antifade (Invitrogen, Molecular Probes, OR, USA, catalogue #P36931), containing 4′,6-Di-amidino-2-phenylindole (DAPI). Slides were washed with TBS twice between all steps. Slides were kept in darkness at room temperature for 48 h and then moved to a −20 °C freezer. Two sections were also stained with NCAM and collagen XXII (made by Manuel Koch) [28], as previously described [29], since it was suspected that the NCAM staining in these sections was due to the presence of myotendinous junction and not denervated muscle fibres.

Table 2. Antibodies used for immunohistochemistry and immunocytochemistry. MHCn: neonatal myosin; MHCe: embryonic myosin heavy chain; NCAM: neural cell adhesion molecule.

Host	Antibody	Primary Antibody Company	Cat. no.	Concentration
Mouse	Dystrophin, IgG2b	Sigma-Aldrich	D8168	1:500
Mouse	Myosin 1, IgG1	Hybridoma Bank	A4.951	1:200
Mouse	MHCe, IgG1	Hybridoma Bank	F1.652	1:100
Mouse	MHCn, IgG1	Novocastra	NCL-MHCn	1:100
Mouse	NCAM, IgG1	Becton Dickinson	347740	1:50
Rabbit	Desmin, IgG	Abcam	AB32362	1:1000
Mouse	Myogenin, IgG1	Hybridoma Bank	F5D-s	1:50
Host	**Antibody**	**Secondary Antibody Company**	**Cat. no.**	**Concentration**
Goat	488, green, IgG1	Invitrogen	A-21121	1:500
Goat	568, red, IgG2b	Invitrogen	A-21144	1:200
Goat	568, red, IgG	Invitrogen	A-11036	1:500
Goat	488, green, IgG	Invitrogen	A-11029	1:500

2.6. Microscopy

All imaging was performed with a ×10/0.30NA objective and a 0.5× camera (Olympus DP71, Olympus Deutschland GmbH, Hamburg, Germany) mounted on a BX51 Olympus microscope, using the Olympus cellSens software (v.1.14). For all analyses, 1.7 × 1.3 mm greyscale images were captured.

Muscle fibre size and muscle fibre type composition analysis was only performed on the control leg. Non-overlapping images of high resolution (4080 × 3072 pixels) were captured to accommodate a semi-automated macro [30], run in ImageJ (v.1.51, U.S. National Institutes of Health, Bethesda, MD, USA). All analyses were conducted by the same person blinded to the age group. All included muscle fibres were manually checked, and fibres were excluded if the dystrophin staining was incomplete or if an area of the biopsy was longitudinally oriented. Fibres at the edge and around holes and folds in the biopsies were always excluded. After delineation of the muscle fibre cross-sectional area (CSA), fibre type was determined based upon the median light intensity. Fibres were classified as type I (positive for myosin type I staining) or type II (negative for myosin type I staining). Hybrid muscle fibres (low levels of type I myosin staining) were excluded from the analysis (a total of 131 fibres from all sections).

For the analysis of embryonic myosin heavy chain (MHCe)-, MHCn-, and NCAM-positive fibres, images at a resolution of 2040 × 1536 pixels were captured. For MHCe, only areas with positive staining were imaged, while for MHCn and NCAM the entire biopsy section was imaged (due to the relatively higher prevalence of positive fibres). Positively stained muscle fibres were determined as fibres with a complete dystrophin staining and a clear staining of one of the three markers. We extended the method used in our previous study [20] by also measuring the CSA of all transversely cut positive muscle fibres in the present study. All analyses were conducted by the same person, blinded to age group and leg of the sample. All values are expressed relative to the total number of fibres in the section. In a sub-analysis, four consecutive sections from two elderly subjects (both the exercised and the control leg) were additionally analysed for MHCn-positive fibres to determine whether small fibres could be found on consecutive sections. Overview images of the sections were initially used to identify areas of the biopsy that were present on all four consecutive sections. Peripherally positioned (at edges or holes) muscle fibres were not included. In total, 31 MHCn-positive muscle fibres were included across the two subjects and followed through the four consecutive sections (see online Supplementary Figure S2 for images).

2.7. Immunocytochemistry

For the cells cultured to differentiate, the fusion index was determined as reported earlier [25]. Briefly, coverslips were stained with the primary antibodies desmin and myogenin (see Table 2 for details) followed by the secondary antibodies goat anti-rabbit 568 (catalogue #A11036) and goat anti-mouse 488 (catalogue # A11029), and mounted with Prolong-Gold-Antifade containing DAPI (catalogue #P36931, Invitrogen), as described [25]. Fusion index was calculated as the percentage of desmin-positive nuclei within myotubes (containing three or more nuclei) divided by the total number of desmin-positive nuclei.

2.8. Statistics

All figures were prepared in GraphPad Prism (v.7.04, GraphPad Software, Inc., La Jolla, CA, USA) and all statistical analyses were conducted in SigmaPlot (v. 13.0, Systat Software Inc, San Jose, CA, USA), except subject characteristics and gene expression of the female subjects, which were analysed using Microsoft Excel 2016 (Microsoft Corporation, Redmond, Washington). p-Values below 0.05 were considered significant, and trends of $p < 0.1$ are also reported. mRNA data were normalized to RPLP0 and log-transformed before statistical analysis. For the female participants, unpaired t-tests (two-tailed) were performed between young and old for subject characteristics, fibre size, fibre type composition, and mRNA data. Paired t-tests (two-tailed) were conducted for the analysis of the exercise response (exercised leg vs. control leg). The Bonferroni correction was applied (multiplying the p-values ×3) to the t-test analyses on the mRNA data to correct for multiple testing. For correlation analyses, mRNA data were log-transformed and then subjected to Pearson's correlation. The number of MHCe-, MHCn-, and NCAM-positive fibres, which was not normally distributed, was subjected to the Mann–Whitney Rank Sum Test and Wilcoxon Signed Rank Test to compare differences between young and old subjects, and control versus exercised leg, respectively. For the male participants, data were analysed by one-way repeated measures analysis of variance, using Dunnett's method for multiple comparisons to compare each time point with baseline, where an overall main effect of time was found. The subject characteristics are presented as means with standard deviation and range, while muscle fibre size and composition are shown as individual values. MHCn- and NCAM-positive muscle fibres are presented as median and individual values.

3. Results

3.1. Subject Characteristics

Age, height, weight, BMI, and Leg Extension 1 RM for all subjects included in the analyses are provided in Table 3. The control muscle biopsy from one elderly woman was found to show irregularities (one fascicle filled with unusually large and small muscle fibres positive for NCAM, MHCn, and MHCe), and this subject was therefore excluded from all analyses.

Table 3. Subject characteristics. Average and standard deviations with ranges (superscript). Abbreviations: BMI, body mass index; 1 RM, one-repetition maximum; yr: years, kg: kilogram.

	Young Women			Old Women			Old Men		
	$n = 12$			$n = 11$			$n = 25$		
Age (yr)	23	± 3	20–28	74	± 3	71–78	70	± 7	64–90
Height (cm)	168	± 7	157–177	166	± 3	162–169	180	± 5	172–189
Weight (kg)	64	± 8	53–75	69	± 10	57–84	82	± 10	67–98
BMI (kg/m^2)	23	± 2	19–26	25	± 4	20–30	26	± 3	21–31
Knee extension 1RM (kg)	39	± 8	30–50	23	± 5	12–28	56	± 14	23–82

3.2. Tissue Immunohistochemistry at Baseline—Young and Elderly Women

On average, the numbers of fibres included in the fibre type and size analysis were 212 (129–352) for type I and 151 (68–247) for type II fibres in the young participants. The corresponding values for the elderly were 169 (85–267) type I and 143 (45–487) type II fibres. The type I fibre percentage was $59 \pm 11\%$ (35%–74%) for the young and $58 \pm 15\%$ (22%–75%) for the elderly, with no difference between them. As seen in Figure 1, the elderly had significantly smaller type II fibres compared to both their own type I fibres (−38%, $p < 0.001$) and the type II fibres in the young (−36%, $p < 0.001$).

On average, the number of fibres included in the immunohistochemical analysis of denervated fibres was 1080 [401–2270]. MHCe-positive fibres were only found in the excluded subject and are therefore not presented. The elderly had significantly more MHCn- and NCAM-positive fibres compared to the young (Figure 2).

No significant differences between the previously exercised and the control leg were found in either the young or the elderly for MHCn or NCAM (online Supplementary Figure S3). We evaluated the fibre size of all transversely cut MHCn- and NCAM-positive fibres from the control leg. A clear majority of the MHCn- and NCAM-positive muscle fibres were smaller than 150 μm^2 (online Supplementary Figure S3).

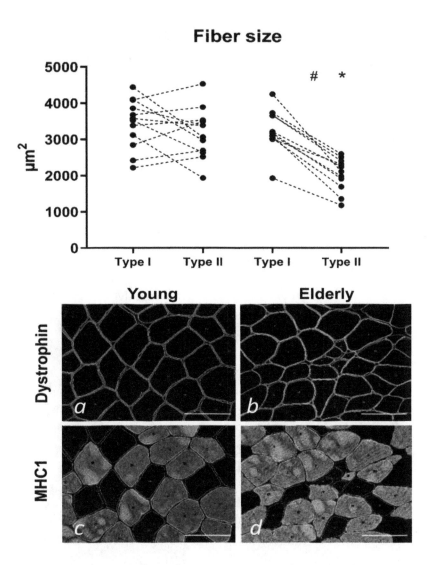

Figure 1. Muscle fibre size analysis in biopsy cross-sections from the control legs of 12 young and 11 elderly women. Individual values are displayed and with type I and II values for an individual connected by a dashed line. The type II fibres of the elderly individuals were significantly smaller than their own type I fibres and the type II fibres of the younger individuals. * $p < 0.001$ vs. young type II, # $p < 0.001$ between fibre types in elderly. Images (**a–d**) illustrate the analysis process. (**b,d**) show representative images of the same area, which has been delineated by the macro in ImageJ. This is an elderly subject with a mean fibre size of 3025 μm^2 and 1688 μm^2 for type I and II fibres, respectively. Similarly, a and c show representative images of the same area in a young subject with a mean fibre size of 3574 μm^2 and 3378 μm^2 for type I and II fibres, respectively. MHC1, myosin heavy chain 1. Scale bars = 100 μm.

One biopsy from the exercised leg of a young subject showed 13 NCAM-positive fibres (1.3% of total fibre count) all located adjacent to a thick band of connective tissue, reminiscent of the myotendinous junction (MTJ). Collagen XXII staining confirmed that this was in fact MTJ, so these fibres were not included in the analysis of this biopsy (see online Supplementary Figure S4 for image). One young subject had 13 (1.45% of total fibre count) NCAM-positive fibres, all of which were located at the edge of the biopsy. This area was not stained by collagen XXII and remained NCAM-positive on additional sections and was therefore not excluded from the analysis. In all other samples MHCn- and NCAM-positive fibres were randomly scattered in between normal muscle fibres.

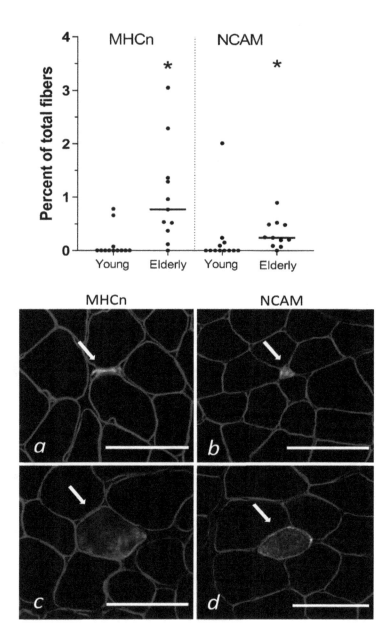

Figure 2. Muscle fibres positive for MHCn or NCAM in biopsy cross-sections from 12 young and 11 elderly women. Only the control leg is shown. Individual values are presented with the median (horizontal line). Panels show examples of small MHCn (**a**) and NCAM (**b**), and large MHCn (**c**) and NCAM (**d**) fibres (arrows). Positive fibres are green, dystrophin, red. * $p < 0.05$ vs. young. MHCn, neonatal myosin heavy chain; NCAM, neural cell adhesion molecule. Scale bars = 100 μm.

3.3. Tissue mRNA at Baseline and in Response to Exercise—Young and Elderly Women

The muscle tissue of the elderly women had significantly lower levels of AChR β1 mRNA compared to the young women, whereas levels of both AChR γ and MHCn mRNA were higher in the elderly compared to the young (Figure 3). Tendencies for differences were seen for gene expression levels of AChR α1 and muscle-specific-kinase (MuSK).

Both the elderly and the young women had a significant upregulation of AChR α1 mRNA in the previously exercised leg compared to the control leg (Figure 3). The exercise response of AChR δ mRNA only reached statistical significance in the elderly. AChR ε mRNA were detected in less than half of the samples at levels very close to detection limit of one molecule and with no preference for any group (data not shown).

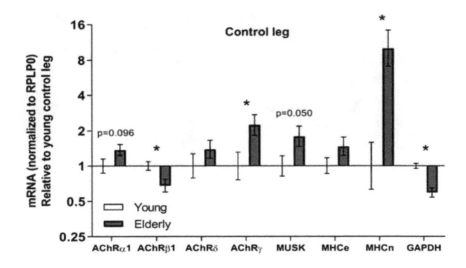

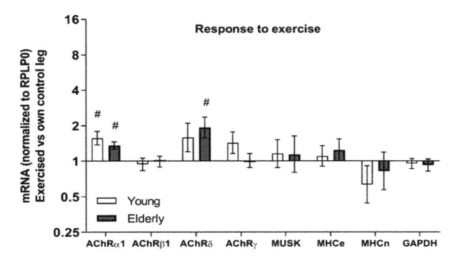

Figure 3. Gene expression in muscle biopsies of healthy young ($n = 12$) and elderly ($n = 11$) women, at rest (control) and five days after a single bout of one-legged exercise. mRNA data were normalized to RPLP0 and are shown as geometric means ± back-transformed SEM, relative to young control legs (control leg) and own control leg (response to exercise). * $p < 0.05$ elderly vs. young. # $p < 0.05$ vs. control leg. Tendencies are written. AChR: acetylcholine receptor; MuSK: muscle-specific-kinase; MHCe: embryonic myosin heavy chain; MHCn, neonatal myosin heavy chain; NCAM, neural cell adhesion molecule; GAPDH: Glyceraldehyde-3-Phosphate Dehydrogenase; RPLP0: Ribosomal Protein Lateral Stalk Subunit P0.

3.4. Cell Culture at Baseline and in Response to Exercise—Young and Elderly Women

The fusion index of the cell cultures from the rested and exercised legs of the elderly women was $36.3 \pm 4.2\%$ and $36.1 \pm 5.0\%$, respectively, with the corresponding values for the young group being $52.2 \pm 1.8\%$ and $49.8 \pm 2.2\%$, respectively (main effect of age, two-way repeated measures ANOVA).

All gene expression targets were more strongly expressed in differentiating compared to proliferating cells (see online Supplementary Figure S5). In the proliferating condition, the cells from the elderly had lower gene expression levels of MHCe and MHCn compared to young (Figure 4). Similarly, we also found a significantly lower level of MHCn gene expression in the differentiating cells in the control leg in the elderly compared to the young. AChR $\beta 1$, δ, and γ all showed age-related tendencies.

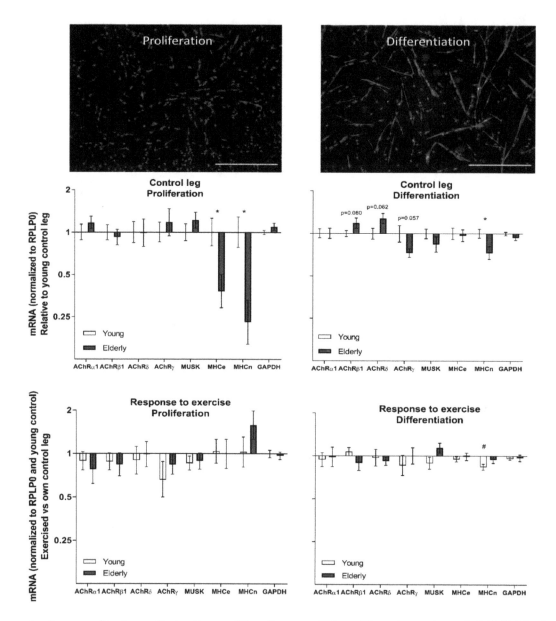

Figure 4. Images display cells in the proliferation condition (Desmin, red, and DAPI, blue) and in the differentiation condition (Desmin, red, Myogenin, green, and DAPI, blue), scale bars = 500 μm. Gene expression in cell cultures from the control and exercised legs of healthy young ($n = 12$) and elderly ($n = 11$) women. mRNA data were normalized to RPLP0 and are shown as geometric means ± back-transformed SEM, relative to young control leg (control leg) and own control leg (response to exercise). * $p < 0.05$ elderly vs. young. # $p < 0.05$ vs. control leg. Tendencies are written. AChR: acetylcholine receptor; MuSK: muscle-specific-kinase; MHCe: embryonic myosin heavy chain; MHCn, neonatal myosin heavy chain; NCAM, neural cell adhesion molecule; GAPDH: Glyceraldehyde-3-Phosphate Dehydrogenase; RPLP0: Ribosomal Protein Lateral Stalk Subunit P0.

Differentiating cells from the previously exercised leg from the young subjects demonstrated a lower gene expression of MHCn versus the control leg (Figure 4).

3.5. Tissue mRNA in Response to Exercise—Elderly Men

In general, gene expression in four out of the five AChR measured demonstrated a response to exercise. AChR α1 mRNA was downregulated 4.5 h and one day after the exercise and returned to baseline in four days (Figure 5). AChR β1 mRNA was downregulated at 1, 4, and 7 days. AChR δ mRNA showed a tendency for a decline 4.5 h after exercise and was upregulated seven days after the exercise. AChR γ mRNA decreased 4.5 h after the exercise bout. No significant exercise-induced changes in gene expression of the AChR ε subunit, MuSK, MHCe, or MHCn were observed.

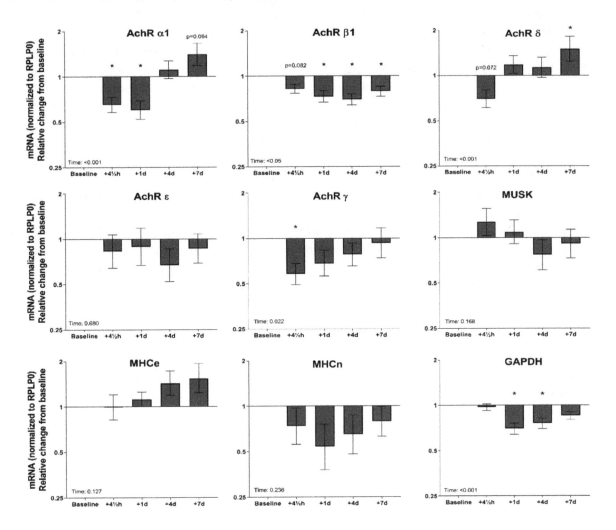

Figure 5. Gene expression in muscle biopsies of 25 healthy elderly men ten days before (baseline) and 4.5 h, one day, four days, and seven days after a single bout of exercise. mRNA data were normalized to RPLP0 and are shown as geometric means ± back-transformed SEM, relative to baseline. * $p < 0.05$ vs. baseline. Tendencies are written. AChR: acetylcholine receptor; MuSK: muscle-specific-kinase; MHCe: embryonic myosin heavy chain; MHCn, neonatal myosin heavy chain; NCAM, neural cell adhesion molecule; GAPDH: Glyceraldehyde-3-Phosphate Dehydrogenase; RPLP0: Ribosomal Protein Lateral Stalk Subunit P0.

4. Discussions

The most notable findings of the present study was that the skeletal muscle of elderly individuals, with morphological signs of ageing as demonstrated by a reduced type II muscle fibre CSA and a heightened number of denervated muscle fibres, has a significantly elevated gene expression level of the denervation-responsive AChR γ subunit and MHCn as compared to young healthy individuals. Our data also suggest an age effect on the capacity of satellite cell-derived myotubes to transcribe AChR genes, which is fundamental for NMJ maintenance. Furthermore, we provide novel insight into the transient changes in gene expression of all five muscle AChR subunits following heavy resistance exercise in healthy elderly human skeletal muscle. Together these data support the role of exercise in stimulating the stability of the NMJ, but also indicate age-related changes, even in healthy elderly individuals.

4.1. Muscle Fibre Denervation in Elderly Humans

Healthy elderly women with clear signs of ageing (lower type II muscle fibre CSA and lower muscle strength), also show a significantly heightened number of denervated muscle fibres compared to young healthy women, as evidenced by a greater proportion of fibres positive for NCAM and MHCn. When a muscle fibre loses its neural input, the plasticity of the peripheral nervous systems allows for adjacent nerve sprouts to attempt to re-innervate denervated muscle fibres through nerve sprouting [31]. It is believed that the increased synthesis of NCAM in denervated muscle fibres facilitates this innervation process [32,33]. Denervated muscle fibres will also revert into an immature myosin heavy chain configuration, as we found more MHCn-positive fibres in old subjects compared to the young. Furthermore, we also observed a substantial 10-fold higher gene expression level of MHCn in the muscle tissue of the elderly compared to the young females, reflecting a persisting synthesis of this distinct myosin isoform. Importantly, it should be noted that there is not a complete overlap between MHCn- and NCAM-positive stained fibres, which suggests that the rate at which these proteins aggregate in the muscle fibres following denervation might differ. In terms of denervated muscle fibre morphology, we observed a persisting MHCn and NCAM protein presence in even the smallest of muscle fibres (<75 μm^2). These miniature fibres are easily missed during regular biopsy assessments and could represent long-term denervated fibres that had atrophied over time [34] and undergone deterioration of muscle proteins [35], but maintained an increased and long-lasting cytoplasmic expression of MHCn [36] and NCAM [32]. The length of these miniature muscle fibres is a matter of uncertainty. We have previously been able to follow such fibres through 400 μm of consecutive biopsy sections in a selected subject [20]. In a sub analysis in the present study, we searched for MHCn-positive fibres through four consecutive sections and found that 13, 32, and 39% of the fibres had disappeared after 1, 2, and 3 sections, respectively. This implies a substantial number of miniature fibres ends, which could indicate that long-term denervated fibres are gradually degraded both transversally and longitudinally.

4.2. Ageing and Exercise Alter Acetylcholine Receptor Gene Expression

One of our most marked findings is that the gene expression of the AChR γ subunit is robustly elevated in the skeletal muscle of elderly compared to young females. This coincides with this subunit being a functionally distinct foetal subunit [37–39], which is increasingly expressed following both denervation [39,40] and neurotransmitter blocking [41]. Interestingly, in our group of male participants the muscle homogenate gene expression of the γ subunit was acutely downregulated after the exercise bout but had already returned to baseline after one day. We were also able to detect this subunit, as well as α1, β1, and δ subunits, in both proliferating and differentiating cell cultures that were devoid of neural presence, meaning that satellite cell derived myonuclei can upregulate AChR gene expression without the presence of a nerve. As satellite cells have been shown to be crucial for maintaining the specialized post-synaptic region of the muscle fibre [23], it is interesting that we observed trends for an age effect in three out of the four subunits. It is worth noting that this is the case even with the conservative Bonferroni correction, but given that the age difference was not always in the same direction, it is possible that this is a real effect of age (and not an effect of general cell culture conditions), potentially reflecting an age-related satellite cell dysfunction that could negatively impact the maintenance of the NMJ. However, it should be noted that the cell cultures derived from satellite cells of the young subjects showed a significantly higher fusion index compared to the old subjects [25], indicative of a higher level of myotube maturity. Furthermore, we also observed a positive correlation between cell fusion index and gene expression levels of AChRγ (R = 0.74), MuSK (R = 0.75), and MHCe (R = 0.66) in the old group (Supplementary Figure S6). This would suggest that AChRγ gene expression in aneural cell cultures is increased concordant with myotube maturity and raises the possibility that the molecular differences we observed between the cell cultures from young and elderly muscle are determined by the extent of fusion. However we cannot rule out the opposite, i.e., that the lower gene expression levels contribute to the lower fusion index values.

Generally, our data show age and exercise effects on AChR γ subunit gene expression, in line with its suggested use in evaluating muscle fibre denervation in healthy individuals. In our previous study, we found a negative correlation between age and the AChR γ subunit in a large group of elderly men [20], which initially might seem to contradict our finding in the present study. However, it is important to acknowledge that a denervated muscle fibre is not in a "stable state", meaning that without the neural input the proteins will be degraded and the structure is gradually lost [34,35]. Ultimately, the muscle fibre completely disappears or is only present as a fraction of its former size and as such its contribution to the whole muscle gene expression profile will also decline.

Since our study includes one data set from males and the other from females, it is worth considering similarities in the pattern of the exercise response between the elderly male and female subjects, given that the day five timepoint of the females can be compared with the four- and seven-day timepoints of the male. In this way it seems that the α, δ, and γ subunits follow a similar pattern between the genders, with the first two subunits being upregulated in both male (α only a tendency) and female subjects after seven and five days, respectively, and the γ subunit being unaffected in both male and female subjects at these timepoints. The β subunit is consistently downregulated in the male subjects whereas this subunit is not affected in the elderly women five days after exercise. Whether this represents a true gender difference and what the functional significance might be however is unknown.

This study is to our knowledge the first to outline the gene expression time course for all AChR subunits following acute heavy resistance exercise and the first to analyse the expression of four out of five AChR subunits in both young and elderly individuals at rest and following acute exercise. The NMJ of humans is challenging to study molecularly since it is difficult to obtain actual human NMJs. Hence, we rely on extra-synaptic expression of various genes that are related to the NMJ. With this approach we observed that most subunits were found to be responsive to exercise, which would suggest that despite having reached an advanced age, there is a sustained tissue plasticity in terms of synthesizing new AChRs following an exercise stimulus. The subunit-specific responses also appear to be time-dependent, as some subunits were acutely reduced after exercise followed by a recovery phase, whereas others were downregulated for longer periods. The root of these widely diverging AChR subunit time courses is puzzling and, given evidence from animal studies that long-term exercise increases the size of the NMJ [11], it would be of interest to investigate the potential of lifelong exercise on NMJ adaptations in humans.

5. Conclusions

Taken together, these data support the concept that the loss of neural signal reverts certain muscle fibre proteins to an embryonic configuration (NCAM/MHCn/AChR γ) and that these markers are useful in evaluating the effectiveness of interventions to counteract the denervation-induced loss of muscle fibres in humans. Gene expression levels of the AChR γ subunit in particular repeatedly demonstrated sensitivity to age and exercise. The trends for age-related differences in the gene expression of AChR subunits in myotubes in cell culture were related to myogenic fusion index and potentially suggest a loss of satellite cell function in relation to the capacity to transcribe key molecules for NMJ stability. Finally, it can be speculated that the temporal manner of the AChR subunit gene expression response following exercise represents a beneficial stimulus for muscle mass preservation through strengthening of the NMJ.

Supplementary Materials:
Figure S1: Gene expression in muscle biopsies of elderly men receiving losartan ($n = 13$) or placebo ($n = 12$). mRNA data were normalized to RPLP0, log-transformed, and are shown as geometric means ± back-transformed SEM, relative to baseline (-10d). Data were analysed with a two-way repeated measures ANOVA (treatment/time). * $p < 0.05$ vs. baseline. Tendencies are written; Figure S2: Panel showing four consecutive biopsy sections of an area with small MHCn-positive muscle fibres (a–d). The dotted squares (b,d) highlight the areas of the inserts (b_{1+2} and d_{1+2}), in which a distinct dystrophin membrane is visible around the small fibre. Note that one of the positive muscle fibres is no longer visible in (c) and (d). MHCn-positive fibres are red, dystrophin, green, and nuclei, blue. MHCn, neonatal myosin heavy chain. Scale bars = 20 µm; Figure S3: Muscle fibre size of MHCn- and NCAM-positive fibres in biopsy cross-sections from the control leg in 12 young and 11 elderly women, pooled

and plotted on a logarithmic scale (a). The majority of the positive fibres were <100 μm^2.Muscle fibres positive for MHCn and NCAM for young and elderly women in control and exercised legs (b). No differences between control and exercised leg was observed for any variable. MHCn, neonatal myosin heavy chain; NCAM, neural cell adhesion molecule; Figure S4: Cross section of a muscle biopsy from one subject stained with NCAM (green) and collagen XXII (red). Nuclei are blue. NCAM-positive fibres are found in close proximity of a tendon-like structure and collagen XXII positivity confirms this is a myotendinous junction. These fibres were excluded from the analysis. Scalebar is 500 μm; Figure S5: Differentiating cells relative to proliferating cells in control leg of young women. mRNA data were normalized to RPLP0 and are shown as geometric means ± SEM. * $p < 0.05$ vs. proliferation; Figure S6: Myogenic fusion index correlates with cell culture mRNA levels of AChRγ, MuSK, and MHCe in rested leg of elderly ($n = 10$) but not young ($n = 11$) subjects. All mRNA data were log transformed and analysed with Pearson's correlation, with R and P values displayed.

Author Contributions: A.L.M., P.S., C.S., J.L.A., C.J.L.B., M.F.H., and M.K. contributed to the design of the project, while A.L.M., P.S., C.S., J.L.A., C.J.L.B., M.F.H., and M.K., S.M.J., E.B., A.K. acquired, analysed or interpreted the data of the project. C.S. and A.L.M. drafted the manuscript, and all authors gave intellectual feedback to the draft. All authors approve the final version of the manuscript to be published in *Cells* and are to be held accountable for all aspects of the work in ensuring that questions related to the accuracy or integrity of any part of the work are appropriately investigated and resolved. All authors have read and agreed to the published version of the manuscript.

Acknowledgments: The authors thank Anja Jokipii-Utzon and Camilla Brink Sørensen for excellent technical assistance with preparation of the muscle biopsies and the mRNA analysis. The monoclonal antibodies F1.652 (developmental MHC) and A4.951 (myosin heavy chain, human slow fibres), developed by Blau, H.M., were obtained from the Developmental Studies Hybridoma Bank, created by the NICHD of the NIH, and maintained at The University of Iowa, Department of Biology, Iowa City, IA 52242.

Abbreviations

MHCe	Embryonic myosin heavy chain
MHCn	Neonatal myosin heavy chain
NCAM	Neural cell adhesion molecule
MHC1	Myosin heavy chain 1
DYST	Dystrophin
AChR	Acetylcholine receptor
DAPI	4′,6-Di-amidino-2-phenylindole
TBS	Tris-buffered saline
BSA	Bovine serum albumin
mTOR	Mammalian target of rapamycin

References

1. Lexell, J.; Taylor, C.C.; Sjöström, M. What is the cause of the ageing atrophy? Total number, size and proportion of different fiber types studied in whole vastus lateralis muscle from 15- to 83-year-old men. *J. Neurol. Sci.* **1988**, *84*, 275–294. [CrossRef]

2. Bean, J.F.; Kiely, D.K.; Herman, S.; Leveille, S.G.; Mizer, K.; Frontera, W.R.; Fielding, R.A. The Relationship Between Leg Power and Physical Performance in Mobility-Limited Older People. *J. Am. Geriatr. Soc.* **2002**, *50*, 461–467. [PubMed]

3. Janssen, I.; Heymsfield, S.B.; Ross, R. Low Relative Skeletal Muscle Mass (Sarcopenia) in Older Persons Is Associated with Functional Impairment and Physical Disability. *J. Am. Geriatr. Soc.* **2002**, *50*, 889–896. [CrossRef] [PubMed]

4. Reid, K.F.; Naumova, E.N.; Carabello, R.J.; Phillips, E.M.; Fielding, R.A. Lower extremity muscle mass predicts functional performance in mobility-limited elders. *J. Nutr. Health Aging* **2008**, *12*, 493. [CrossRef] [PubMed]

5. Porter, M.M.; Vandervoort, A.A.; Lexell, J. Aging of human muscle: Structure, function and adaptability. *Scand. J. Med. Sci. Sports* **1995**, *5*, 129–142. [CrossRef]

6. Campbell, M.J.; McComas, A.J.; Petito, F. Physiological changes in ageing muscles. *J. Neurol. Neurosurg. Psychiatry* **1973**, *36*, 174–182. [CrossRef]

7. Tomlinson, B.E.; Irving, D. The numbers of limb motor neurons in the human lumbosacral cord throughout life. *J. Neurol. Sci.* **1977**, *34*, 213–219. [CrossRef]

8. Hepple, R.T.; Rice, C.L. Innervation and neuromuscular control in ageing skeletal muscle. *J. Physiol. (Lond.)* **2016**, *594*, 1965–1978. [CrossRef]

9. Snijders, T.; Leenders, M.; de Groot, L.C.P.G.M.; van Loon, L.J.C.; Verdijk, L.B. Muscle mass and strength gains following 6 months of resistance type exercise training are only partly preserved within one year with autonomous exercise continuation in older adults. *Exp. Gerontol.* **2019**, *121*, 71–78. [CrossRef]

10. Bechshøft, R.L.; Malmgaard-Clausen, N.M.; Gliese, B.; Beyer, N.; Mackey, A.L.; Andersen, J.L.; Kjær, M.; Holm, L. Improved skeletal muscle mass and strength after heavy strength training in very old individuals. *Exp. Gerontol.* **2017**, *92*, 96–105. [CrossRef]

11. Nishimune, H.; Stanford, J.A.; Mori, Y. ROLE of exercise in maintaining the integrity of the neuromuscular junction: Invited Review: Exercise and NMJ. *Muscle Nerve* **2014**, *49*, 315–324. [CrossRef]

12. Baehr, L.M.; West, D.W.D.; Marcotte, G.; Marshall, A.G.; De Sousa, L.G.; Baar, K.; Bodine, S.C. Age-related deficits in skeletal muscle recovery following disuse are associated with neuromuscular junction instability and ER stress, not impaired protein synthesis. *Aging* **2016**, *8*, 127–146. [CrossRef] [PubMed]

13. Hughes, D.C.; Marcotte, G.R.; Marshall, A.G.; West, D.W.D.; Baehr, L.M.; Wallace, M.A.; Saleh, P.M.; Bodine, S.C.; Baar, K. Age-related Differences in Dystrophin: Impact on Force Transfer Proteins, Membrane Integrity, and Neuromuscular Junction Stability. *J. Gerontol. Ser. A Biol. Sci. Med. Sci.* **2016**, *72*, 640–648. [CrossRef] [PubMed]

14. Sonjak, V.; Jacob, K.; Morais, J.A.; Rivera-Zengotita, M.; Spendiff, S.; Spake, C.; Taivassalo, T.; Chevalier, S.; Hepple, R.T. Fidelity of muscle fibre reinnervation modulates ageing muscle impact in elderly women. *J. Physiol.* **2019**, *597*, 5009–5023. [CrossRef] [PubMed]

15. Fambrough, D.M.; Drachman, D.B.; Satyamurti, S. Neuromuscular junction in myasthenia gravis: Decreased acetylcholine receptors. *Science* **1973**, *182*, 293–295. [CrossRef] [PubMed]

16. Merlie, J.P.; Sanes, J.R. Concentration of acetylcholine receptor mRNA in synaptic regions of adult muscle fibres. *Nature* **1985**, *317*, 66–68. [CrossRef] [PubMed]

17. Fambrough, D.M. Control of acetylcholine receptors in skeletal muscle. *Physiol. Rev.* **1979**, *59*, 165–227. [CrossRef] [PubMed]

18. Gundersen, K.; Rabben, I.; Klocke, B.J.; Merlie, J.P. Overexpression of myogenin in muscles of transgenic mice: Interaction with Id-1, negative crossregulation of myogenic factors, and induction of extrasynaptic acetylcholine receptor expression. *Mol. Cell. Biol.* **1995**, *15*, 7127–7134. [CrossRef]

19. Pestronk, A.; Drachman, D.B. Motor Nerve Sprouting and Acetylcholine Receptors. *Science* **1978**, *199*, 1223–1225. [CrossRef]

20. Soendenbroe, C.; Heisterberg, M.F.; Schjerling, P.; Karlsen, A.; Kjaer, M.; Andersen, J.L.; Mackey, A.L. Molecular indicators of denervation in aging human skeletal muscle. *Muscle Nerve* **2019**, *60*, 453–463. [CrossRef]

21. Sanes, J.R.; Lichtman, J.W. Induction, assembly, maturation and maintenance of a postsynaptic apparatus. *Nat. Rev. Neurosci.* **2001**, *2*, 791–805. [CrossRef] [PubMed]

22. Reist, N.E.; Werle, M.J.; McMahan, U.J. Agrin released by motor neurons induces the aggregation of acetylcholine receptors at neuromuscular junctions. *Neuron* **1992**, *8*, 865–868. [CrossRef]

23. Liu, W.; Klose, A.; Forman, S.; Paris, N.D.; Wei-LaPierre, L.; Cortés-Lopéz, M.; Tan, A.; Flaherty, M.; Miura, P.; Dirksen, R.T.; et al. Loss of adult skeletal muscle stem cells drives age-related neuromuscular junction degeneration. *Elife* **2017**, *6*, e26464. [CrossRef] [PubMed]

24. Liu, W.; Wei-LaPierre, L.; Klose, A.; Dirksen, R.T.; Chakkalakal, J.V. Inducible depletion of adult skeletal muscle stem cells impairs the regeneration of neuromuscular junctions. *Elife* **2015**, *4*, e09221. [CrossRef] [PubMed]

25. Bechshøft, C.J.L.; Jensen, S.M.; Schjerling, P.; Andersen, J.L.; Svensson, R.B.; Eriksen, C.S.; Mkumbuzi, N.S.; Kjær, M.; Mackey, A.L. Age and prior exercise in vivo determine the subsequent in vitro molecular profile of myoblasts and nonmyogenic cells derived from human skeletal muscle. *Am. J. Physiol. Cell Physiol.* **2019**, *316*, C898–C912. [CrossRef] [PubMed]

26. Heisterberg, M.F.; Andersen, J.L.; Schjerling, P.; Bülow, J.; Lauersen, J.B.; Roeber, H.L.; Kjær, M.; Mackey, A.L. Effect of Losartan on the Acute Response of Human Elderly Skeletal Muscle to Exercise. *Med. Sci. Sports Exerc.* **2018**, *50*, 225–235. [CrossRef]

27. Bergstrom, J. Percutaneous needle biopsy of skeletal muscle in physiological and clinical research. *Scand. J. Clin. Lab. Investig.* **1975**, *35*, 609–616. [CrossRef]

28. Koch, M.; Schulze, J.; Hansen, U.; Ashwodt, T.; Keene, D.R.; Brunken, W.J.; Burgeson, R.E.; Bruckner, P.; Bruckner-Tuderman, L. A novel marker of tissue junctions, collagen XXII. *J. Biol. Chem.* **2004**, *279*, 22514–22521. [CrossRef]

29. Jakobsen, J.R.; Mackey, A.L.; Knudsen, A.B.; Koch, M.; Kjaer, M.; Krogsgaard, M.R. Composition and adaptation of human myotendinous junction and neighboring muscle fibers to heavy resistance training. *Scand. J. Med. Sci. Sports* **2017**, *27*, 1547–1559. [CrossRef]

30. Karlsen, A.; Bechshøft, R.L.; Malmgaard-Clausen, N.M.; Andersen, J.L.; Schjerling, P.; Kjaer, M.; Mackey, A.L. Lack of muscle fibre hypertrophy, myonuclear addition, and satellite cell pool expansion with resistance training in 83-94-year-old men and women. *Acta Physiol. (Oxf.)* **2019**, *227*, e13271. [CrossRef]

31. Brown, M.C.; Holland, R.L.; Hopkins, W.G. Motor Nerve Sprouting. *Annu. Rev. Neurosci.* **1981**, *4*, 17–42. [CrossRef] [PubMed]

32. Covault, J.; Sanes, J.R. Neural cell adhesion molecule (N-CAM) accumulates in denervated and paralyzed skeletal muscles. *Proc. Natl. Acad. Sci. USA* **1985**, *82*, 4544–4548. [CrossRef] [PubMed]

33. Gillon, A.; Sheard, P. Elderly mouse skeletal muscle fibres have a diminished capacity to upregulate NCAM production in response to denervation. *Biogerontology* **2015**, *16*, 811–823. [CrossRef] [PubMed]

34. Viguie, C.A.; Lu, D.-X.; Huang, S.-K.; Rengen, H.; Carlson, B.M. Quantitative study of the effects of long-term denervation on the extensor digitorum longus muscle of the rat. *Anat. Rec.* **1997**, *248*, 346–354. [CrossRef]

35. Gosztonyi, G.; Naschold, U.; Grozdanovic, Z.; Stoltenburg-Didinger, G.; Gossrau, R. Expression of Leu-19 (CD56, N-CAM) and nitric oxide synthase (NOS) I in denervated and reinnervated human skeletal muscle. *Microsc. Res. Tech.* **2001**, *55*, 187–197. [CrossRef] [PubMed]

36. Doppler, K.; Mittelbronn, M.; Bornemann, A. Myogenesis in human denervated muscle biopsies. *Muscle Nerve* **2008**, *37*, 79–83. [CrossRef]

37. Mishina, M.; Takai, T.; Imoto, K.; Noda, M.; Takahashi, T.; Numa, S.; Methfessel, C.; Sakmann, B. Molecular distinction between fetal and adult forms of muscle acetylcholine receptor. *Nature* **1986**, *321*, 406–411. [CrossRef]

38. Gu, Y.; Hall, Z.W. Immunological evidence for a change in subunits of the acetylcholine receptor in developing and denervated rat muscle. *Neuron* **1988**, *1*, 117–125. [CrossRef]

39. Missias, A.C.; Chu, G.C.; Klocke, B.J.; Sanes, J.R.; Merlie, J.P. Maturation of the acetylcholine receptor in skeletal muscle: Regulation of the AChR gamma-to-epsilon switch. *Dev. Biol.* **1996**, *179*, 223–238. [CrossRef]

40. Goldman, D.; Staple, J. Spatial and temporal expression of acetylcholine receptor RNAs in innervated and denervated rat soleus muscle. *Neuron* **1989**, *3*, 219–228. [CrossRef]

41. Witzemann, V.; Brenner, H.R.; Sakmann, B. Neural factors regulate AChR subunit mRNAs at rat neuromuscular synapses. *J. Cell Biol.* **1991**, *114*, 125–141. [CrossRef] [PubMed]

4

The Diversity of Muscles and their Regenerative Potential across Animals

Letizia Zullo [1,2,*], Matteo Bozzo [3], Alon Daya [4], Alessio Di Clemente [1,5],
Francesco Paolo Mancini [6], Aram Megighian [7,8], Nir Nesher [4], Eric Röttinger [9], Tal Shomrat [4],
Stefano Tiozzo [10], Alberto Zullo [6,*] and Simona Candiani [3]

[1] Istituto Italiano di Tecnologia, Center for Micro-BioRobotics & Center for Synaptic Neuroscience and Technology (NSYN), 16132 Genova, Italy; Alessio.DiClemente@iit.it
[2] IRCCS Ospedale Policlinico San Martino, 16132 Genova, Italy
[3] Laboratory of Developmental Neurobiology, Department of Earth, Environment and Life Sciences, University of Genova, Viale Benedetto XV 5, 16132 Genova, Italy; matteo.bozzo@edu.unige.it (M.B.); candiani@unige.it (S.C.)
[4] Faculty of Marine Sciences, Ruppin Academic Center, Michmoret 40297, Israel; alond@ruppin.ac.il (A.D.); nirn@ruppin.ac.il (N.N.); talsh@ruppin.ac.il (T.S.)
[5] Department of Experimental Medicine, University of Genova, Viale Benedetto XV, 3, 16132 Genova, Italy
[6] Department of Science and Technology, University of Sannio, 82100 Benevento, Italy; mancini@unisannio.it
[7] Department of Biomedical Sciences, University of Padova, 35131 Padova, Italy; aram.megighian@unipd.it
[8] Padova Neuroscience Center, University of Padova, 35131 Padova, Italy
[9] Institute for Research on Cancer and Aging (IRCAN), Université Côte d'Azur, CNRS, INSERM, 06107 Nice, France; eric.rottinger@univ-cotedazur.fr
[10] Laboratoire de Biologie du Développement de Villefranche-sur-Mer (LBDV), Sorbonne Université, CNRS, 06230 Paris, France; tiozzo@obs-vlfr.fr
* Correspondence: letizia.zullo@iit.it (L.Z.); albzullo@unisannio.it (A.Z.)

Abstract: Cells with contractile functions are present in almost all metazoans, and so are the related processes of muscle homeostasis and regeneration. Regeneration itself is a complex process unevenly spread across metazoans that ranges from full-body regeneration to partial reconstruction of damaged organs or body tissues, including muscles. The cellular and molecular mechanisms involved in regenerative processes can be homologous, co-opted, and/or evolved independently. By comparing the mechanisms of muscle homeostasis and regeneration throughout the diversity of animal body-plans and life cycles, it is possible to identify conserved and divergent cellular and molecular mechanisms underlying muscle plasticity. In this review we aim at providing an overview of muscle regeneration studies in metazoans, highlighting the major regenerative strategies and molecular pathways involved. By gathering these findings, we wish to advocate a comparative and evolutionary approach to prompt a wider use of "non-canonical" animal models for molecular and even pharmacological studies in the field of muscle regeneration.

Keywords: myogenesis; evolution; metazoans; differentiation; transdifferentiation; muscle precursors; regenerative medicine

1. Introduction

One particular challenge in regenerative biology concerns the development of reconstructive strategies after muscle-related injuries, but also the treatments of degenerative myopathies for which no reliable clinical strategy exists such as muscle dystrophy, sarcopenia, cachexia, to mention just a few [1,2]. In mammals regenerative capacities are restricted to only a small number of organs [3], yet, in other metazoans, the ability to respond to environmental injuries ranges from "simple" wound healing to complete anatomical and functional restoration of the lost or damaged part of the body, including muscles [4]. The musculature is a tissue specialized in contraction and cells with contractile functions are present in almost all metazoans but, despite their structural similarity, the origin of muscles is considered to be the outcome of a process of convergent evolution [5]. Indeed, typical muscle protein core sets are present even in unicellular organisms and in early diverged organisms like sponges, which lacks a proper tissue organization and therefore "true" muscles, and in cnidarians, where muscle-like cells are present but lack almost all molecular hallmarks of bilaterian striated muscles thus suggesting evolution from cells with ancient contractile machinery [5]. The processes of myogenesis and muscle homeostasis have also various degrees of conservation among different clades, and so is the extent of muscle regenerative capabilities [5–10].

Animals adopt different basic strategies of regeneration that include the activation of adult stem cells, the dedifferentiation of preexisting cells, and/or the proliferation of differentiated cells. This diversity of mechanisms is still widely understudied and underexploited for biomedical applications.

In this review, we provide an outline of main animals' clades (see Figure 1), muscle types, their development, homeostasis, and regeneration abilities highlighting what is known of their molecular mechanisms. We emphasize some potential contributions of comparative studies into the biomedical fields, therefore advocating deeper employment of 'non-canonical' animals as models for muscle regeneration studies.

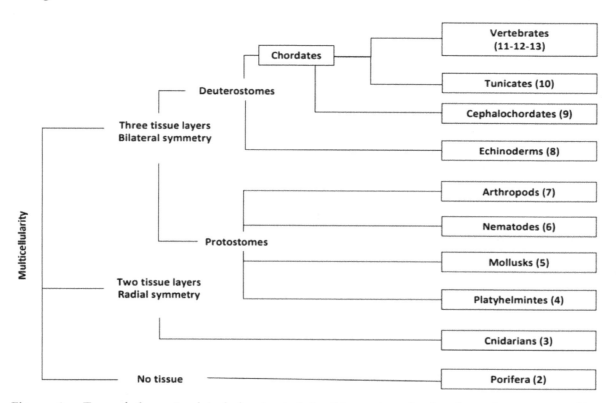

Figure 1. Tree of the animals' clades treated in this review (in brackets the corresponding section numbers).

Understanding the molecular pathways and mechanistic underlying regenerative events may offer insights into potential methods to unlock regeneration in animals where the regenerating capabilities are more restricted, e.g., mammals. Indeed, regeneration is greatly attenuated in mammals although portions of major organs, such as the liver, retain event-triggered regenerative potentials for the entire animal's life [2]. Interestingly, recent pieces of evidence suggest that regeneration can be induced even in non-regenerating species by altering specific signaling pathways [11–13]. This might be also the case for mammals and thus the principles underlying the induction of regeneration in non-regenerating species may be transferred to humans to trigger regeneration [3,14].

Elucidating muscle regeneration in metazoans also provides opportunities to 'model' a complex biological process relevant to human health and offers a window into fundamental principles underpinning this important response.

2. Porifera: Low Body Complexity with High Regenerative Capabilities

The phylum Porifera includes mainly sponges, aquatic multicellular organisms with relatively simple anatomy, lacking an organization of tissues and organs.

They have a very simple functioning relying on water circulating throughout a system of canals and chambers, called a water-current system. Circulatory, digestive, nervous, and muscular systems are completely absent. Their body is composed of a few types of cells [15,16]. For instance, in demosponges we found pinacocytes (the skin cells), mesenchymal cells, choanocytes (lining in the interior body walls), archaeocytes (totipotent cells), sclerocytes, myocytes, and porocytes (surrounding canal openings). Two types of contractile cells can be identified: the pinacocytes, and the myocytes. Pinacocytes form a functional contractile epithelium. They are composed of actin networks and actin-dense plaques allowing a coordinated contraction in adjacent pinacocytes but their mechanism of contractility remains to be further elucidated [17].

Most sponge species have an extraordinary capacity to regenerate lost body parts. Four cell types have been identified as stem-cell-like in sponge: choanocytes and archaeocytes, also referred to as adult stem cells (ASCs), pinacocytes, and particular ameboid vacuolar cells [18,19].

Muscle-Like Cells

Myocytes are spindle-shaped, smooth muscle-like cells containing microtubules lying parallel to peripheral microfilaments. They contract similarly to muscle cells thanks to a non-muscle myosin type II with high homology to that found in bilaterians and vertebrates. They allow the sponge to change shape and expel sediments even without the presence of a nervous system as their contraction is entirely controlled at a cellular level through variation of calcium (Ca^{2+}) concentration [20,21]. In particular, channels located at the plasma membrane allow the control of intracellular Ca^{2+} concentration that, in turn, regulates cell contractility. This mechanism is believed to be rely on the activation of type II myosin by Ca^{2+}-dependent protein kinases [20,22]. Myocytes allow only movement internal to the sponge but these animals remain essentially sessile. Predation and physical injuries are events very common during the entire adult life of sessile organisms that had to develop efficient strategies of repair and replacement of lost structures to survive [23,24].

Very limited information is currently available on the molecular pathways involved in body regeneration. The activity of ADP-ribosyl cyclase (ADPRC) is related to physiological activities in sponges, such as stem cell duplication and regeneration events [25]. Sponges regenerate using diverse and complex morphogenetic mechanisms involving different cell sources depending on the species. Regeneration can occur through epimorphosis and morphallaxis. The first process involves the formation of a mass of undifferentiated cells (blastema) at the wound site. Pluripotent cells such as archaeocytes and choanocytes from sites adjacent to the injury, undergo a process of epithelial-to-mesenchymal transition (EMT) and migrate to the injured area. Here they actively proliferate and form a typical blastema with dedifferentiated cells. Thereafter a process of mesenchymal-to-epithelial transition (MET) re-establish the differentiated cell identity. Different members of the transforming growth factor (TGF) superfamily are also involved in these processes [26]. In morphallaxis, of particular importance is cell transdifferentiation, the conversion of a differentiated cell to another type of differentiated cell [18]. During this process, spreading and fusion of the epithelia surrounding the wound is accompanied by the transdifferentiation of the choanocytes and exopinacocytes without the formation of a blastema. This supports the hypothesis that these cells combine properties of somatic and stem cells.

Taken together, Porifera represents, for their exceptional regenerative capacities and low body complexity, a promising model for investigating mechanisms of cell recognition, adhesion, migration, and cell type transition during regeneration.

3. Cnidarians: The Starlet Sea Anemone, *Nematostella vectensis* (Anthozoa)

Cnidarians (*Hydra*, jellyfish, corals, sea anemones) are aquatic animals that are the sister group to the bilaterian clade [27] and hold a key phylogenetic position for understanding the evolution of common biological processes and mechanisms [28]. The two main groups of the phylum Cnidaria are Medusozoa (jellyfish, hydroids, *Hydra*) and Anthozoa (corals, sea anemones) (Figure 2A). Cnidarians are structurally simple animals with remarkable regeneration capacity. They can regenerate amputated head, foot, and intact animals can even regenerate grouping single dissociated cells [29].

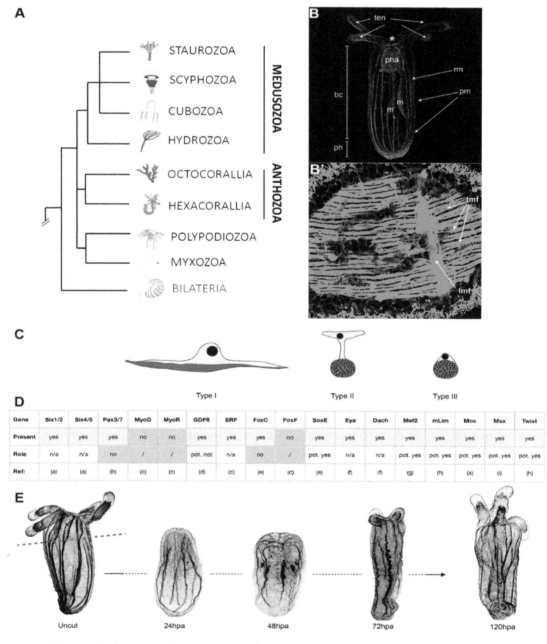

Gene	Six1/2	Six4/5	Pax3/7	MyoD	MyoR	GDF8	SRF	FoxC	FoxF	SoxE	Eya	Dach	Mef2	mLim	Mox	Msx	Twist
Present	yes	yes	yes	no	no	yes	yes	yes	no	yes	yes	yes	yes	yes	yes	yes	yes
Role	n/a	n/a	no	/	/	pot. not	n/a	no	/	pot. yes	n/a	n/a	pot. yes	pot. yes	pot. yes	pot. yes	pot. yes
Ref:	(a)	(a)	(b)	(c)	(c)	(d)	(c)	(e)	(c)	(e)	(f)	(f)	(g)	(h)	(a)	(i)	(h)

Figure 2. The epitheliomuscular system and regenerative capacity of the anthozoan cnidarian *Nematostella vectensis*. (**A**) Schematic representation of the relationship between the main cnidarian lineages and the phylogenetic position of *Nematostella vectensis* (Anthozoa, Hexacorallia). (**B**) The upper

panel shows the muscle network of nematostella in a fixed MyHC1::mCherry transgene [30] labeling the retractor muscles, co-stained with phalloidin thus showing the entire muscle network in green. (ten) tentacles, (*) mouth, (pha) pharynx, (bc) body column, (ph) physa, (m) mesenteries, (rm) retractor muscles, (pm) parietal muscles. (**B′**) Magnification of a body column region to highlight the orientation of the muscle fibers. (tmf) transverse muscle fibers, (lmf) longitudinal muscle fibers. (**C**) Three epitheliomuscular cell types have been identified in nematostella; they vary in their apical and basal cell junctions as well as their localizations within the body [31]. (**D**) Overview of the known bilateral myogenic factors identified in nematostella. (Present) indicates that the gene has been identified in the genome, (Role) indicates a myogenic role (or not) of this gene in nematostella; (pot. yes), indicates evidence of a myogenic role based on functional experiments or gene expression. (pot. not), indicates evidence of a non-myogenic role based on functional experiments or gene expression. (n/a) data not available. References cited: (a) [32], (b) [33], (c) [34], (d) [35], (e) [36], (f) [37], (g) [38], (h) [39], (i) [40]. (**E**) Oral regeneration of lost body parts after sub-pharyngeal amputation (red dashed line) is completed after 120 h post amputation and reforms a fully functional organism. Animals were fixed at various time points during regeneration and stained with phalloidin to show f-actin filaments (black). Elements of the figure are extracted from [28,41].

The present section focuses on the sea anemone *Nematostella vectensis* that belongs to the Anthozoa, mostly sessile cnidarians that are represented by individual or colony-forming polyps.

The sea anemone *Nematostella vectensis* (Anthozoa, Figure 2B), was initially employed for studying the evolution of embryonic developmental mechanisms [42] and is now emerging as a novel complementary whole-body regeneration model [41]. Nematostella possesses a range of fundamental advantages, such as the access to biological material, a relatively short life-cycle, an annotated genome that revealed astonishing similarities with the one from vertebrates [34], a wealth of -omics data [43,44] and well developed functional genomics and genome editing approaches [45–47].

Nematostella is a rather small sea anemone (juveniles ~0.5 mm, adults ~3 cm), translucent, and well suited for imaging purposes (Figure 2B). It is a diploblastic animal formed by a bifunctional internal endomesoderm and an outer ectoderm. On the oral extremity are the tentacles that surround the mouth and the so-called physa on the opposite. Food caught by the tentacles is ingested via a muscular and neuron-rich pharynx and digested within the body cavity. While most of the digestive enzymes are secreted by the mesenteries that also store nutrients [37], these internal structures play another role as they harbor the gonads that are crucial for sexual reproduction [42] and for inducing a regenerative response [48].

3.1. Muscle Types, Organization, and Myogenic Genes

Cnidarians display a large diversity of muscle types and organizations that are involved in multiple crucial physiological functions such as feeding, locomotion, or defense [28]. Although this group of marine invertebrates lacks a large part of the molecular hallmarks of striated muscles [5], jellyfish present some ultrastructural and functional features (such as striated myonemes, thick and thin myofilaments, desmosomes as well as a mechanism of excitation–contraction coupling based on intracellular calcium stores [49]) resembling the structure and function of striated muscles [50–53].

For a global overview of cnidarian muscle diversity, their development, and regeneration, please refer to [28]. Most anthozoan muscle cells, and nematostella is no exception, are epitheliomuscular; they contain smooth myofilaments [28] forming a transverse and longitudinal muscle fiber network clearly visible using a MyHC1::mCherry transgenic line [30] and phalloidin/actin staining (Figure 2B′). The epitheliomuscular cells, whose actin fibers form more or less condensed muscle fibers are responsible for various functions of the animal such as feeding or locomotion.

A recent study has characterized three epitheliomuscular cell types (Figure 2C); two types (I and II) with elongated cytoplasmic bridges present in the endodermal parietal and retractor muscles (Figure 2B) and one type III corresponding to basiepithelial muscle cells encountered in the ectoderm of the tentacles [31]. While the known bilaterian myogenic regulatory factors (MRFs [54]) are missing in nematostella (e.g., MyoD, MyoR), a large part of the conserved myogenic gene regulatory network (e.g., Pax3, Pax7, Six1 [55]) has been identified (Figure 2D, reviewed in [28]). However, their exact roles in the formation of the epitheliomuscular cells in nematostella are yet to be understood.

3.2. Muscle Regeneration and Role of Epitheliomuscular Cells in the Regenerative Process

Like cnidarians in general, nematostella possesses proliferation-dependent whole-body regenerative capacities and can regrow fully functional animals from isolated body pieces within less than a week (Figure 2E) [56–59]. In addition, nematostella is very well suited to compare embryonic development and whole-body regeneration within the same organism [43,57,60], one of the long-lasting questions in regenerative biology [61].

By assessing the MyHC1::mCherry transgenic gene expression after bisection, Renfer and colleagues have observed that the retractor muscles retract from the wound site immediately after amputation. In later steps of the regenerative process, mCherry positive cells accumulate in the regenerating body part suggesting active cellular re-organization and differentiation to reform the retractor muscles [30]. However, the cellular and molecular mechanisms underlying retractor muscle regeneration remain unknown.

On the other hand, there are shreds of evidence suggesting an active role of muscle fibers in the regenerative process. Bossert and colleagues have shown that muscular contractions are involved in reducing the epithelia of the wound site and potentially favoring the wound-healing process [62]. In addition, a stereotyped tissue dynamics that may reflect the above-mentioned observation of MyHc1::mCherry positive cells retracting from the amputation site, supports the idea that muscle contractions play also a crucial role during various phases of the regenerative process [59]. A recent study has shown that the retractor-muscle containing mesenteries are fundamental in inducing regeneration in nematostella [48]. Based on data from planarian [63] and mammalian myoepithelial cells [64], one could thus speculate that the epitheliomuscular cells that form the retractor muscle are also involved in the regeneration process via contraction-independent biochemical signals. However, additional work is required to further support those evidences and to determine the cellular and molecular mechanisms involved.

4. Platyhelminthes: The Freshwater Planarian

Since the beginning of the 21st century, the freshwater, free-living, flatworm planarian, has become a leading model for the study of development and regeneration mechanisms [65]. As a model organism, it possesses a set of clear advantages. 1. Reductionism: although its relative simplicity, planarians exhibits much of the "complexity" of vertebrate systems, including a well-differentiated nervous system, simple eyes, central brain, triploblastic organization, and bilateral symmetry. 2. Planarians are inexpensive and very easy to rear and maintain in the lab, therefore ideal for primary high-throughput screening processes [66]. 3. Planarians are molecularly-tractable model organisms, easily manipulated by RNAi interference [67] and their thin and somewhat transparent body allows whole-mount in situ hybridization in an intact worm [68].

However, there is no doubt that the most astounding feature is its regeneration capability. Planarians are considered as the "Masters of Regeneration". Adult pluripotent stem cells that are called neoblasts and are the only proliferating cells, account for 25–30% of all cells distributed in the planarian body, and give them remarkable regenerative abilities. Whole worms can regenerate from only a small proportion of the adult worm, within 1–2 weeks. Consequently, full results from regeneration experiments are revealed in a relatively short time. For a broad review of planarian as a model system for regeneration see Ivankovic et al. [69].

4.1. Muscle Types

The planarian's muscle cells combine features common to both skeletal and smooth muscles [63]. The planarian contains two main muscular systems, somatic and pharyngeal, that differ in their myosin heavy-chain (MHC) muscle isoforms along with their function and location possibly due to their different biological functions [63]. Without a supportive skeleton, the maintenance of body shape, posture, movements, and defense (strength for their soft bodies) depends on the somatic muscular system. Locomotion is mainly executed by ciliary gliding. The muscular body wall, organized beneath the epithelium, is arranged in a grid work of 4 layers of fibers lying in different orientations and linked to an extracellular network of filaments associated with the body's organs [63]. Moreover, recent works [70–72] revealed that in planarian, the muscles also provide patterning signals essential to regeneration and guidance of tissue turnover and regrowth after injury. Interestingly, this resembles what has been suggested to be a function of the connective tissues in vertebrates [73]. The somatic muscular system provides regeneration guidance through the expression of position control genes (PCGs) differing over time, body region, and types of genes expressed.

In addition to the somatic muscular system, planarians possess a separate pharyngeal musculature system. Planarians have an incomplete digestive system with pharynx (proboscis and anus) connected to the intestine duct by its anterior thus providing a single opening that functions as both, anus and mouth. The pharynx is composed of a muscular tube and demonstrates repertoires of movement capabilities. It is extruded from the body center during feeding and can direct itself toward the food by bending and stretching till it reaches the food; it thus swallows the food and transfers it to the intestine by peristaltic movements. The pharynx does not contain neoblasts [74] and therefore is incapable to regenerate the rest of the worm when amputated. However, a worm losing its pharynx can regenerate it in a few days [75]. The pharynx can thus serve as a module of organ regeneration where stem cells differentiate into distinct cell types to form an organ that integrates within the rest of the body [76].

4.2. Muscle Regeneration and Homeostasis

Upon regeneration, planarian muscle cells, as all other tissue components, arise from the large reservoir of the existent neoblasts population that migrate to the wound area and start proliferate, thus creating a blastema where they differentiate to form the missing body parts. Irradiation protocols applied to the whole body or to specific areas allows neoblasts ablation [77]. Further transplantation of a single pluripotent neoblast can restore regenerative ability and the whole process can be monitored from scratch [78]. Therefore, planarian is an ideal model for deciphering the mystery of stem cell differentiation [79], allowing experimental approaches that are unavailable in any other model organism. Research on planarian muscle regeneration is still limited but provides some interesting perspectives.

One other unique feature of the planarian model (e.g., *Dugesia japonica* and *Schmidtea mediterranea*) is the ability to shift from growing (up to few centimeters) to de-growing (down to few millimeters) by food deprivation and vice versa. The process depends on the balance between cell proliferation and cell death and by keeping stable body shape and proportions through constant remodeling mechanisms [80]. Therefore, it is a perfect model system for the study of tissue homeostasis (for a broad overview of the subject see [81]).

In spite of their exceptional features and their growing popularity as a model for basic research on regeneration, planarians are not yet considered as a conventional organism for studying human pathologies and diseases, maybe it is time to rethink [82].

5. Mollusks: The Cephalopods

Cephalopods represent one the main and most evolved mollusk class. They are the most intelligent, mobile, and the largest of all mollusks and include very diverse species such as squid, octopus, cuttlefish and the chambered nautilus.

Regeneration is a frequent event occurring during cephalopods' lifetime. Wild animals often lose body parts such as portions of arms and fins and as a consequence, it is common to find signs of traumatic events on their bodies [83,84]. These events can dramatically impair their capacity to swim, capture, and manipulate preys [85], and therefore they can seriously impact their survival in the natural environment. Indeed, cephalopods can regenerate their cornea, peripheral nerves, and body limb (arms and tentacles) [86]. Cephalopod limbs are complex organs composed of a tightly packed three-dimensional array of muscle fibers controlled by a sophisticated peripheral nervous system (PNS). The arm PNS is composed of three distinct parts: the arm nerve cord (composed of axial nerve cords and the ganglionic core), the sucker ganglia, and the intramuscular nerves. This assembly allows the transmission of a large amount of sensory and motor information to and from the brain [87–90]. All of these structures are fully and functionally recovered during regeneration.

5.1. Muscle Types

Similar to vertebrates, muscle cells in cephalopods can be found in a variety of different organs that differ dramatically in structure and function. Indeed, muscle cells are in the mantle and appendages (arms and tentacles) but also in eyes, hearts, viscera and chromatophores. Such diversity is paralleled by specific adaptations in muscular organization and physiology.

The majority of the musculature of arms and tentacles is composed by uninucleate transverse or obliquely striated muscle fibers with shared morphological and physiological characteristics. When oblique striation is present, this pattern is uniform and continuous among adjacent cells. Generally, these muscle cells do not exceed 8–20 μm in diameter and 0.8–1 mm in length. The nucleus is in the central portion of the cell whose transverse section is usually round or polygonal, with a mitochondria-rich core and a contractile apparatus in the cortical zone. The contractile apparatus lies along the main axis of the fiber and is organized in sarcomeres with identifiable acto-myosin striations. Cephalopod muscle actin and myosin heavy chain, show strong sequence identity to other invertebrates and vertebrate gene orthologs suggesting a similar contraction mechanism [91,92]. On the contrary, regulatory proteins are very cephalopod-specific [93] suggesting that specific control kinetics and cross-bridge cycle regulation might be developed in cephalopods (for a review see [94,95]). Different from typical skeletal muscles, cephalopod arm muscle cells do not possess a proper T-tubules system, but smaller sarcoplasmic structures named "terminal cisternae" that take contacts with plasma membrane invaginations thus forming "dyads" at the level of the Z-disks. In contrast to the muscle cells of other invertebrates, they are isopotential, and thus each synaptic input can control the membrane potential of the entire muscle cell (for a review see [94]).

Among cephalopods, muscle cells can differ in their activation properties. As an example, in octopus arm, muscle action potentials rely on Ca^{2+} spikes [96,97] generating a massive entrance of Ca^{2+} that activates a calcium-induced calcium release (CICR) process from the internal stores [98]. An intriguing analogy here can be found with vertebrate cardiac muscle cells that represent an important target of regeneration medicine [99,100].

In contrast to the octopus arm muscles, transverse muscles of squid tentacles show 'graded' Na^+ based action potentials different from the typical 'all or nothing' action potentials of squid giant axon or vertebrate muscle fibers. Interestingly, the transverse muscle of the squid arms lacks Na^+-based action potentials [101]. All the above-mentioned characteristics co-evolved with the complex brain to body adaptation and limb specialization [102–104] whose integrity is essential to the animal survival.

Several myogenic genes have been identified in some (but not all) cephalopod species. As an example myoblast-specific Myf5 and MyoD proteins have been identified in *Sepia officinalis* tentacles during late stage development and NK4 is found to be involved in cephalopod striated muscle formation just as in vertebrate cardiac cells [94,105,106]. In addition, an hh-homolog signaling molecule and its receptor Patched (Ptc) have been found to be expressed during myoblast differentiation in *Sepia officinalis* [107].

5.2. Muscle Regeneration

Cephalopod mollusks are a powerful model of limb regeneration due to their similarities in early arm development to vertebrate models and their fast and efficient regenerative abilities (for a review see [94]) and, among regeneration studies of other body parts, rather ample literature is currently available on the regeneration of their limbs (for a review see [84]). However, very little is known about the molecular pathways controlling the regenerative process.

Hereafter, we will employ the octopus arm as a template to describe the step of a regeneration process. Morphologically, a sequence of events can be identified during arm regeneration: (1) wound healing; (2) formation of a knob at the stump tip; (3) elongation of the knob and formation of a hook-like structure; and (4) elongation of the regenerating arm till complete restoration of a functional structure [85,94,108,109].

At early steps of regeneration, a mixture of extracellular matrix (ECM), vesicles, and mucus are present at the plug region, and only subsequently the connective tissue is deposited by fibrocytes migrating to this region [109]. The presence of ECM and connective fibers might be relevant for the correct reorganization of the regenerating structure, a role that has been also suggested in octopus pallial nerve regeneration [84]. Cephalopods might have evolved fine mechanisms of regulating ECM composition and organization during regeneration that favor the tissue competency to regrow. Interestingly, similar fibrillary elements are the ones limiting vertebrates skeletal muscle regeneration as their accumulation at the injury site negatively interferes with regeneration and drives instead scarring and fibrosis of the tissues [94].

At a cellular level, cells composing the stump are first characterized by a layer of undifferentiated cells together with diffuse vascular components forming a typical blastemal region. This structure then disappears, and cells start differentiating [110]. Cell proliferation remains active throughout the entire regeneration process, but while at an early step is primarily localized at the blastema, at later stages it is present within differentiating tissues such as the axial nerve cord and the musculature.

Unfortunately, no study reported so far could reveal the molecular identity of muscle cell precursor during regeneration. It has been speculated that new muscles and nerve cells can originate from dedifferentiated cells of the same type (for a review see [84]) but due to the lack of species-specific molecular markers, we are currently not able to assess the existence of pluripotent vs. lineage-committed progenitor cells, as well as vertebrate satellite-like cells associated with adult muscles. From a mechanicistic viewpoint it has been shown that after an arm lesion, muscles close to the injury site degenerate fast, and large cells containing little protoplasm and a large nucleus appear within the same area. These cells are supposed to be sarcoblasts that later migrate to the most distal part of the wound and undergo active proliferation. Sarcoblasts will then differentiate into the arm and sucker muscle fibers in different time intervals [108]. This process is possibly paralleled by the recovery of the arm functional capacity.

Few data are available on the molecular pathways underlying muscle formation during regeneration in cephalopods. It is known that cephalopods muscle development rely on MRFs, however, still, no data are available on their expression during muscle regeneration in octopus. Several studies suggested that acetylcholinesterase (AChE), a conserved molecule between vertebrates and invertebrates, may orchestrate the formation of the octopus arm during regeneration [110,111] similarly to what happens in regeneration phenomena occurring in other animal phyla such as Platyhelminthes, Mollusca, Arthropoda, and even Chordata (for a review see [94]).

6. Nematodes: The *Caenorabditis elegans* Model

Nematodes are one of the most diverse animal phyla. They occupy a large variety of environments, and many species are parasitic. Nematodes are relatively small animals (~1 mm long adults), and, given their size, a heart and a closed circulatory system are not required.

C. elegans has been employed as a model to study extrinsic and intrinsic factors crucial for axon regeneration and wound healing. In particular it have disclosed important aspects of the mechanisms of wound healing and cellular plasticity, axon regeneration and transdifferentiation in vivo [112].

Muscle Type and Homeostasis

The majority of muscles of the animal body wall are used for the animal's locomotion [113]. *C. elegans* body wall muscle cells are spindle-shaped mononuclear cells with multiple sarcomeres per cell [114]. Muscle cells are obliquely striated and form body-wall muscles running along the length of the body underneath the epidermis [115,116]. Unlike most other animals, their innervation is unusual in that the nerves do not branch out into the muscles but the muscle cells send extensions (muscle arms) to the nerve cord to receive *en passant* synapses from the motor neurons [117,118].

Embryonic development of body wall muscle is controlled by maternally expressed genes initially, but then there is a switch to control by zygotically expressed genes. Several molecular players (e.g., Wnt/Mitogen-Activated Protein (MAP) kinase signaling, Myogenic regulatory factors (MRFs) as many others) act during muscle development and differentiation. For a detailed description please refer to [119,120].

C. elegans muscles lack satellite cells (muscle stem cells) and therefore muscles cannot regenerate. Adult worms only carry post-mitotic body wall muscles [119]. It is interesting to notice that, although lacking an open circulatory system, proteins and structures composing the body wall muscles manifest a high homology with that of human heart muscle. In addition, many molecules involved in sarcomere assembly and maintenance are in common with other animals. A dystrophin ortholog, dys-1 gene, has been identified in *C. elegans* with a key role in the sarcomere structural regulation [121]. The mechanism of assembly of sarcomeres into functional muscles have been extensively investigated in *C. elegans* within the context of repair following activity-induced muscle stress and muscle degeneration [117].

For the reasons listed above, *C. elegans* has become a model study for muscle diseases such as Duchenne's Muscular Dystrophy (DMD) [122] and cardiomyopathies [113]. A more explanatory and detailed list of advantages and disadvantages of this animal as a model of human heart pathologies can be found in [113].

Interestingly, the lack of regeneration capacity of *C. elegans* muscles has been key to the use of this animal as a model of DMD. Indeed, as *C. elegans* adult muscle cells are mono-nucleated and post-mitotic, they can be individually tracked during the process of muscle degeneration and do not undergo fibrosis and chronic inflammation, processes that are common in vertebrate models [121].

7. Artropods: The Insect *Drosophila melanogaster*

Insects have a reduced lifespan and events related to degeneration/regeneration processes following physical, pathological or aging damage are less frequent. Hence, the establishment of a real physiological regenerative mechanism have been under a lower evolutionary pressure. However insects manifest adult muscle hypertrophy, which can be viewed as a degeneration/regeneration-like process, in response to particular hormones as well as to environmental factors, population density, food availability, or mating [123,124].

Drosophila melanogaster is a model organism in which genetic and molecular techniques, coupled with physiological and structural approaches, have been used to unravel specific issues of invertebrates and vertebrates muscle biology, including regeneration processes.

Muscle Type and Homeostasis

In *D. melanogaster* larvae and adults, three types of muscles can be recognized: (1) Tubular muscles, including most of the adult skeletal muscles. They are striated with a centrally located nucleus and are synchronous muscles because each nerve stimulation evokes calcium release from internal stores which triggers a mechanical contraction of the muscle similarly to vertebrate skeletal muscles [125]. (2) Adult indirect flight muscles, or "fibrillar" muscles. In these muscles individual myofibrils can be identified by light microscopy; they are striated and asynchronous muscles as their mechanical response is activated both by calcium following nerve impulse and by stretch-activation due to the elastic recoil of thorax cuticle [125,126]. (3) Supercontractile striated visceral and heart muscles, and larval body wall muscles. Supercontractile muscles are called "supercontractile" because they can contract to a length well below 50% of their resting length [127–131]. They contract in response to caffeine also in the absence of external calcium, showing that a functional store of calcium is present in the sarcoplasmic reticulum and that it is sufficient for muscle contraction [132]. Interestingly, a similar activation property has been also found in the octopus arm muscles [98].

Larval and adult muscle cells and fibers derive from progenitor cells of the embryonic mesoderm. Signaling crosstalk between ectoderm and mesoderm (for instance Decantaplegic and Wingless) and gene (e.g., *twist*, *even-skipped*, and *floppy-paired*) dynamic temporal expression, regulate the muscle cell fate of these cells [133,134]. Cardiac and visceral muscle cell progenitors are formed from these generic muscle cell progenitors by their compartmentalization in segmental regions with low Twist high Even-skipped domains. High Twist high Sloppy-paired domains are, on the other hand, a key point for the development of somatic cell progenitors [134,135]. Both these muscle cell progenitors undergo then asymmetric cell divisions, which generate low Twist cells that fuse to form embryonic myoblasts and subsequently embryonic muscles. Some, but not all, asymmetric division give rise also to a single founder cell and to an adult muscle precursor (AMP), an adult muscle stem cell that remains in quiescence.

Larval muscles degenerate throughout metamorphosis. In some cases (indirect flight muscles in the thorax) larval muscles are utilized as templates for the formation of adult muscles. In other cases, peripheral nerve fibers and the space between larval muscle fibers drive adult muscle fibers development and differentiation. Adult muscle fibers origin from AMP precursors which proliferate, differentiate, and fuse to form myotubes and then adult fibers. This process was deeply studied in indirect flight muscles that are the main power source for flight. From these studies, however, it was found that only a small number of AMPs descendent stem cells remain associated with the adult differentiated indirect flight muscle fibers. These cells resemble mammalian satellite cells which are associated with the adult skeletal muscle fibers and retain the competence to proliferate and differentiate in myoblasts and then adult myofibers when stimulated (for example following skeletal muscle fiber degeneration). It is interesting to note also that these "fly satellite cells" undergo a proliferation/differentiation program leading to the generation of myoblasts which fuse with a damaged indirect flight muscle fiber. This process, similarly to what was observed in vertebrate satellite cells of skeletal muscle fibers, points to repair the damaged fibers, and it is activated by Notch-Delta signaling [136]. In the absence of tissue damage, satellite cells are maintained, not differentiated, and "quiescent" probably by the transcription factor Zhf1 [137].

Other authors claim that there are probably no "satellite cells" in adult flies' muscles. Indeed, almost all of these studies were investigating the indirect flight muscles (IFMs) that are considered the most similar to mammalian skeletal muscles. In these, regeneration processes are triggered by damage consequent to physical or pathological injuries as well as damages related to aging. Considering fly lifespan, these events are less frequent and therefore they should have exerted a minor pressure from the evolutionary point of view to establish a real regenerative mechanism in adult muscles. Moreover, a regeneration-like process is considered for adult skeletal muscles as regarded as muscle hypertrophy. Again, in flies, differently from other invertebrates, the small dimension of IFMs could have been a factor against a "pressure" from an evolutionary perspective.

8. Echinoderms: A Compendium of Regeneration Strategies

Echinodermata is a phylum consisting of radially symmetrical marine animals. All larval and adult echinoderms exhibit high regenerative capacities of entire lost parts following predation or traumatic events [138]. Echinoderms manifest all the regenerative strategies identified in other animals, such as epimorphosis and morphallaxis, and have an impressive high genetic homology with Chordates. They can show epimorphic processes, by which a blastemal is formed through active proliferation of migratory undifferentiated cells. They can also show morphallaxis, where cells derive from differentiation, transdifferentiation, or migration of existing tissues. Most classical and bio-molecular tools currently available have been successfully employed in this animal species giving rise to a large body of literature on Echinoderms regeneration from molecular, cellular, and tissue level. These features make them interesting models in translational research [139].

8.1. Echinoderm Muscles

Movements in echinoderms are assured by a muscular and a water vascular system; two main muscular systems, the visceral and the somatic, are present. Similar to what happens in nematodes and amphioxus, echinoderm visceral muscles may extend cytoplasmic prolongations towards the nerve fibers that they make contact with. Echinoderm muscles retain some epithelial features. Indeed, the epithelial cell of coelom can give rise to peritoneocytes, myoepithelial cells, and myocytes through successive stages of specialization. Despite differences in anatomical location, echinoderm muscles share a similar structure. They are made up of numerous contractile bundles and each of them is composed of several myocytes containing myofilaments of variable thickness [140].

Two main types of muscle fibers can be identified, the first (and most common) in which individual bundles are composed of myocytes of fusiform shape and resemble vertebrate smooth muscle fibers. These fibers are embedded in the extracellular matrix of connective tissue composed of a network of thick striated (collagenous) and thin unstriated fibers and an amorphous component; it also comprises fibroblasts, nerve cells, and different coelomocytes (the immune effector cells of sea urchins). A second muscle type, typical of crinoid arms, consists of obliquely striated fibers with each muscle bundle composed of 8–20 myocytes and surrounded by a basal lamina.

8.2. Echinoderm Muscle Regeneration

Several signaling pathways are involved in regeneration. These include the bone morphogenetic protein/transforming growth factor (BMP/TGFB)-signaling pathway, the homeobox (HOX) signaling pathway and the Ependymin pathway. Nonetheless, it is not directly possible to associate these pathways with the specific process of muscle regeneration. To provide this information, it would be necessary to screen for genes expressed by muscle cells such as cytoskeletal genes, actin, and myosin genes. Interestingly, their expressions are known to be modulated during different stages of the regeneration process [141–143].

Upon injury, echinoderm muscles undergo processes of de-differentiation and myogenesis. In the wound region damaged myocytes degenerate and muscle bundles disintegrate. De-differentiation of the coelomic epithelial cells represents an early regeneration event occurring already during wound healing and continuing at different rates during the regenerative period.

These cells dedifferentiate and start migrating toward the region occupied by the injured muscle, here they form clusters of muscle bundle rudiments. Then, they increase in number and start developing the contractile filaments of future muscle cells. The process of myogenesis goes on in parallel with many other regenerative events and brings to the restoration of a functional muscular tissue [142,144].

In conclusion, echinoderms represent an interesting model with a high potential for muscle regeneration studies (for extended reviews see also [138,142,144]). Their close phylogenetic relation to vertebrates makes them attractive models to determine what cellular and molecular processes are required for successful muscle regeneration to occur.

9. Cephalochordates, the Basal Chordates: Amphioxus

The cephalochordate amphioxus is the sister group of the tunicate–vertebrate clade [145] (Figure 1) and represents a new emerging model for studies on cell and tissue regeneration and in particular for muscle regeneration. Its phylogenetic position also offers insights into the evolution of regenerative capacity in vertebrates.

As demonstrated in other organisms, amphioxus regeneration can vary among body parts and several variables affect the speed of healing such as species, animal age, and body size [146–149].

In amphioxus, two districts show the highest regenerative capacity: the oral cirri, skeletal structures surrounding the mouth, and the post-anal tail.

9.1. Structure of Amphioxus Muscles

The adult amphioxus possesses almost exclusively striated muscles, the most prominent of which are the segmental axial muscles providing force for burrowing and swimming, the notochord and the pterygial muscle. The axial musculature is composed of the myomeres thatare segmentally repeated in dozens of pairs throughout the entire length of the body. Myomeres are composed of flattened striated muscle cells 0.8 μm thick [150], 100 μm wide and at least 500 μm long. They are similar to vertebrate skeletal muscle cells in banding and in the arrangement of the myofilaments [151]. Moreover, the sarcoplasmic reticulum, although not arranged to form the typical T-tubule system, is present and, as in vertebrate striated muscles, might serve as calcium storage [152]. Despite these similarities, amphioxus axial muscle cells are mononucleated, in contrast to the fused myofibers of vertebrate skeletal muscles. The notochord, a modified muscle structure extending from the tail to the most anterior tip of the rostrum, consists of a row of coin-shaped striated muscle cells plus other non-muscle cells known as Müller cells. The pterygial muscle is constituted by striated fibers [153] responsible for the contraction of the branchial cavity, which results in gamete emission from the atriopore.

9.2. Muscle Regeneration in the Amphioxus Tail

Due to its ability to regenerate skin, nerve cord, and muscles after amputation, the post-anal tail is the most studied system for understanding regeneration in amphioxus (see Figure 3 for timing and principal steps of regeneration in *B. lanceolatum* and *B. japonicum*). Indeed, the tail contains the two most prominent striated muscle structures: the myomeres and the notochord.

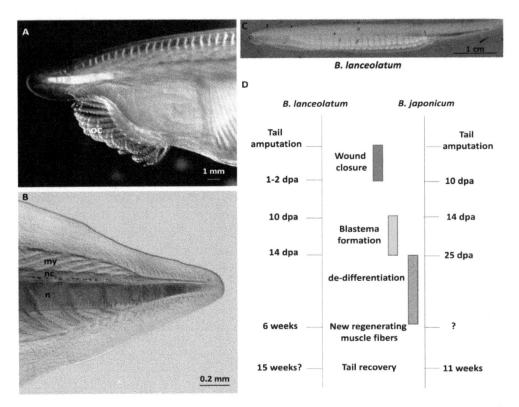

Figure 3. Timing and principal steps of regeneration in *B. lanceolatum* and *B. japonicum*. (**A**) Enlargement of the most anterior end of a *Branchiostoma lanceolatum* adult showing the oral cirri (oc). (**B**) Post-anal tail of the same animal. my, myomeres; nc, nerve cord; n, notochord. (**C**) *B. lanceolatum* individual collected in Banyuls-sur-Mer, France. (**D**) Schematic overview of the series of events occurring during tail regeneration in the *B. lanceolatum* and *B. japonicum*. dpa, days post-amputation.

While little data are available on the role of myogenic factors during tail regeneration in amphioxus, much more is known on muscle development formation in the embryo. Like vertebrates, amphioxus axial muscles derive from the myotomal portion of the somites. Here, the Six1/2-Pax3/7 myogenic program is activated [154] and regulates the differential expression of members of the myogenic regulatory factors (MRFs) gene family, which underwent independent expansion in the amphioxus lineage [155]. Amphioxus somitic mesoderm, which extends for the whole length of the body, is divided into three portions, each induced by a unique combination of transcription factors [154]. The most anterior somites depend on fibroblast growth factor (FGF) signaling [156]. The signals regulating the other two populations are yet to be identified but it has been shown that the most posterior somites, arising from the tail bud as the embryo elongates, do not require FGF nor retinoic acid signaling [156] and that Notch is required for correct separation of contiguous somites [157].

From a mechanistic viewpoint, Somorjai and coworkers [146,147] described a blastema-like structure in the amputated tail of *B. lanceolatum*, with proliferating cells from notochord, myotomes and nerve cord positive for phospho-histone H3. Subsequently, Liang and coworkers [148] confirmed cell proliferation in blastemal cells of the regenerating tail of *B. japonicum* by Bromodeoxyuridine (BrdU) labeling. Conversely, Kaneto and Wada [149] identified in the amputated oral cirri of *Branchiostoma belcheri* a large number of mesenchymal cells able to reform the skeleton, but most likely without the influence of a proliferating cell population, as phospho-histone H3 was not detected. Thus, oral cirri seem to undergo tissue remodeling by morphallaxis, whereas the tail can respond to amputation injury by epimorphic regeneration. In addition, de-differentiation of existing structures but not trans-differentiation or lineage reprogramming seems to occur during amphioxus tail regeneration, as seen in amphibians [146,147].

10. Tunicates: The Sister Group of Vertebrates

Tunicates (Phylum Chordata) encompass a large group of ubiquitous and diverse animals that occupy a wide variety of marine habitats and ecosystems around the world [158]. Despite their appearance, these animals are the sister group of vertebrates, with whom they share a common ancestor [159]. Most of the tunicate species have a biphasic life cycle, with a swimming larva, with the chordate synapomorphies, and either a benthic (like the group of ascidians) or a planktonic (in the order thaliaceans) post-metamorphic phase. During this phase, the chordate features are lost and the larva turns into a filter feeder sac-like body structure with two tubular openings, known as inhalant and exhalant siphons (Figure 4). While solitary tunicates reproduce strictly sexually and have limited regenerative capabilities, colonial species can also reproduce asexually and regenerate an entire body via diverse modes of budding, also referred to as non-embryonic development. The result is often a colony of connected, genetically identical zooids [160,161]. Budding can be part of the life cycle, which accounts for colony growth, replication and reproduction, or regeneration, i.e., passive forms triggered by injury [162].

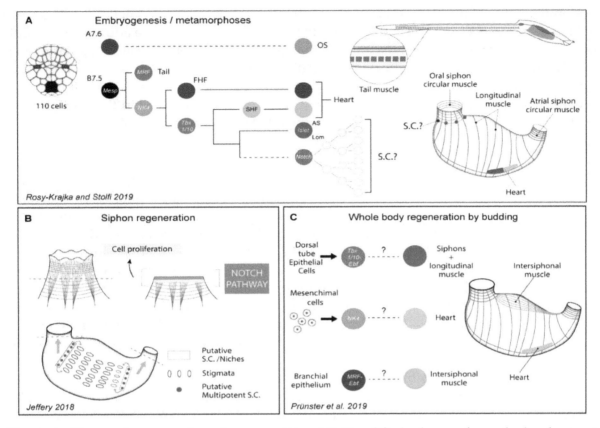

Figure 4. Ciona embryogenesis and regeneration. (**A**) Simplified scheme of muscle development during ciona embryogenesis and metamorphoses. (modified from [163]). (**B**) Scheme of oral siphon regeneration in ciona (modified from [164]). (**C**) Simplified scheme of myogenesis during budding in *Botryllus schlosseri*. FHF: first heart field; SHF: second heart field; OS: oral siphon; AS: atrial siphon; LoM: longitudinal muscles; SC: stem cells.

10.1. Myogenesis during Embryogenesis and Metamorphoses

The typical tunicate larva carries in the tail two bands of mononucleated muscle cells, one on each side of the notochord. The myofibrils of each cell are connected through intercellular junctions, similarly to the vertebrate cardiomyocytes. Each row of cells behaves as a syncytium, allowing the swimming movement. The myocytes are arranged in a striated manner and express myosin heavy chain. After metamorphosis, the sarcomere organized musculature gets reabsorbed along with the tail, and the musculature of the formed zooid generally consists of longitudinal and circular multinucleated fibers that run throughout the mantle along the body and around the two siphons (Figure 4). While ultrastructural studies show unstriated morphology, the adult body musculature seems to have intermediate characteristics between the vertebrate smooth and striated muscles [165]. For instance, the post-metamorphic musculature uses a troponin-tropomyosin complex similar to vertebrate striated muscles, their myocytes are specified via MRFs that generally controls vertebrate skeletal muscle development, and lacks on smooth muscle specification [165,166]. Post metamorphic zooids also develop a tubular heart, which consists of a single chamber formed from two epithelial monolayers. The pericardium is a non-contractile epithelium, whereas the myocardium is a single layer epithelium of mononucleated striated cardiomyocytes.

Most of the information on the molecular bases of muscle cell specification and differentiation comes from a copious amount of studies focused on few solitary model species namely *Ciona intestinalis*, *Halocynthia roretzi*, and Molgula, and have been recently summarized in a comprehensive review by Razy-Krajka and Stolfi (2019) [163]. Briefly, during embryogenesis, the maternal deposition of a zinc finger family member (Zic-r.ca) and the activation of a T-box transcription factor is necessary to induce the development of tail muscles. At the stage of 110-cells, a couple of blastomeres, the B7.5, acquire a cardiopharyngeal mesodermal fate and give rise to both heart and part of the adult body musculature, specifically the exhalant siphon and the longitudinal muscles (Figure 4). The gene regulatory network that governs this cell lineage specification is highly conserved between tunicates and vertebrates cardiopharyngeal myogenesis [167]. Another couple of blastomeres (the A7.6) follow a different fate but are partially regulated by the same transcription factors involved in the cardiopharyngeal specification [107] and give rise to the muscles of the inhalant siphon (Figure 4A).

10.2. Myogenesis during Budding and Regeneration

Many solitary ascidians can repair and regenerate efficiently both the exhalant and inhalant siphons, including the associated muscle fibers [168]. Interestingly, during its progressive differentiation, the B7.5 cell lineage gives rise also to a population of cells that do not express the MRF, but seems to maintain an undifferentiated state and settle around the exhalant siphon [169,170]. These muscle precursors maintain a stem cell-like state via a Notch-mediated lateral inhibition, a mechanism that has been also reported in drosophila and vertebrates to control muscle differentiation [170]. In addition, the A7.6 is multi-lineage, but it is not clear if such multipotency is retained in the fully developed adult. So far, the link between the B7.5 and A7.6 myogenic lineage and the siphon muscle regeneration has not yet been explored. Recently, Jeffery (2018) suggested that, in *Ciona intestinalis*, the siphons repair and regeneration are triggered by the mobilization of multipotent progenitors that migrates from niches located in the branchial sac rather than around the very same siphon [164]. The very same stem cells are also responsible for the regeneration of the central nervous system. In addition, the nature and the dynamics of these stem cells have not been yet described (Figure 4B). While there are no recent studies on *bona fide* heart regeneration in tunicates, growth regions have been reported in the ciona myocardium [167,171]. In these area, clusters of proliferating undifferentiated cells start to accumulate myofilaments and eventually mature into cardiomyocytes. The nature of these precursors, i.e., transdifferentiating cells or cardiac stem cells, remains to be studied.

Although way less studied, the embryogenesis of most colonial tunicates seems to occur in the same way than the solitary ones [172,173] and, at least in the model *Botryllus schlosseri* the myogenic regulative modules and mechanisms appears to be conserved [174]. The blastozooid, the adult produced by non-embryonic development, generally has a bauplan and a muscle architecture that is comparable to the oozooids, i.e., the individuals formed by embryonic development [165,174]. However, budding bypass fertilization, embryogenesis, larval stage, and metamorphosis [24,160,171]. Contrary to their embryonic development, which displays a remarkable level of conservation among almost all the tunicate orders, non-embryonic development encompasses a clade-specific assortment of cells, tissues, and ontogenesis, all displaying different degrees of interaction between epithelial and mesenchymal cells [161].

In *Botryllus schlosseri*, the blastozooid musculature is formed de novo during morphogenesis by partially co-opting and re-wiring the embryonic cardiopharyngeal regulatory network [174]. The body muscle fate seems to be regulated by a kernel of genes expressed in progenitor cells located in a transitory structure, the dorsal tube, which has also neurogenic potential [173]. Instead, the hierarchy of the expression of specific cardiomyogenic transcription factors suggests that the heart is specified by different mesenchymal precursors, located in another domain of the developing bud. Therefore, the reshuffling of the embryonic cardiopharyngeal regulatory modules is also linked with uncoupling of the body muscle and heart muscle precursors [174]. It does remain unclear if these populations of precursors are renewed every budding cycle or persist and pass over asexual generations, or if the same precursor is responsible for the myogenesis during other forms of partial or total regeneration [175] (Figure 4C).

In the other two ascidian species, *Botrylloides leachii* and *Perophora viridis*, a population of adult pluripotent stem cells circulating in the hemolymph seems to be responsible of the regeneration of the whole body, including the entire musculature [176,177]. As for solitary species, the study of these cell populations is still in its infancy.

11. Vertebrates: The Zebrafish

The zebrafish (*Danio rerio*) is one of the most widely used vertebrate model for regeneration studies. Zebrafish are capable of regenerating many of their organs and tissues, including heart, central nervous system, retina, lateral line hair cells, caudal fin, kidney, pancreas, liver, and skeletal muscle (reviewed in [178–180]; Figure 5).

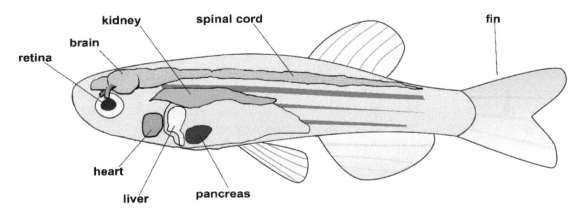

Figure 5. Regeneration in zebrafish. Schematic drawing of a zebrafish adult showing organs used for regeneration studies.

11.1. Zebrafish Skeletal Muscle Regeneration

Zebrafish trunk is composed of spatially separated slow and fast muscle fibers, and slow myofibers are embryonically mononucleated (reviewed in [181,182]). The trunk muscles are arranged in repeated chevron-shaped segments, along the head-to-tail axis. The thin partition between each pair of adjacent somites is named 'vertical myoseptum' and the one between the dorsal and ventral halves is named 'horizontal myoseptum'. The myosepta are anchoring structures for muscle fibers, enabling force transmission [183]. Two main Pax7-positive muscle stem cell populations were characterized in zebrafish. The first population is formed after somitogenesis at the external surface of the myotome, the external cell layer (ECL), expresses Pax3 and Pax7, and contributes to muscle growth throughout the zebrafish lifespan by secondary myogenesis [184]. The second population is functionally equivalent to the amniote satellite-cell population, scattered between myofibers throughout most of the myotome and serves as a source of new muscle fibers during adult zebrafish muscle repair and regeneration. These satellite-cells are mainly enriched in slow muscle near the myosepta, have dense heterochromatin and express Pax7, Pax3, and Met. In response to muscle injury, they divide asymmetrically to form two distinct cell pools: proliferative cells that fuse to form de novo myofibers or repair damaged muscle fibers, and proliferative cells that self-renew to ensure the preservation of a satellite stem cell pool [180,185]. Zebrafish skeletal muscle is a heterogeneous tissue, composed of slow, fast, and intermediate myofibers. However, at variance with mammals' intermixed muscle bundles, zebrafish trunk is composed of spatially separated slow and fast muscle fibers, and slow myofibers are embryonically mononucleated (reviewed in [181,182]). The trunk muscles are arranged in repeated chevron-shaped segments, along the head-to-tail axis. The thin partition between each pair of adjacent somites is named 'vertical myoseptum' and the one between the dorsal and ventral halves is named 'horizontal myoseptum'. The myosepta are anchoring structures for muscle fibers, enabling force transmission [183].

Myogenesis events are fundamentally common to all vertebrates. The myogenic regulatory factors (MRFs) that direct myogenic lineage development and muscle differentiation (i.e., Myf5, MyoD, Myogenin, Mrf4) are highly conserved in fish and mammals (reviewed in [178–180,186]). Two main

Pax7-positive muscle stem cell populations were characterized in zebrafish. The first population, the external cell layer (ECL), is formed after somitogenesis at the external surface of the myotome. It expresses Pax3 and Pax7 and contributes to hyperplastic muscle growth throughout the zebrafish lifespan by secondary myogenesis [184]. The second population is functionally equivalent to the amniote satellite-cell population, scattered between myofibers throughout most of the myotome and serves as a source of new muscle fibers during adult zebrafish muscle repair and regeneration. These satellite-cells are mainly enriched in slow muscle near the myosepta, have dense heterochromatin and express Pax7, Pax3, and Met. In response to muscle injury, they divide asymmetrically to form two distinct cell pools: proliferative cells that fuse to form de novo myofibers or repair damaged muscle fibers, and proliferative cells that self-renew to ensure the preservation of a satellite stem cell pool [180,185].

11.2. Zebrafish Heart Regeneration

The zebrafish heart is simpler than the mammalian heart and is composed of a single atrium and a single ventricle. Blood exits the heart through the *bulbous arteriosus*, an elastic, non-contractile chamber composed of smooth muscle. The wall of the zebrafish ventricle is lined by the epicardium, an outer mesothelial lining, and an inner endothelial lining, the endocardium. The wall is composed mainly by muscle cells, it is vascularized and innervated, and contain also fibroblast and several other type of cells [187].

Poss et al., in 2002, described for the first time that zebrafish is able to regenerate up to ~20% of its heart ventricle after amputation, thus showing the most robust cardiac regenerative response in a vertebrate [188]. The injury leads to a blood clot formation that is subsequently replaced by fibrin and collagen to preserve the ventricular wall and seal the wound. From 7–9 days post-injury (dpi) to the next following weeks, this fibrotic tissue is replaced by new cardiomyocytes (CM). After 60 dpi the size and shape of the ventricle, as well as the heart beating contractile capability, gets back to normal [189]. The use of genetic fate-mapping approaches allowed establishing that the source of the new muscle cells is from pre-existing muscle cells, stimulated by injury to divide [190,191] but, it is not completely clear what molecular signals are involved in this process. Few insights came from a study of Sande-Melon et al. that identified a subset of sox10-positive cardiomyocytes within the uninjured heart with a high capacity to contribute to the new myocardium [192]. Ablation of these cardiomyocytes confirmed that they play an essential role during the heart regeneration.

The induction of CM proliferation is triggered and controlled by various cells and factors. The first responders to heart injury are inflammatory cells like neutrophils, macrophages, and T-cells [193–195]. The cryoinjury procedure revealed that early macrophage invasion, rapid appearance of angiogenic sprouts into the wound, and transient fibrosis are required for robust cardiomyocyte proliferation [182, 196–199].

Several works assessed that the epicardium is involved in multiple aspects of cardiac repair after injury with the ability to regulate heart regeneration through secretion of soluble growth factors. Indeed, when activated, cells from the epicardium are able to proliferate and migrate to the injury area where they can secrete extracellular matrix components and molecules able to regulate cell proliferation and heart regeneration [189,200–202]. Furthermore, genetic ablation of the epicardium and its derivatives, disrupts CM proliferation and muscle regeneration, but the process renews following epicardium recovery [202].

Information available on the signaling pathways underlying cardiac regeneration in zebrafish is not very extensive but some of the identified factors, e.g., the Hippo pathway and its downstream effectors, the transcriptional co-activators Yes-associated protein (YAP) and transcriptional co-activator with PDZ-binding motif (TAZ), seems to be important in enhancing cardiac regeneration. Hereafter we summarize the main signaling pathways know and their specific functional involvement in cardiac regeneration.

The FGF family is fundamental in regeneration as they initiate a downstream signaling cascade through Ras/MAPK, Akt, and Stat signaling. Impaired heart regeneration was observed in blocked FGF-signaling transgenic fish [203]. Additionally, FGFs stimulate neovascularization and epicardial cell activation during the zebrafish heart regeneration [203,204]. However, the exact role of FGF ligands directly on zebrafish cardiomyocyte proliferation remains to be determined.

The Nrg1 is an extracellular ligand that also activates Ras/MAPK signaling. It is secreted from perivascular and epicardial cells at 7 dpi and has fundamental roles in regulating cardiomyocyte proliferation in both zebrafish and mice. Overexpression of Nrg1 increased cardiomyocytes proliferation after injury and inhibition of Nrg1 receptor caused reduction in cardiomyocyte proliferation after injury [179].

Growth factors are important modulators of zebrafish heart regeneration. The insulin growth factor (IGF) binds to receptors Igf1r and activates downstream signaling pathways that contribute to cell growth, differentiation, and anti-apoptotic pathways. Studies have shown that Igf signaling is a critical stimulator of cardiomyocyte proliferation [205]. Another growth factor, the platelet-derived growth factor (PDGF) is also important in cardiac regeneration as it activates downstream pathways involved in wound healing and proliferation. Studies have shown that PDGF ligands and receptors play an important role in heart regeneration and they are required in coronary vasculature formation during heart regeneration [206]. Apparently, their direct and main function in vivo is to support angiogenesis of the regenerating heart.

Transforming growth Factor-β (TGF-β) family ligands, such as TGF-β, BMPs, and activins seem to be key regulators in cardiomyocyte proliferation and scar formation. These factors operate through two different classes of receptors to phosphorylate distinct Smad transcription factors, which then complex with each other, and additional co-factors that regulate gene expression. Blocking TGF-β receptor activin Receptor-like Kinase 5/4 (Alk5/4) resulted with a significant decrease in pSmad3 and BrdU+ cardiomyocytes near the infarct suggesting that TGF-β is required for cardiomyocyte proliferation [207,208]. Further genetic loss-of-function mutations in activin A (*inhbaa*) showed a significant decrease in cardiomyocyte proliferation after cryoinjury [209].

BMP plays also an important role as chemical inhibition or overexpression of BMP-inhibitor *noggin3* delayed muscle repair, limited CM de-differentiation and cell cycle entry, while Induced global overexpression of *bmp2b* decreased the wound size [210].

Notch signaling pathway is also involved in heart development and cardiomyocyte maturation and proliferation. In zebrafish, following amputation of ventricular apex, Notch receptor expression becomes activated specifically in the endocardium and epicardium. Using a dominant-negative approach, Long Zhao et al. show the exquisite sensitivity of regenerative cardiomyocyte proliferation to perturbations in Notch signaling. They discovered that suppression of Notch signaling profoundly impairs cardiac regeneration and induces scar formation at the amputation site. Unexpectedly, hyperactivation of Notch signaling also suppressed cardiomyocyte proliferation and heart regeneration [211].

Additional regeneration effectors, such as miRNAs, are suggested being able to affect cardiomyocytes proliferation by inhibiting or activating the cell cycle [212]. Epigenetic regulation through chromatin remodeling or histone modification has also been shown to be involved in zebrafish heart regeneration [213] and seem to be important for cardiomyocyte regeneration.

11.3. Zebrafish as a Model of Human Regeneration

Zebrafish is a useful model for studying molecular mechanisms of regeneration [179] due to the availability of genetic data, fully sequenced genome, readiness for genetic manipulations and biosensor and reporter zebrafish lines [214,215]. In addition, the muscle structure and muscle-related gene expression are highly conserved between human and zebrafish and over 70% of human genes have a true ortholog in the zebrafish genome [216]. From a methodological viewpoint, many study on zebrafish regeneration employ larval stages whose transparent body allows easy tracking of structural changes during development and regeneration of the skeletal and heart muscle tissue.

Injured human heart does not regenerate and results in irreversible loss of myocardial cells. The damaged myocardium is replaced by fibrotic scar tissue that undermines pump function and leads to congestive heart failure and arrhythmia. Although several works suggest cardiomyocytes proliferation ability in the human heart [217], this process is not significant in response to injury [218] thus not providing a complete restoration of its functions. The zebrafish is probably one of the most important vertebrate model for studying heart developmental and regenerative properties relevant also to mammalian heart for its impressive regeneration ability following different forms of injury [187] that it is not based on stem cells or transdifferentiation of other cells but on the proliferation of preexisting cardiomyocytes [190,191]. Hence, studying the zebrafish model could expand the knowledge on cardiac regenerative processes and may contribute to the identification of specific molecules able to regulate the proliferation of these cells. This may provide insights for the design of future therapies for cardiac repair after myocardial infarction (MI) and other cardiac injuries in humans.

Concerning skeletal muscles, zebrafish and human share a high similarity at cellular, molecular, histological, and ultrastructural levels. In addition to the genetic tools for the expression of pathological phenotypes such as muscular dystrophy [219], both adult and larval zebrafish muscle have been shown to be a valuable models to study regeneration events by exploiting the possibility of performing selective injury of muscles while imaging morphogenetic processes using for example fluorescent reporter lines [178,220,221]. Notably, these studies also shed light on possible factors limiting mammalians regeneration abilities. Indeed, it has been shown that in order to allow a proper regeneration, and differently from mammals, zebrafish heart and skeletal muscles maintain the ability to activate specific gene regulatory networks (GNRs) in response to injury and perform epigenetic modifications necessary to trigger regeneration. In addition, a fundamental role is also played by the immune system whose harnessing has been shown to promote cardiac regeneration (for a review see [178]).

12. Mammals: Cell Therapy for Skeletal Muscle Regeneration

Mammalian skeletal muscle possesses a certain potential to regenerate, but this process can be compromised in several pathological conditions (e.g., neuromuscular disease, cancer-associated cachexia, or age-dependent sarcopenia) and following trauma the extended loss of muscle fibers cannot be fully recovered. These events lead to a weak regeneration and formation of fibrotic scar tissue, and result in loss of functional muscle mass. Consequently, the ability to perform intense muscular efforts and even easy, daily-life tasks may be impaired [222–224].

In the last decades, the scientific community devoted increasing efforts to develop therapies for the regeneration of damaged tissues in humans. This section aims at providing an overview of the cellular strategies that have been developed for improving skeletal muscle regeneration in mammals, particularly humans. As for the methods employed to study skeletal muscle regeneration, readers can refer to more comprehensive reviews [7,223,225–227].

Regenerative medicine aims at promoting the formation of new functional tissue by delivering precursor cells or bio-engineered tissue patches into the injured area. Indeed, therapeutic cells are isolated from the donor subject, expanded in culture (if needed), integrated into an acellular synthetic scaffold (in case of bio-engineered tissue patches), and transplanted into the recipient tissue. Although this general procedure looks simple, the choice of the specific therapeutic strategy is very complex due to the large number of different cell sources and implantation technologies. As for the cell source, the immunological compatibility between donor and recipient should be taken into account. Therefore, in the clinical setting, autologous transplantation is often preferred over the heterologous or xenologous one [223].

Focusing on skeletal muscle regeneration, the following types of cells have been employed: satellite cells, muscle-derived stem cells, myoblasts, mesoangioblasts, hTERT/Bmi-1- or hTERT/CD4-immortalized muscle precursor cells, pericytes, CD133+ cells, hematopoietic stem cells, mesenchymal stem cells, myoendothelial cells, side-population interstitial cells, myogenic precursor cells, dental pulp pluripotent-like stem cells, and eventually induced pluripotent stem cells (iPSCs) [228,229]. In mammalian animal models, these cells demonstrated a certain ability to proliferate both in vitro and in vivo, and to generate functional, integrated skeletal muscle tissue [228,230]. However, the ideal source of myogenic cells is still debated, due to a number of limitations such as the availability of bioptic biological material, the tumorigenic risk of immortalized cells, the capacity of cells to proliferate and graft into the host tissue, etc.

The possibility to artificially reprogram fully differentiated mammalian cells into iPSCs provides a virtually unlimited source of pluripotent stem cells for almost every individual. Nowadays, iPSCs represent a very useful tool for developing patient-specific regenerative therapies, thanks to the effective and reliable protocols for the expansion and differentiation of these cells both in vitro and in vivo [231–233]. Moreover, the opportunity to generate myoblasts, as well as different types of cells from iPSCs, such as neurons, endothelial cells, pericytes, and to edit their genome through CRISPR/CAS9 and TALEN technologies, further enhances their possible use for therapeutic applications [234,235]. IPSCs are stem-like cells generated by the reprogramming of fully differentiated somatic cells. Reprogramming strategies involve either the delivery of genetic material encoding reprogramming factors (e.g., Oct4, Sox2, Nanog, c-Myc, Klf4, and Lin28) or the administration of specific miRNAs or cocktail of proteins and small molecules into the somatic cells. In the latter case, reprogramming is triggered by direct activation of the endogenous stem-cell factors. The integration of exogenous DNA into the host genome relies on retroviruses, lentiviruses, and piggy Bac transposons; the non-integrating DNA and RNA procedures use adenoviruses, Sendai virus, plasmids, episomal vectors, and mRNA. Once generated, iPSCs can proliferate indefinitely in culture and differentiate into any kind of adult somatic cell by administering the appropriate growth or differentiation factors. In particular, the induction of myogenesis can be achieved either by expressing exogenous muscle-specific transcription factors, such as MYOD, PAX7, and PAX3, into the cells, or by activating endogenous pro-myogenic differentiation pathways (e.g., Wnt and BMPs signaling) by supplying, in the culture media, specific molecules, such as GSK3b inhibitors, bFGF, FGF-2, epidermal growth factor (EGF), DAPT, forskolin, BMP inhibitors, hepatocyte growth factor (HGF), and IGF-1 [236].

From a clinical perspective, the use of genetic manipulation, although more effective, is not safe, due to the risk of genetic recombination. Methods based on the supplementation in the culture media of chemical compounds prompting cell reprogramming and differentiation toward a skeletal muscle phenotype, are preferred. It should also be considered that in vitro, the differentiation process has not a 100% efficiency. Therefore, besides myogenic cells, other cell types, such as neural cells and fibroblasts, originate within the culture. In addition, myogenic cell at different stages of differentiation coexist in the entire cell population and a cell sorting strategy (by means of a fluorescence-activated cell sorter) is required to obtain a pure pool of myogenic precursor cells [237–239]. The selected population of progenitor cells can be transplanted into the host via different methods, such as intramuscular injection, systemic cell delivery, and microsurgical implants. Each of these methods has pros and cons and a unique optimal strategy has not been defined yet. Indeed, systemic delivery results in a highly variable success rate, intramuscular injection requires multiple local treatments, and implants involve more invasive procedures.

The efficacy of these regenerative therapies strictly depends on the capacity of the transplanted cells to engraft the injured site, survive, proliferate, differentiate, and integrate within the native skeletal muscles. To promote the success of these therapies, specific strategies have been developed: artificial co-administration of small molecules and growth factors such as TGF-b and myostatin inhibitors, IGF-I, fibrin, keratin, collagen; tissue engineering and bioprinting for the generation of synthetic scaffolds embedding myogenic cells [228]. The composition and the three-dimensional architecture of the synthetic scaffold provide structural and functional support to the cells and promote the formation of new, functional skeletal muscle tissue, as well as the establishment of a pool of self-renewing stem cells [240–244].

Although regenerative medicine applied to muscle disorders has greatly advanced, a standard for cell-based therapeutic interventions is still lacking. At the moment, we are far away from effective treatments promoting skeletal muscle regeneration in mammals. However, cell therapies, benefiting from the great potential of iPSCs, genome editing, tissue engineering, and cell biology methods, hold great promise for successful skeletal muscle regeneration.

13. Conclusions and Future Perspectives

Model organisms have always been playing a fundamental role to uncover general biological mechanisms common also to humans and historically they have a key role in translational medicine. In the last decades, deeper mechanistic studies of animal diversity have been made possible by the availability of a broader and affordable toolbox of technical resources such as genomics, transcriptomic, connectomics, and many other molecular biology techniques [245]. One emblematic example is the introduction of CRISPR/Cas9 genome editing, which made functional approaches possible in a wider range of so-called non-canonical model organisms. These techniques are allowing scientists to address a broader spectrum of biological problems exploiting the diversity of animal biology [246]. For instance, "simple" model organisms like Planarians and Echinoderms greatly benefited from these advancements and are nowadays considered *bona fide* models in translational research for the possibility of performing cell tracking and expression profiling of their tissue.

Nonetheless, the number and variety of animal species currently used in biomedical research are still rather limited. The reason is certainly not the suitability of particular species to a specific scientific question, but rather to the laboratory amenability (due for example to the flexibility and cost of breeding, the animal availability, the length of life cycles, the optical transparency, the possibility to perform genetic manipulations, etc.) and the familiarity of a critical mass of researchers with established animal models. The result is a scenario where only a few species retain a legitimate biomedical interest, while many others are left aside.

Nowadays, only few animal models (mainly rodents, chicken, and to some extent zebrafish) have been suitably exploited in muscle regeneration studies and various injury protocols (e.g., surgery, chemically induced muscle damage, genetic ablation, denervation-devascularization, intensive exercise, etc.) have been employed [178,225,226,247–249]. Except for zebrafish, none of the animal species presented in this review have been systematically tested for the efficacy and utility of the diverse injury models; indeed, the main methods employed to stimulate regeneration are based on physically- (by surgery or irradiation) and chemically-induced muscle damage, and genetic ablation.

It is important to point out that the application of a specific injury protocol in different animal species, given their diversity in body morphology, physiology and regeneration mechanisms, may not lead to directly comparable results. Thus, a comparative experimental approach taking into account animal diversity is fundamental to explain the variation in regenerative capacity through phylogeny, ontogeny, and even aging [250]. This may provide hallmarks of molecular homology between regenerative events in the metazoans [251] as well as an explanation of the loss or restriction of regeneration abilities occurring in some animals like *D. melanogaster* and *C. elegans*. Notably, even with their limited regeneration abilities, these animals may supply important insights into the negative regulation of this supposedly advantageous attribute.

In this review, we wished to provide the researchers interested in muscle regeneration with a lookout of muscle diversity across animals, and a prospect on their regenerating potentials (see Table 1). This work was not meant to provide 'guidelines' into animal selection when addressing specific regeneration issue but to offer 'insights' on open questions and new standpoints. We thus gave an overview of how cell precursors and regeneration strategies are adopted to partially or completely restore muscular components in various clades or even in different species within a single clade.

Table 1. Overview of muscle cell types and regenerative potentials of the animals treated in this review. * Muscle type discussed in this review in the context of regeneration, ** Induced pluripotent stem cells, can be derived from various species, *** Mostly repair.

Animal Species	Muscle Type *	REG	Cell Precursor	Known Signaling Pathways and Molecular Players
IPSC **	Any	n/a	n/a	MyoD, Pax7/3, Wnt and BMPs
Vertebrates	Striated; Cardiac	yes	Satellite stem cell; Pre-existing muscle cells	Notch, BMP, TGF-β, IGF, FGF family, Ngr1; Pax3/7, Met
Tunicates	Striated, smooth-like, cardiac	yes	Stem cells-like precursors (?)	Notch, Nk4, Tbx1/10, MRF
Cephalocordates	Striated, mononucleated	yes	De-differentiation, Multipotent cells	Pax3/7, Wnt/β-catenin and BMP
Echinoderms	Smooth-like, striated, mononucleated	yes	De-differentiation	BMP/TGFB, HOX, Ependymin, etc.
Arthropods	Striated	no ***	Adult muscle precursor (AMP)	Notch-Delta, Transcription factor Zhf1
Nematodes	Striated, mononucleated	no	—	—
Mollusks	Striated, mononucleated	yes	Sarcoblasts (?)	AChE, Growth factors (EGF, FGFs and VEGF)??
Platyhelmintes	Combine features of both vertebrate skeletal and smooth muscle cells	yes	Neoblasts: Adult pluripotent stem cells	Many known signaling pathways such as PCGs, Wnt/β-catenin, FGF family, insulin/IGF-1, Pax3/7, TGF-β, Hox genes, etc. (see text for references)
Cnidarians	Epitheliomuscular, smooth	yes	Hydrozoan: i-cells in Hydractinia, epithelial stem cells in Hydra Anthozoan: yet to be determined	The myogenic gene repertoire is present in cnidarians, but no experimental evidence relate them to the myogenic trajectory
Porifera	Myocytes	yes	Adult stem cells (ASC) Totypotent, pluripotent cells	ADPRC (ADP-ribosyl cyclase), TGF-β

We showed that the presence and nature of cell precursors giving rise to new muscles have been addressed in most of the clades and seem to be rather heterogeneous although a proper cell fate mapping has in many cases not yet been disclosed. In Tunicates, the sister-group of vertebrates, we saw the involvement of putative pluri- or multipotent stem cells during regenerative processes, and the partial co-option of embryonic myogenesis (the latter highly conserved in vertebrates) during muscle regeneration.

We saw that cell migration and tissue re-organization are crucial for regeneration and, given their rather 'simplicity', animals like Porifera, Cnidarians, and Planarians may represent valuable model to investigate these aspects. Moreover, we saw that animals use different regeneration strategies, e.g., epimorphosis and morphallaxis, that are equally successful and that may also coexist within the same organism, as it happens in amphioxus, to meet tissue specific regeneration requirements. From a translational perspective, these examples reinforce the idea that regenerative medicine should not seek out a 'regeneration blueprint' but rather a set of 'context-dependent' regeneration strategies.

We highlighted how the gene regulation aspect has been studied to various extents in many clades and is particularly well assessed for Echinoderms. On the other hand, the range of epigenetic controls has been investigated only in few species, such as zebrafish. Indeed, epigenetic studies are still at their dawn in non-vertebrates.

Comparing the architectures of a "regeneration permissive" vs. a "non-permissive" gene regulatory network (GRN) between closely related species, or finding signatures of epigenetic control of regeneration can fuel the expanding field of synthetic biology or allow for an ample testing of new classes of drug, targeting molecular and cellular mechanisms conserved in human but more functionally testable in other animal models. In this sense, regenerative therapies might greatly benefit from these comparative studies.

We also showed that, besides genetics and epigenetics, another key factor for a successful regeneration in metazoans is the 'environmental qualification', i.e., the extracellular matrix (ECM) structure, remodeling, composition, collagen content, cytoarchitecture, and secreted factors influencing the heterogeneous population of cells present within the regenerating environment [2,223]. Environmental qualification is currently considered a fundamental aspect of cell engraftment during transplantation and the lack of knowledge on this topic represent one of the current bottlenecks in regenerative medicine. Indeed, to improve regeneration of muscle tissues, transplantation of cells can be done through scaffolds ideally mimicking native tissues. Scaffolds can be made by natural polymers, synthetic polymers, or even decellularized ECM that can be filled after implantation by stem cells to restore muscle morphology. They are used to provide chemical and physical cues to transplanted cells and to create a microenvironment niche that favor survival of the resident cells and engraftment of the transplanted cells [223]. These study are at the forefront of tissue engineering and aim at providing a structural and biochemical framework for regeneration. In this regard, animals such as octopus and zebrafish can be useful models to study the cytological and histological architecture of the regenerating environment thus providing information on how to model and enrich the regenerating niche [109,189,251].

From a more clinical perspective, the information provided by studying and comparing different animal models, without forgetting their phylogenetic framework, can help to address the problem of lack of regeneration in human tissues and might eventually be used to overcome the limits of muscle regenerative therapy.

Author Contributions: L.Z. conceptualized the study; all authors wrote the original draft, reviewed and edited the text. Figures have been assembled by E.R., S.C., S.T. and L.Z. and Tables reviewed and edited by all authors. All authors have read and agreed to the published version of the manuscript.

Acknowledgments: We would like to thank M. Khamla for his contribution to the artwork (Figure 3). S.C. and M.B. are thankful to H. Escriva and M. Schubert for help obtaining *B. lanceolatum* adults.

References

1.   Ciciliot, S.; Schiaffino, S. Regeneration of mammalian skeletal muscle. Basic mechanisms and clinical implications. *Curr. Pharm. Des.* **2010**, *16*, 906–914. [CrossRef] [PubMed]
2.   Musaro, A. The basis of muscle regeneration. *Adv. Biol.* **2014**, *2014*, 1–16. [CrossRef]
3.   Maden, M. The evolution of regeneration—Where does that leave mammals? *Int. J. Dev. Biol.* **2018**, *62*, 369–372. [CrossRef] [PubMed]
4.   Tiozzo, S.; Copley, R. Reconsidering regeneration in metazoans: An evo-devo approach. *Front. Ecol. Evol.* **2015**, *3*, 67. [CrossRef]

5. Steinmetz, P.R.; Kraus, J.E.; Larroux, C.; Hammel, J.U.; Amon-Hassenzahl, A.; Houliston, E.; Worheide, G.; Nickel, M.; Degnan, B.M.; Technau, U. Independent evolution of striated muscles in cnidarians and bilaterians. *Nature* **2012**, *487*, 231–234. [CrossRef]

6. Li, Q.; Yang, H.; Zhong, T. Regeneration across metazoan phylogeny: Lessons from model organisms. *J. Genet. Genom.* **2015**, *42*. [CrossRef]

7. Baghdadi, M.; Tajbakhsh, S. Regulation and phylogeny of skeletal muscle regeneration. *Dev. Biol.* **2017**, *433*. [CrossRef]

8. Hejnol, A. Muscle's dual origins. *Nature* **2012**, *487*, 181–182. [CrossRef]

9. Telford, M.J.; Moroz, L.L.; Halanych, K.M. Evolution: A sisterly dispute. *Nature* **2016**, *529*, 286–287. [CrossRef]

10. Brunet, T.; Fischer, A.H.L.; Steinmetz, P.R.H.; Lauri, A.; Bertucci, P.; Arendt, D. The evolutionary origin of bilaterian smooth and striated myocytes. *eLife* **2016**, *5*, e19607. [CrossRef]

11. Sikes, J.M.; Newmark, P.A. Restoration of anterior regeneration in a planarian with limited regenerative ability. *Nature* **2013**, *500*, 77–80. [CrossRef] [PubMed]

12. Liu, S.Y.; Selck, C.; Friedrich, B.; Lutz, R.; Vila-Farré, M.; Dahl, A.; Brandl, H.; Lakshmanaperumal, N.; Henry, I.; Rink, J.C. Reactivating head regrowth in a regeneration-deficient planarian species. *Nature* **2013**, *500*, 81–84. [CrossRef] [PubMed]

13. Umesono, Y.; Tasaki, J.; Nishimura, Y.; Hrouda, M.; Kawaguchi, E.; Yazawa, S.; Nishimura, O.; Hosoda, K.; Inoue, T.; Agata, K. The molecular logic for planarian regeneration along the anterior-posterior axis. *Nature* **2013**, *500*, 73–76. [CrossRef] [PubMed]

14. Mokalled, M.H.; Poss, K.D. A Regeneration Toolkit. *Dev. Cell* **2018**, *47*, 267–280. [CrossRef] [PubMed]

15. Ruppert, E.E.; Fox, R.S.; Barnes, R.D. *Invertebrate Zoology: A Functional Evolutionary Approach*, 7th ed.; Thomson-Brooks/Cole: Pacific Grove, CA, USA, 2004; pp. 662–664.

16. Dorit, R.L.; Walker, W.F.; Barnes, R.D. *Zoology*; Saunders College Publishers: New York, NY, USA, 1991; pp. 154–196.

17. Nickel, M.; Scheer, C.; Hammel, J.U.; Herzen, J.; Beckmann, F. The contractile sponge epithelium sensu lato–body contraction of the demosponge Tethya wilhelma is mediated by the pinacoderm. *J. Exp. Biol.* **2011**, *214*, 1692–1698. [CrossRef]

18. Borisenko, I.; Adamska, M.; Tokina, D.; Ereskovsky, A. Transdifferentiation is a driving force of regeneration in Halisarca dujardini (Demospongiae, Porifera). *PeerJ* **2015**, *3*, e1211. [CrossRef]

19. Funayama, N. The stem cell system in demosponges: Insights into the origin of somatic stem cells. *Dev. Growth Differ.* **2010**, *52*, 1–14. [CrossRef]

20. Lorenz, B.; Bohnensack, R.; Gamulin, V.; Steffen, R.; Muller, W.E. Regulation of motility of cells from marine sponges by calcium ions. *Cell. Signal.* **1996**, *8*, 517–524. [CrossRef]

21. Katz, A.M. Review of calcium in muscle contraction, cellular, and molecular physiology, by J. C. Rüegg. *J. Mol. Cell. Cardiol.* **1994**, *26*. [CrossRef]

22. Müller, W. *Sponges (Porifera)*; Springer: New York, NY, USA, 2003; Volume 3, pp. 154–196.

23. Padua, A.; Klautau, M. Regeneration in calcareous sponges (Porifera). *J. Mar. Biol. Assoc. UK* **2015**, *96*, 553–558. [CrossRef]

24. Kürn, U.; Rendulic, S.; Tiozzo, S.; Lauzon, R. Asexual propagation and regeneration in colonial ascidians. *Biol. Bull.* **2011**, *221*, 43–61. [CrossRef] [PubMed]

25. Basile, G.; Cerrano, C.; Radjasa, O.K.; Povero, P.; Zocchi, E. ADP-ribosyl cyclase and abscisic acid are involved in the seasonal growth and in post-traumatic tissue regeneration of Mediterranean sponges. *J. Exp. Mar. Biol. Ecol.* **2009**, *381*, 10–17. [CrossRef]

26. Pozzolini, M.; Gallus, L.; Ghignone, S.; Ferrando, S.; Candiani, S.; Bozzo, M.; Bertolino, M.; Costa, G.; Bavestrello, G.; Scarfi, S. Insights into the evolution of metazoan regenerative mechanisms: Roles of TGF superfamily members in tissue regeneration of the marine sponge Chondrosia reniformis. *J. Exp. Biol.* **2019**, *222*, jeb207894. [CrossRef] [PubMed]

27. Zapata, F.; Goetz, F.; Smith, S.; Howison, M.; Siebert, S.; Church, S.; Sanders, S.; Ames, C.L.; McFadden, C.; France, S.; et al. Phylogenomic analyses support traditional relationships within cnidaria. *PLoS ONE* **2015**, *10*, e0139068. [CrossRef] [PubMed]

28. Leclere, L.; Rottinger, E. Diversity of cnidarian muscles: Function, Anatomy, development and regeneration. *Front. Cell Dev. Biol.* **2016**, *4*, 157. [CrossRef]

29. Holstein, T.W.; Hobmayer, E.; Technau, U. Cnidarians: An evolutionarily conserved model system for regeneration? *Dev. Dyn. Off. Publ. Am. Assoc. Anat.* **2003**, *226*, 257–267. [CrossRef]

30. Renfer, E.; Amon-Hassenzahl, A.; Steinmetz, P.R.; Technau, U. A muscle-specific transgenic reporter line of the sea anemone, nematostella vectensis. *Proc. Natl. Acad. Sci. USA* **2010**, *107*, 104–108. [CrossRef]

31. Jahnel, S.M.; Walzl, M.; Technau, U. Development and epithelial organisation of muscle cells in the sea anemone Nematostella vectensis. *Front. Zool.* **2014**, *11*, 44. [CrossRef]

32. Ryan, J.F.; Mazza, M.E.; Pang, K.; Matus, D.Q.; Baxevanis, A.D.; Martindale, M.Q.; Finnerty, J.R. Pre-bilaterian origins of the Hox cluster and the Hox code: Evidence from the sea anemone, nematostella vectensis. *PLoS ONE* **2007**, *2*, e153. [CrossRef]

33. Matus, D.Q.; Pang, K.; Daly, M.; Martindale, M.Q. Expression of Pax gene family members in the anthozoan cnidarian, Nematostella vectensis. *Evol. Dev.* **2007**, *9*, 25–38. [CrossRef]

34. Putnam, N.H.; Srivastava, M.; Hellsten, U.; Dirks, B.; Chapman, J.; Salamov, A.; Terry, A.; Shapiro, H.; Lindquist, E.; Kapitonov, V.V.; et al. Sea anemone genome reveals ancestral eumetazoan gene repertoire and genomic organization. *Science* **2007**, *317*, 86–94. [CrossRef] [PubMed]

35. Saina, M.; Genikhovich, G.; Renfer, E.; Technau, U. BMPs and chordin regulate patterning of the directive axis in a sea anemone. *Proc. Natl. Acad. Sci. USA* **2009**, *106*, 18592–18597. [CrossRef] [PubMed]

36. Magie, C.R.; Pang, K.; Martindale, M.Q. Genomic inventory and expression of Sox and Fox genes in the cnidarian Nematostella vectensis. *Dev. Genes Evol.* **2005**, *215*, 618–630. [CrossRef] [PubMed]

37. Steinmetz, P.R.H.; Aman, A.; Kraus, J.E.M.; Technau, U. Gut-like ectodermal tissue in a sea anemone challenges germ layer homology. *Nat. Ecol. Evol.* **2017**, *1*, 1535–1542. [CrossRef]

38. Genikhovich, G.; Technau, U. Complex functions of Mef2 splice variants in the differentiation of endoderm and of a neuronal cell type in a sea anemone. *Development* **2011**, *138*, 4911–4919. [CrossRef]

39. Martindale, M.Q.; Pang, K.; Finnerty, J.R. Investigating the origins of triploblasty: 'mesodermal' gene expression in a diploblastic animal, the sea anemone Nematostella vectensis (phylum, Cnidaria; class, Anthozoa). *Development* **2004**, *131*, 2463–2474. [CrossRef]

40. Ryan, J.F.; Burton, P.M.; Mazza, M.E.; Kwong, G.K.; Mullikin, J.C.; Finnerty, J.R. The cnidarian-bilaterian ancestor possessed at least 56 homeoboxes: Evidence from the starlet sea anemone, Nematostella vectensis. *Genome Biol.* **2006**, *7*, R64. [CrossRef]

41. Layden, M.J.; Rentzsch, F.; Rottinger, E. The rise of the starlet sea anemone nematostella vectensis as a model system to investigate development and regeneration. *Wiley Interdiscip. Rev. Dev. Biol.* **2016**, *5*, 408–428. [CrossRef]

42. Hand, C.; Uhlinger, K.R. The culture, sexual and asexual reproduction, and growth of the sea anemone nematostella vectensis. *Biol. Bull.* **1992**, *182*, 169–176. [CrossRef]

43. Warner, J.F.; Guerlais, V.; Amiel, A.R.; Johnston, H.; Nedoncelle, K.; Rottinger, E. NvERTx: A gene expression database to compare embryogenesis and regeneration in the sea anemone nematostella vectensis. *Development* **2018**, *145*. [CrossRef]

44. Sebe-Pedros, A.; Saudemont, B.; Chomsky, E.; Plessier, F.; Mailhe, M.P.; Renno, J.; Loe-Mie, Y.; Lifshitz, A.; Mukamel, Z.; Schmutz, S.; et al. Cnidarian Cell type diversity and regulation revealed by whole-organism single-cell RNA-Seq. *Cell* **2018**, *173*, 1520–1534. [CrossRef] [PubMed]

45. Rottinger, E.; Dahlin, P.; Martindale, M.Q. A framework for the establishment of a cnidarian gene regulatory network for "endomesoderm" specification: The inputs of ss-catenin/TCF signaling. *PLoS Genet.* **2012**, *8*, e1003164. [CrossRef] [PubMed]

46. Layden, M.J.; Rottinger, E.; Wolenski, F.S.; Gilmore, T.D.; Martindale, M.Q. Microinjection of mRNA or morpholinos for reverse genetic analysis in the starlet sea anemone, nematostella vectensis. *Nat. Protoc.* **2013**, *8*, 924–934. [CrossRef] [PubMed]

47. Ikmi, A.; McKinney, S.A.; Delventhal, K.M.; Gibson, M.C. TALEN and CRISPR/Cas9-mediated genome editing in the early-branching metazoan Nematostella vectensis. *Nat. Commun.* **2014**, *5*, 5486. [CrossRef]

48. Amiel, A.R.; Foucher, K.; Ferreira, S. Synergic coordination of stem cells is required to induce a regenerative response in anthozoan cnidarians. *bioRxiv* **2019**. [CrossRef]

49. Lin, Y.C.J.; Spencer, A. Localisation of intracellular calcium stores in the striated muscles of the jellyfish Polyorchis penicillatus: Possible involvement in excitation-contraction coupling. *J. Exp. Biol.* **2001**, *204*, 3727–3736.

50. Hyman, L. The invertebrates. (Scientific books: The invertebrates: Protozoa through ctenophora). *Science* **1940**, *92*, 219–220.

51. Boero, F.; Gravili, C.; Pagliara, P.; Piraino, S.; Bouillon, J.; Schmid, V. The cnidarian premises of metazoan evolution: From triploblasty, to coelom formation, to metamery. *Ital. J. Zool.* **1998**, *65*, 5–9. [CrossRef]

52. Satterlie, R.; Thomas, K.; Gray, C. Muscle organization of the cubozoan jellyfish tripedalia cystophora conant 1897. *Biol. Bull.* **2005**, *209*, 154–163. [CrossRef]

53. Helm, R.; Tiozzo, S.; Lilley, M.; Fabien, L.; Dunn, C. Comparative muscle development of scyphozoan jellyfish with simple and complex life cycles. *EvoDevo* **2015**, *6*, 11. [CrossRef]

54. Davis, R.L.; Weintraub, H.; Lassar, A.B. Expression of a single transfected cDNA converts fibroblasts to myoblasts. *Cell* **1987**, *51*, 987–1000. [CrossRef]

55. Andrikou, C.; Pai, C.Y.; Su, Y.H.; Arnone, M.I. Logics and properties of a genetic regulatory program that drives embryonic muscle development in an echinoderm. *eLife* **2015**, *4*. [CrossRef] [PubMed]

56. Hand, C.; Uhlinger, K.R. Asexual reproduction by transverse fission and some anomalies in the sea anemone nematostella vectensis. *Invertebr. Biol.* **1995**, *114*, 9–18. [CrossRef]

57. Reitzel, A.; Burton, P.; Krone, C.; Finnerty, J. Comparison of developmental trajectories in the starlet sea anemone Nematostella vectensis: Embryogenesis, regeneration, and two forms of asexual fission. *Invertebr. Biol.* **2007**, *126*, 99–112. [CrossRef]

58. Passamaneck, Y.; Martindale, M. Cell proliferation is necessary for the regeneration of oral structures in the anthozoan cnidarian nematostella vectensis. *Bmc Dev. Biol.* **2012**, *12*, 34. [CrossRef] [PubMed]

59. Amiel, A.; Johnston, H.; Nedoncelle, K.; Warner, J.; Ferreira, S.; Röttinger, E. Characterization of morphological and cellular events underlying oral regeneration in the sea anemone, nematostella vectensis. *Int. J. Mol. Sci.* **2015**, *2015*, 28449–28471. [CrossRef]

60. Warner, J.; Amiel, A.; Johnston, H.; Röttinger, E. Regeneration is a partial Redeployment of the embryonic Gene Network. *bioRxiv* **2019**. [CrossRef]

61. Morgan, T.H. Regeneration and liability to injury. *Science* **1901**, *14*, 235–248. [CrossRef]

62. Bossert, P.E.; Dunn, M.P.; Thomsen, G.H. A staging system for the regeneration of a polyp from the aboral physa of the anthozoan Cnidarian Nematostella vectensis. *Dev. Dyn. Off. Publ. Am. Assoc. Anat.* **2013**, *242*, 1320–1331. [CrossRef]

63. Cebria, F. Planarian body-wall muscle: Regeneration and function beyond a simple skeletal support. *Front. Cell Dev. Biol.* **2016**, *4*, 8. [CrossRef]

64. Moumen, M.; Chiche, A.; Cagnet, S.; Petit, V.; Raymond, K.; Faraldo, M.M.; Deugnier, M.A.; Glukhova, M.A. The mammary myoepithelial cell. *Int. J. Dev. Biol.* **2011**, *55*, 763–771. [CrossRef]

65. Newmark, P.; Sánchez Alvarado, A. Not your father's planarian: A classic model enters the era of functional genomics. *Nat. Rev. Genet.* **2002**, *3*, 210–219. [CrossRef]

66. Giacomotto, J.; Ségalat, L. High-throughput screening and small animal models, where are we? *Br. J. Pharmacol.* **2010**, *160*, 204–216. [CrossRef] [PubMed]

67. Chan, J.D.; Marchant, J.S. Pharmacological and functional genetic assays to manipulate regeneration of the planarian Dugesia japonica. *J. Vis. Exp.* **2011**. [CrossRef] [PubMed]

68. King, R.S.; Newmark, P.A. Whole-mount in situ hybridization of planarians. *Methods Mol. Biol.* **2018**, *1774*, 379–392. [CrossRef] [PubMed]

69. Ivankovic, M.; Haneckova, R.; Thommen, A.; Grohme, M.A.; Vila-Farré, M.; Werner, S.; Rink, J.C. Model systems for regeneration: Planarians. *Development* **2019**, *146*. [CrossRef] [PubMed]

70. Scimone, M.L.; Cote, L.E.; Reddien, P.W. Orthogonal muscle fibres have different instructive roles in planarian regeneration. *Nature* **2017**, *551*, 623–628. [CrossRef]

71. Witchley, J.N.; Mayer, M.; Wagner, D.E.; Owen, J.H.; Reddien, P.W. Muscle cells provide instructions for planarian regeneration. *Cell Rep.* **2013**, *4*, 633–641. [CrossRef]

72. Cote, L.E.; Simental, E.; Reddien, P.W. Muscle functions as a connective tissue and source of extracellular matrix in planarians. *Nat. Commun.* **2019**, *10*, 1592. [CrossRef]

73. Baguñà, J. The planarian neoblast: The rambling history of its origin and some current black boxes. *Int. J. Dev. Biol.* **2012**, *56*, 19–37. [CrossRef]

74. Kreshchenko, N.D. Pharynx regeneration in planarians. *Ontogenez* **2009**, *40*, 3–18. [CrossRef] [PubMed]

75. Adler, C.E.; Seidel, C.W.; McKinney, S.A.; Sanchez Alvarado, A. Selective amputation of the pharynx identifies a FoxA-dependent regeneration program in planaria. *eLife* **2014**, *3*, e02238. [CrossRef] [PubMed]

76. Guedelhoefer, O.C., IV; Alvarado, A.S. Planarian immobilization, partial irradiation, and tissue transplantation. *JoVE* **2012**. [CrossRef] [PubMed]

77. Zeng, A.; Li, H.; Guo, L.; Gao, X.; McKinney, S.; Wang, Y.; Yu, Z.; Park, J.; Semerad, C.; Ross, E.; et al. Prospectively isolated tetraspanin. *Cell* **2018**, *173*, 1593–1608. [CrossRef] [PubMed]

78. Dattani, A.; Sridhar, D.; Aziz Aboobaker, A. Planarian flatworms as a new model system for understanding the epigenetic regulation of stem cell pluripotency and differentiation. *Semin. Cell Dev. Biol.* **2019**, *87*, 79–94. [CrossRef]

79. Felix, D.; Gutiérrez-Gutiérrez, Ó.; Espada, L.; Thems, A.; González-Estévez, C. It is not all about regeneration: Planarians striking power to stand starvation. *Semin. Cell Dev. Biol.* **2018**, *87*. [CrossRef]

80. Pellettieri, J.; Sánchez Alvarado, A. Cell turnover and adult tissue homeostasis: From humans to planarians. *Annu. Rev. Genet.* **2007**, *41*, 83–105. [CrossRef]

81. Karami, A.; Tebyanian, H.; Goodarzi, V.; Shiri, S. Planarians: An in vivo model for regenerative medicine. *Int. J. Stem. Cells* **2015**, *8*, 128–133. [CrossRef]

82. Guzmán, L.; Alejo-Plata, C. Arms regeneration in lolliguncula panamensis (Mollusca: Cephalopoda). *Lat. Am. J. Aquat. Res.* **2019**, *47*, 356–360. [CrossRef]

83. Imperadore, P.; Fiorito, G. Cephalopod tissue regeneration: Consolidating over a century of knowledge. *Front. Physiol.* **2018**, *9*. [CrossRef]

84. Tressler, J.; Maddox, F.; Goodwin, E.; Zhang, Z.; Tublitz, N. Arm regeneration in two species of cuttlefish Sepia officinalis and Sepia pharaonis. *Invertebr. Neurosci.* **2013**, *14*. [CrossRef] [PubMed]

85. Zullo, L.; Imperadore, P. Regeneration and healing. In *Handbook of Pathogens and Diseases in Cephalopods*; Gestal, C., Pascual, S., Guerra, Á., Fiorito, G., Vieites, J.M., Eds.; Springer International Publishing: Cham, Switzerland, 2019; pp. 193–199. [CrossRef]

86. Fossati, S.; Benfenati, F.; Zullo, L. Morphological characterization of the Octopus vulgaris arm. *Front. Cell Dev. Biol.* **2011**, *61*, 191–195.

87. Zullo, L.; Fossati, S.M.; Benfenati, F. Transmission of sensory responses in the peripheral nervous system of the arm of Octopus vulgaris. *Front. Cell Dev. Biol.* **2011**, *61*, 197–201.

88. Kier, W.; Stella, M. The arrangement and function of octopus arm musculature and connective tissue. *J. Morphol.* **2007**, *268*, 831–843. [CrossRef]

89. Zullo, L.; Eichenstein, H.; Maiole, F.; Hochner, B. Motor control pathways in the nervous system of Octopus vulgaris arm. *Front. Cell Dev. Biol.* **2019**. [CrossRef]

90. Nödl, M.T.; Fossati, S.M.; Domingues, P.; Sánchez, F.J.; Zullo, L. The making of an octopus arm. *Front. Cell Dev. Biol.* **2015**, *6*. [CrossRef]

91. Ochiai, Y. Structural and phylogenetic profiles of muscle actins from cephalopods. *J. Basic Appl. Sci.* **2013**. [CrossRef]

92. Motoyama, K.; Ishizaki, S.; Nagashima, Y.; Shiomi, K. Cephalopod tropomyosins: Identification as major allergens and molecular cloning. *Food Chem. Toxicol.* **2007**, *44*, 1997–2002. [CrossRef]

93. Zullo, L.; Fossati, S.M.; Imperadore, P.; Nödl, M.-T. Molecular determinants of cephalopod muscles and their implication in muscle regeneration. *Front. Cell Dev. Biol.* **2017**, *5*, 53. [CrossRef]

94. Kier, W.M. The musculature of coleoid cephalopod arms and tentacles. *Front. Cell Dev. Biol.* **2016**, *4*, 10. [CrossRef]

95. Matzner, H.; Gutfreund, Y.; Hochner, B. Neuromuscular system of the flexible arm of the octopus: Physiological characterization. *J. Neurophysiol.* **2000**, *83*, 1315–1328. [CrossRef] [PubMed]

96. Rokni, D.; Hochner, B. Ionic currents underlying fast action potentials in the obliquely striated muscle cells of the octopus arm. *J. Neurophysiol.* **2003**, *88*, 3386–3397. [CrossRef] [PubMed]

97. Nesher, N.; Maiole, F.; Shomrat, T.; Hochner, B.; Zullo, L. From synaptic input to muscle contraction: Arm muscle cells of Octopus vulgaris show unique neuromuscular junction and excitation-contraction coupling properties. *Proc. R. Soc. B* **2019**, *286*. [CrossRef]

98. Taylor, D.; Sampaio, L.; Gobin, A. Building new hearts: A review of trends in cardiac tissue engineering. *Am. J. Transplant.* **2014**, *14*. [CrossRef] [PubMed]

99. Sommese, L.; Zullo, A.; Schiano, C.; Mancini, F.; Napoli, C. Possible muscle repair in the human cardiovascular system. *Stem. Cell Rev. Rep.* **2017**, *13*. [CrossRef] [PubMed]

100. Gilly, W.; Renken, C.; Rosenthal, J.; Kier, W. Specialization for rapid excitation in fast squid tentacle muscle involves action potentials absent in slow arm muscle. *J. Exp. Biol.* **2020**, *223*, jeb.218081. [CrossRef]

101. Kang, R.; Guglielmino, E.; Zullo, L.; Branson, D.T.; Godage, I.; Caldwell, D.G. Embodiment design of soft continuum robots. *Adv. Mech. Eng.* **2016**, *8*, 1–13. [CrossRef]

102. Zullo, L.; Hochner, B. A new perspective on the organization of an invertebrate brain. *Commun. Integr. Biol.* **2011**, *4*, 26–29. [CrossRef]

103. Zullo, L.; Sumbre, G.; Agnisola, C.; Flash, T.; Hochner, B. Nonsomatotopic organization of the higher motor centers in octopus. *Curr. Biol.* **2009**, *19*, 1632–1636. [CrossRef]

104. Grimaldi, A.; Tettamanti, G.; Rinaldi, L.; Brivio, M.; Castellani, D.; Eguileor, M. Muscle differentiation in tentacles of Sepia officinalis (Mollusca) is regulated by muscle regulatory factors (MRF) related proteins. *Dev. Growth Differ.* **2004**, *46*, 83–95. [CrossRef]

105. Albertin, C.B.; Simakov, O.; Mitros, T.; Wang, Z.Y.; Pungor, J.R.; Edsinger-Gonzales, E.; Brenner, S.; Ragsdale, C.W.; Rokhsar, D.S. The octopus genome and the evolution of cephalopod neural and morphological novelties. *Nature* **2015**, *524*, 220–224. [CrossRef] [PubMed]

106. Grimaldi, A.; Tettamanti, G.; Acquati, F.; Bossi, E.; Guidali, M.L.; Banfi, S.; Monti, L.; Valvassori, R.; de Eguileor, M. A hedgehog homolog is involved in muscle formation and organization of Sepia officinalis (mollusca) mantle. *Dev. Dyn.* **2008**, *237*, 659–671. [CrossRef] [PubMed]

107. Lange, M.M. On the regeneration and finer structure of the arms of the cephalopods. *J. Exp. Zool.* **1920**, *31*, 1–57. [CrossRef]

108. Shaw, T.J.; Osborne, M.; Ponte, G.; Fiorito, G.; Andrews, P.L.R. Mechanisms of wound closure following acute arm injury in Octopus vulgaris. *Zool. Lett.* **2016**, *2*, 8. [CrossRef]

109. Fossati, S.M.; Carella, F.; De Vico, G.; Benfenati, F.; Zullo, L. Octopus arm regeneration: Role of acetylcholinesterase during morphological modification. *J. Exp. Mar. Biol. Ecol.* **2013**, *447*, 93–99. [CrossRef]

110. Fossati, S.M.; Candiani, S.; Nödl, M.T.; Maragliano, L.; Pennuto, M.; Domingues, P.; Benfenati, F.; Pestarino, M.; Zullo, L. Identification and expression of acetylcholinesterase in octopus vulgaris arm development and regeneration: A conserved role for ACHE? *Mol. Neurobiol.* **2015**, *52*, 45–56. [CrossRef]

111. Vibert, L.; Daulny, A.; Jarriault, S. Wound healing, cellular regeneration and plasticity: The elegans way. *Int. J. Dev. Biol.* **2018**, *62*, 491–505. [CrossRef]

112. Benian, G.; Epstein, H. Caenorhabditis elegans muscle A Genetic and molecular model for protein interactions in the heart. *Circ. Res.* **2011**, *109*, 1082–1095. [CrossRef]

113. Moerman, D.; Fire, A. *Muscle: Structure, Function, and Development*, 2nd ed.; Springer: New York, NY, USA, 1997; Volume 33, pp. 154–196.

114. Kiontke, K.; Sudhaus, W. Ecology of caenorhabditis species. *WormBook* **2006**. [CrossRef]

115. Bird, A.; Bird, J. *The Structure of Nematodes*, 2nd ed.; Academic Press: Boston, MA, USA, 1991; pp. 10–317.

116. Corsi, A.; Wightman, B.; Chalfie, M. A transparent window into biology: A primer on caenorhabditis elegans. *WormBook* **2015**, *200*, 1–31. [CrossRef]

117. White, J.G.; Southgate, E.; Thomson, J.N.; Brenner, S. The structure of the nervous system of the nematode caenorhabditis elegans. *Philos. Trans. R. Soc.* **1986**, *275*, 327–348.

118. Gieseler, K.; Qadota, H.; Benian, G. Development, structure, and maintenance of *C. elegans* body wall muscle. *WormBook* **2016**, *2017*, 1–59. [CrossRef] [PubMed]

119. Stetina, S.E. *Brenner's Encyclopedia of Genetics*, 2nd ed.; Academic Press: Boston, MA, USA, 2013; pp. 469–476.

120. Brouilly, N.; Lecroisey, C.; Martin, E.; Pierson, L.; Mariol, M.C.; Qadota, H.; Labouesse, M.; Streichenberger, N.; Mounier, N.; Gieseler, K. Ultra-structural time-course study in the C. elegans model for Duchenne muscular dystrophy highlights a crucial role for sarcomere-anchoring structures and sarcolemma integrity in the earliest steps of the muscle degeneration process. *Hum. Mol. Genet.* **2015**, *24*, 6428–6445. [CrossRef] [PubMed]

121. Chamberlain, J.S.; Benian, G.M. Muscular dystrophy: The worm turns to genetic disease. *Curr. Biol. CB* **2000**, *10*, R795–R797. [CrossRef]

122. Marden, J.H. Variability in the size, composition, and function of insect flight muscles. *Annu. Rev. Physiol.* **2000**, *62*, 157–178. [CrossRef] [PubMed]

123. Bhakthan, N.; Nair, K.; Borden, J. Fine structure of degenerating and regenerating flight muscles in a bark beetle, Ips confusus. II. Regeneration. *Can. J. Zool.* **1971**, *49*, 85–89. [CrossRef]

124. Bernstein, S.; O'Donnell, P.; Cripps, R. Molecular genetic analysis of muscle development, structure, and function in drosophila. *Int. Rev. Cytol.* **1993**, *143*, 63–152. [CrossRef]

125. Josephson, R.; Malamud, J.; Stokes, D. Asynchronous muscle: A primer. *J. Exp. Biol.* **2000**, *203*, 2713–2722.

126. Osborne, M.P. Supercontraction in the muscles of the blowfly larva: An ultrastructural study. *J. Insect Physiol.* **1967**, *13*, 1471–1482. [CrossRef]

127. Goldstein, M.; Burdette, W. Striated visceral muscle of Drosophila melanogaster. *J. Morphol.* **1971**, *134*, 315–334. [CrossRef]

128. Goldstein, M.A. An ultrastructural study of supercontraction in the body wall muscles of Drosophila melanogaster larvae. *Anat. Rec.* **1971**, *169*, 326.

129. Hardie, J. The tension/length relationship of an insect (Calliphora erythrocephala) supercontracting muscle. *Cell. Mol. Life Sci. CMLS* **1976**, *32*, 714–716. [CrossRef]

130. Herrel, A.; Meyers, J.; Aerts, P.; Nishikawa, K. Functional implications of supercontracting muscle in the chameleon tongue retractors. *J. Exp. Biol.* **2001**, *204*, 3621–3627. [PubMed]

131. Beramendi, A.; Peron, S.; Megighian, A.; Reggiani, C.; Cantera, R. The IκB ortholog cactus is necessary for normal neuromuscular function in drosophila melanogaster. *Neuroscience* **2005**, *134*, 397–406. [CrossRef]

132. Staehling, K.; Hoffmann, F.; Baylies, M.; Rushton, E.; Bate, M. Dpp induces mesodermal gene expression in drosophila. *Nature* **1994**, *372*, 783–786. [CrossRef]

133. Azpiazu, N.; Lawrence, P.A.; Vincent, J.-P.; Frasch, M. Segmentation and specification of the drosophila mesoderm. *Genes Dev.* **1997**, *10*, 3183–3194. [CrossRef]

134. Baylies, M.; Bate, M. twist: A Myogenic Switch in Drosophila. *Science* **1996**, *272*, 1481–1484. [CrossRef]

135. Chaturvedi, D.; Reichert, H.; Gunage, R.; Vijayraghavan, K. Identification and functional characterization of muscle satellite cells in Drosophila. *eLife* **2017**, *6*. [CrossRef]

136. Postigo, A.A.; Ward, E.; Skeath, J.B.; Dean, D.C. zfh-1, the Drosophila homologue of ZEB, is a transcriptional repressor that regulates somatic myogenesis. *Mol. Cell. Biol.* **1999**, *19*, 7255–7263. [CrossRef]

137. Carnevali, M.D.C. Regeneration in echinoderms: Repair, regrowth, cloning. *Invertebr. Surviv. J.* **2006**, *3*, 64–76.

138. Dupont, S.; Thorndyke, M. Bridging the regeneration gap: Insights from echinoderm models. *Nat. Rev. Genet.* **2007**, *8*, 320. [CrossRef]

139. Ziegler, A.; Schröder, L.; Ogurreck, M.; Faber, C.; Stach, T. Evolution of a Novel Muscle Design in Sea Urchins (Echinodermata: Echinoidea). *PLoS ONE* **2012**, *7*, e37520. [CrossRef] [PubMed]

140. Ortiz-Pineda, P.; Ramirez-Gomez, F.; Pérez-Ortiz, J.; González-Díaz, S.; Jesús, F.; Hernández-Pasos, J.; Avila, C.; Rojas-Cartagena, C.; Suárez-Castillo, E.; Tossas, K.; et al. Gene expression profiling of intestinal regeneration in the sea cucumber. *BMC Genom.* **2009**, *10*, 262. [CrossRef]

141. García-Arrarás, J.E.; Dolmatov, I.Y. Echinoderms: Potential model systems for studies on muscle regeneration. *Curr. Pharm. Des.* **2010**, *16*, 942–955. [CrossRef] [PubMed]

142. Quiñones, J.L.; Rosa, R.; Ruiz, D.L.; García-Arrarás, J.E. Extracellular matrix remodeling and metalloproteinase involvement during intestine regeneration in the sea cucumber holothuria glaberrima. *Dev. Biol.* **2002**, *250*, 181–197. [CrossRef]

143. Dolmatov, I.Y.; Eliseikina, M.G.; Ginanova, T.T.; Lamash, N.E.; Korchagin, V.P.; Bulgakov, A.A. Muscle regeneration in the holothurian *Stichopus japonicus. Roux's Arch. Dev. Biol.* **1996**, *205*, 486–493. [CrossRef]

144. Holland, L.; Albalat, R.; Azumi, K.; Benito Gutierrez, E.; Blow, M.; Bronner-Fraser, M.; Brunet, F.; Butts, T.; Candiani, S.; Dishaw, L.; et al. The amphioxus genome illuminates vertebrate origins and cephalochordate biology. *Genome Res.* **2008**, *18*, 1100–1111. [CrossRef]

145. Somorjai, I.; Escrivà, H.; GarciaFernandez, J. Amphioxus makes the cut—Again. *Commun. Integr. Biol.* **2012**, *5*, 499–502. [CrossRef]

146. Somorjai, I.; Somorjai, R.; GarciaFernandez, J.; Escrivà, H. Vertebrate-like regeneration in the invertebrate chordate amphioxus. *Proc. Natl. Acad. Sci. USA* **2011**, *109*, 517–522. [CrossRef]

147. Liang, Y.; Rathnayake, D.; Huang, S.; Pathirana, A.; Xu, Q.; Zhang, S. BMP signaling is required for amphioxus tail regeneration. *Development* **2019**, *146*, dev.166017. [CrossRef]

148. Kaneto, S.; Wada, H. Regeneration of amphioxus oral cirri and its skeletal rods: Implications for the origin of the vertebrate skeleton. *J. Exp. Zool. Part. B Mol. Dev. Evol.* **2011**, *316*, 409–417. [CrossRef] [PubMed]

149. Flood, P.; Guthrie, D.; Banks, J. Paramyosin muscle in the notochord of amphioxus. *Nature* **1969**, *222*, 87–88. [CrossRef] [PubMed]

150. Peachey, L. Structure of the longitudinal body muscles of Amphioxus. *J. Biophys. Biochem. Cytol.* **1961**, *10*, 159–176. [CrossRef] [PubMed]

151. Hagiwara, S.; Henkart, M.; Kidokoro, Y. Excitation-contraction coupling in amphioxus muscle cells. *J. Physiol.* **1972**, *219*, 233–251. [CrossRef] [PubMed]

152. Welsch, U. The fine structure of the pharynx, cyrtopodocytes and digestive caecum of amphioxus (*Branchiostoma lanceolatum*). *Symp. Zool. Soc. Lond.* **1975**, *36*, 17–41.

153. Aldea, D.; Subirana, L.; Keime, C.; Meister, L.; Maeso, I.; Marcellini, S.; Gómez-Skarmeta, J.; Bertrand, S.; Escrivà, H. Genetic regulation of amphioxus somitogenesis informs the evolution of the vertebrate head mesoderm. *Nat. Ecol. Evol.* **2019**, *3*. [CrossRef]

154. Meulemans, D.; Bronner-Fraser, M.; Holland, L.; Holland, N. Differential mesodermal expression of two amphioxus MyoD family members (AmphiMRF1 and AmphiMRF2). *Gene Expr. Patterns GEP* **2003**, *3*, 199–202. [CrossRef]

155. Bertrand, S.; Camasses, A.; Somorjai, I.; Belgacem, M.; Chabrol, O.; Escande, M.-L.; Pontarotti, P.; Escrivà, H. Amphioxus FGF signaling predicts the acquisition of vertebrate morphological traits. *Proc. Natl. Acad. Sci. USA* **2011**, *108*, 9160–9165. [CrossRef]

156. Onai, T.; Aramaki, T.; Inomata, H.; Hirai, T.; Kuratani, S. On the origin of vertebrate somites. *Zool. Lett.* **2015**, *1*. [CrossRef]

157. Shenkar, N.; Swalla, B. Global Diversity of Ascidiacea. *PLoS ONE* **2011**, *6*, e20657. [CrossRef]

158. Delsuc, F.; Brinkmann, H.; Chourrout, D.; Philippe, H. Tunicates and not cephalochordates are the closest living relatives of vertebrates. *Nature* **2006**, *439*, 965–968. [CrossRef] [PubMed]

159. Tiozzo, S.; Brown, F.; de Tomaso, A. Regeneration and stem cells in ascidians. In *Stem Cells*; Springer: New York, NY, USA, 2008; pp. 95–112.

160. Alié, A.; Hiebert, L.; Scelzo, M.; Tiozzo, S. The eventful history of non-embryonic development in tunicates. *J. Exp. Zool. Part. B Mol. Dev. Evol.* **2020**. [CrossRef] [PubMed]

161. Nakauchi, M. Asexual development of ascidians: Its biological significance, diversity, and morphogenesis. *Am. Zool.* **1982**, *22*. [CrossRef]

162. Razy-Krajka, F.; Stolfi, A. Regulation and evolution of muscle development in tunicates. *EvoDevo* **2019**, *10*. [CrossRef]

163. Jeffery, W. Progenitor targeting by adult stem cells in ciona homeostasis, injury, and regeneration. *Dev. Biol.* **2018**, *448*. [CrossRef]

164. Degasperi, V.; Gasparini, F.; Shimeld, S.; Sinigaglia, C.; Burighel, P.; Manni, L. Muscle differentiation in a colonial ascidian: Organisation, gene expression and evolutionary considerations. *BMC Dev. Biol.* **2009**, *9*, 48. [CrossRef]

165. Meedel, T.; Chang, P.; Yasuo, H. Muscle development in Ciona intestinalis requires the b-HLH myogenic regulatory factor gene Ci-MRF. *Dev. Biol.* **2007**, *302*, 333–344. [CrossRef]

166. Anderson, H.E.; Christiaen, L. Ciona as a simple chordate model for heart development and regeneration. *J. Cardiovasc. Dev. Dis.* **2016**, *3*, 25. [CrossRef]

167. Jeffery, W. Closing the wounds: One hundred and twenty five years of regenerative biology in the ascidian ciona intestinalis. *Genesis* **2015**, *53*. [CrossRef]

168. Christiaen, L.; Tolkin, T. Rewiring of an ancestral Tbx1/10-Ebf-Mrf network for pharyngeal muscle specification in distinct embryonic lineages. *BioRxiv* **2016**. [CrossRef]

169. Razy-Krajka, F.; Lam, K.; Wang, W.; Stolfi, A.; Joly, M.; Bonneau, R.; Christiaen, L. Collier/OLF/EBF-dependent transcriptional dynamics control pharyngeal muscle specification from primed cardiopharyngeal progenitors. *Dev. Cell* **2014**, *29*. [CrossRef] [PubMed]

170. Davidson, B. Ciona intestinalis as a model for cardiac development. *Semin. Cell Dev. Biol.* **2007**, *18*, 16–26. [CrossRef] [PubMed]

171. Ricci, L.; Cabrera, F.; Lotito, S.; Tiozzo, S. Re-deployment of germ layers related TFs shows regionalized expression during two non-embryonic developments. *Dev. Biol.* **2016**, *416*. [CrossRef] [PubMed]

172. Prünster, M.M.; Ricci, L.; Brown, F.; Tiozzo, S. De novo neurogenesis in a budding chordate: Co-option of larval anteroposterior patterning genes in a transitory neurogenic organ. *Dev. Biol.* **2018**, *448*. [CrossRef]

173. Prünster, M.M.; Ricci, L.; Brown, F.; Tiozzo, S. Modular co-option of cardiopharyngeal genes during non-embryonic myogenesis. *EvoDevo* **2019**, *10*. [CrossRef]

174. Voskoboynik, A.; Simon-Blecher, N.; Soen, Y.; de Tomaso, A.; Ishizuka, K.; Weissman, I. Striving for normality: Whole body regeneration through a series of abnormal generations. *FASEB J.* **2007**, *21*, 1335–1344. [CrossRef]

175. Freeman, G. The role of blood cells in the process of asexual reproduction in the tunicate Perophora. *J. Exp. Zool.* **1964**, *156*, 157–183. [CrossRef]

176. Kassmer, S.; Langenbacher, A.; de Tomaso, A. *Primordial Blasts, a Population of Blood Borne Stem Cells Responsible for Whole Body Regeneration in a basal Chordate*; Springer: New York, NY, USA, 2019. [CrossRef]

177. Marques, I.J.; Lupi, E.; Mercader, N. Model systems for regeneration: Zebrafish. *Development* **2019**, *146*. [CrossRef]

178. Gemberling, M.; Bailey, T.; Hyde, D.; Poss, K. The zebrafish as a model for complex tissue regeneration. *TIG* **2013**, *29*. [CrossRef]

179. Berberoglu, M.; Gallagher, T.; Morrow, Z.; Talbot, J.; Hromowyk, K.; Tenente, I.; Langenau, D.; Amacher, S. Satellite-like cells contribute to pax7-dependent skeletal muscle repair in adult zebrafish. *Dev. Biol.* **2017**, *424*. [CrossRef]

180. Keenan, S.R.; Currie, P.D. The developmental phases of zebrafish myogenesis. *J. Dev. Biol.* **2019**, *7*, 12. [CrossRef] [PubMed]

181. Lai, S.L.; Marin-Juez, R.; Moura, P.L.; Kuenne, C.; Lai, J.K.H.; Tsedeke, A.T.; Guenther, S.; Looso, M.; Stainier, D.Y. Reciprocal analyses in zebrafish and medaka reveal that harnessing the immune response promotes cardiac regeneration. *eLife* **2017**, *6*. [CrossRef] [PubMed]

182. Charvet, B.; Malbouyres, M.; Pagnon-Minot, A.; Ruggiero, F.; le Guellec, D. Development of the zebrafish myoseptum with emphasis on the myotendinous junction. *Cell Tissue Res.* **2011**, *346*, 439–449. [CrossRef] [PubMed]

183. Hammond, C.L.; Hinits, Y.; Osborn, D.P.; Minchin, J.E.; Tettamanti, G.; Hughes, S.M. Signals and myogenic regulatory factors restrict pax3 and pax7 expression to dermomyotome-like tissue in zebrafish. *Dev. Biol.* **2007**, *302*, 504–521. [CrossRef]

184. Gurevich, D.B.; Nguyen, P.D.; Siegel, A.L.; Ehrlich, O.V.; Sonntag, C.; Phan, J.M.; Berger, S.; Ratnayake, D.; Hersey, L.; Berger, J.; et al. Asymmetric division of clonal muscle stem cells coordinates muscle regeneration in vivo. *Science* **2016**, *353*, aad9969. [CrossRef]

185. Rossi, G.; Messina, G. Comparative myogenesis in teleosts and mammals. *Cell. Mol. Life Sci.* **2014**, *71*, 3081–3099. [CrossRef]

186. González-Rosa, J.M.; Burns, C.; Burns, C. Zebrafish heart regeneration: 15 years of discoveries. *Regeneration* **2017**, *4*. [CrossRef]

187. Poss, K.D.; Wilson, L.G.; Keating, M.T. Heart regeneration in zebrafish. *Science* **2002**, *298*, 2188–2190. [CrossRef]

188. Beffagna, G. Zebrafish as a smart model to understand regeneration after heart injury: How fish could help humans. *Front. Cardiovasc. Med.* **2019**, *6*. [CrossRef]

189. Kikuchi, K.; Holdway, J.; Werdich, A.; Anderson, R.; Fang, Y.; Egnaczyk, G.; Evans, T.; Macrae, C.; Stainier, D.; Poss, K. Primary contribution to zebrafish heart regeneration by Gata4 cardiomyocytes. *Nature* **2010**, *464*, 601–605. [CrossRef]

190. Jopling, C.; Sleep, E.; Raya, M.; Marti, M.; Raya, A.; Izpisua Belmonte, J.C. Zebrafish heart regeneration occurs by cardiomyocyte dedifferentiation and proliferation. *Nature* **2010**, *464*, 606–609. [CrossRef] [PubMed]

191. Sande-Melón, M.; Marques, I.; Galardi-Castilla, M.; Langa Oliva, X.; Pérez-López, M.; Botos, M.-A.; Sánchez-Iranzo, H.; Guzmán-Martínez, G.; Francisco, D.; Pavlinic, D.; et al. Adult sox10+ Cardiomyocytes Contribute to Myocardial Regeneration in the Zebrafish. *Cell Rep.* **2019**, *29*, 1041–1054. [CrossRef] [PubMed]

192. Huang, W.-C.; Yang, C.-C.; Chen, I.H.; Liu, L.Y.-m.; Chang, S.J.; Chuang, Y.-J. Treatment of glucocorticoids inhibited early immune responses and impaired cardiac repair in adult zebrafish. *PLoS ONE* **2013**, *8*, e66613. [CrossRef] [PubMed]

193. de Preux Charles, A.-S.; Bise, T.; Baier, F.; Marro, J.; Jazwinska, A. Distinct effects of inflammation on preconditioning and regeneration of the adult zebrafish heart. *Open Biol.* **2016**, *6*, 160102. [CrossRef] [PubMed]

194. Harrison, M.; Bussmann, J.; Huang, Y.; Zhao, L.; Osorio, A.; Burns, C.; Burns, C.; Sucov, H.; Siekmann, A.; Lien, C.-L. Chemokine-guided angiogenesis directs coronary vasculature formation in zebrafish. *Dev. Cell* **2015**, *33*, 442–454. [CrossRef]

195. González-Rosa, J.M.; Martín, V.; Peralta, M.; Torres, M.; Mercader, N. Extensive scar formation and regression during heart regeneration after cryoinjury in zebrafish. *Development* **2011**, *138*, 1663–1674. [CrossRef]

196. Schnabel, K.; Wu, C.C.; Kurth, T.; Weidinger, G. Regeneration of cryoinjury induced necrotic heart lesions in zebrafish is associated with epicardial activation and cardiomyocyte proliferation. *PLoS ONE* **2011**, *6*, e18503. [CrossRef]

197. Marín-Juez, R.; Marass, M.; Gauvrit, S.; Rossi, A.; Lai, S.-L.; Materna, S.; Black, B.; Stainier, D. Fast revascularization of the injured area is essential to support zebrafish heart regeneration. *Proc. Natl. Acad. Sci. USA* **2016**, *113*. [CrossRef]

198. Sánchez-Iranzo, H.; Galardi-Castilla, M.; Sanz-Morejón, A.; González-Rosa, J.M.; Costa, R.; Ernst, A.; Sainz de Aja, J.; Langa Oliva, X.; Mercader, N. Transient fibrosis resolves via fibroblast inactivation in the regenerating zebrafish heart. *Proc. Natl. Acad. Sci. USA* **2018**, *115*, 201716713. [CrossRef]

199. Cao, J.; Poss, K. The epicardium as a hub for heart regeneration. *Nat. Rev. Cardiol.* **2018**, *15*. [CrossRef]

200. Lavine, K.; Yu, K.; White, A.; Zhang, X.; Smith, C.; Partanen, J.; Ornitz, D. Endocardial and epicardial derived FGF signals regulate myocardial proliferation and differentiation in vivo. *Dev. Cell* **2005**, *8*, 85–95. [CrossRef] [PubMed]

201. Wang, J.; Cao, J.; Dickson, A.; Poss, K. Epicardial regeneration is guided by cardiac outflow tract and Hedgehog signalling. *Nature* **2015**, *522*. [CrossRef] [PubMed]

202. Lepilina, A.; Coon, A.N.; Kikuchi, K.; Holdway, J.E.; Roberts, R.W.; Burns, C.G.; Poss, K.D. A dynamic epicardial injury response supports progenitor cell activity during zebrafish heart regeneration. *Cell* **2006**, *127*, 607–619. [CrossRef] [PubMed]

203. González-Rosa, J.M.; Peralta, M.; Mercader, N. Pan-epicardial lineage tracing reveals that epicardium derived cells give rise to myofibroblasts and perivascular cells during zebrafish heart regeneration. *Dev. Biol.* **2012**, *370*, 173–186. [CrossRef] [PubMed]

204. Huang, Y.; Harrison, M.; Osorio, A.; Kim, J.; Baugh, A.; Duan, C.; Sucov, H.; Lien, C.-L. Igf Signaling is required for cardiomyocyte proliferation during zebrafish heart development and regeneration. *PLoS ONE* **2013**, *8*, e67266. [CrossRef]

205. Kim, J.; Wu, Q.; Zhang, Y.; Wiens, K.; Huang, Y.; Rubin, N.; Shimada, H.; Handin, R.; Chao, M.; Tuan, T.-L.; et al. PDGF signaling is required for epicardial function and blood vessel formation in regenerating zebrafish hearts. *Proc. Natl. Acad. Sci. USA* **2010**, *107*, 17206–17210. [CrossRef]

206. Chablais, F.; Jazwinska, A. The regenerative capacity of the zebrafish heart is dependent on TGFβ signaling. *Development* **2012**, *139*, 1921–1930. [CrossRef]

207. Chablais, F.; Jazwinska, A. Induction of myocardial infarction in adult zebrafish using cryoinjury. *J. Vis. Exp. JoVE* **2012**, *62*. [CrossRef]

208. Dogra, D.; Ahuja, S.; Kim, H.-T.; Rasouli, S.J.; Stainier, D.; Reischauer, S. Opposite effects of Activin type 2 receptor ligands on cardiomyocyte proliferation during development and repair. *Nat. Commun.* **2017**, *8*. [CrossRef]

209. Wu, C.C.; Kruse, F.; Dalvoy, M.; Junker, J.; Zebrowski, D.C.; Fischer, K.; Noel, E.; Grün, D.; Berezikov, E.; Engel, F.; et al. Spatially resolved genome-wide transcriptional profiling identifies BMP signaling as essential regulator of zebrafish cardiomyocyte regeneration. *Dev. Cell* **2015**, *36*. [CrossRef]

210. Zhao, L.; Borikova, A.; Ben-Yair, R.; Guner-Ataman, B.; Macrae, C.; Lee, R.; Burns, C.; Burns, C. Notch signaling regulates cardiomyocyte proliferation during zebrafish heart regeneration. *Proc. Natl. Acad. Sci. USA* **2014**, *111*, 1403–1408. [CrossRef] [PubMed]

211. Yin, V.; Thomson, J.; Thummel, R.; Hyde, D.; Hammond, S.; Poss, K. Fgf-dependent depletion of microRNA-133 promotes appendage regeneration in zebrafish. *Genes Dev.* **2008**, *22*, 728–733. [CrossRef] [PubMed]

212. Xiao, C.-L.; Hou, Y.; Xu, C.; Chang, N.; Wang, F.; Hu, K.; He, A.; Luo, Y.; Wang, J.; Peng, J.; et al. Chromatin-remodelling factor Brg1 regulates myocardial proliferation and regeneration in zebrafish. *Nat. Commun.* **2016**, *7*, 13787. [CrossRef] [PubMed]

213. Keßler, M.; Rottbauer, W.; Just, S. Recent progress in the use of zebrafish for novel cardiac drug discovery. *Expert Opin. Drug Discov.* **2015**, *10*. [CrossRef] [PubMed]

214. Moro, E.; Vettori, A.; Porazzi, P.; Schiavone, M.; Rampazzo, E.; Casari, A.; Ek, O.; Facchinello, N.; Astone, M.; Zancan, I.; et al. Generation and application of signaling pathway reporter lines in zebrafish. *Mol. Genet. Genom.* **2013**, *288*, 231–242. [CrossRef]

215. Howe, K.; Clark, M.D.; Torroja, C.F.; Torrance, J.; Berthelot, C.; Muffato, M.; Collins, J.E.; Humphray, S.; McLaren, K.; Matthews, L.; et al. The zebrafish reference genome sequence and its relationship to the human genome. *Nature* **2013**, *496*, 498–503. [CrossRef]

216. Beltrami, A.P.; Urbanek, K.; Kajstura, J.; Yan, S.-M.; Finato, N.; Bussani, R.; Nadal-Ginard, B.; Silvestri, F.; Leri, A.; Beltrami, C.A.; et al. Evidence that human cardiac myocytes divide after myocardial infarction. *N. Engl. J. Med.* **2001**, *344*, 1750–1757. [CrossRef]

217. Pasumarthi, K.B.; Field, L.J. Cardiomyocyte cell cycle regulation. *Circ. Res.* **2002**, *90*, 1044–1054. [CrossRef]

218. Bassett, D.I.; Currie, P.D. The zebrafish as a model for muscular dystrophy and congenital myopathy. *Hum. Mol. Genet.* **2003**, *12*, R265–R270. [CrossRef]

219. Otten, C.; Abdelilah-Seyfried, S. Laser-inflicted injury of zebrafish embryonic skeletal muscle. *JoVE* **2013**. [CrossRef]

220. Saera-Vila, A.; Kish, P.E.; Kahana, A. Fgf regulates dedifferentiation during skeletal muscle regeneration in adult zebrafish. *Cell. Signal.* **2016**, *28*, 1196–1204. [CrossRef] [PubMed]

221. Naranjo, J.; Dziki, J.; Badylak, S. Regenerative medicine approaches for age-related muscle loss and sarcopenia: A mini-review. *Gerontology* **2017**, *63*. [CrossRef] [PubMed]

222. Liu, J.; Saul, D.; Böker, K.; Ernst, J.; Lehmann, W.; Schilling, A. Current methods for skeletal muscle tissue repair and regeneration. *Biomed. Res. Int.* **2018**, *2018*. [CrossRef] [PubMed]

223. Zullo, A.; Mancini, F.P.; Schleip, R.; Wearing, S.; Yahia, L.H.; Klingler, W. The interplay between fascia, skeletal muscle, nerves, adipose tissue, inflammation and mechanical stress in musculo-fascial regeneration. *J. Gerontol. Geriatr.* **2017**, *65*, 271–283.

224. Forcina, L.; Cosentino, M.; Musaro, A. Mechanisms regulating muscle regeneration: Insights into the interrelated and time-dependent phases of tissue healing. *Cells* **2020**, *9*, 1297. [CrossRef]

225. Sicherer, S.; Grasman, J. Recent trends in injury models to study skeletal muscle regeneration and repair. *Bioengineering* **2020**, *7*, 76. [CrossRef]

226. Khodabukus, A.; Prabhu, N.; Wang, J.; Bursac, N. In vitro tissue-engineered skeletal muscle models for studying muscle physiology and disease. *Adv. Healthc. Mater.* **2018**, *7*, 1701498. [CrossRef]

227. Mueller, A.; Bloch, R. Skeletal muscle cell transplantation: Models and methods. *J. Muscle Res. Cell Motil.* **2019**. [CrossRef]

228. Marg, A.; Escobar, H.; Karaiskos, N.; Grunwald, S.; Metzler, E.; Kieshauer, J.; Sauer, S.; Pasemann, D.; Malfatti, E.; Mompoint, D.; et al. Human muscle-derived CLEC14A-positive cells regenerate muscle independent of PAX7. *Nat. Commun.* **2019**, *10*, 5776. [CrossRef]

229. Lingjun, R.; Qian, Y.; Khodabukus, A.; Ribar, T.; Bursac, N. Engineering human pluripotent stem cells into a functional skeletal muscle tissue. *Nat. Commun.* **2018**, *9*. [CrossRef]

230. Chan, S.S.-K.; Arpke, R.; Filareto, A.; Xie, N.; Pappas, M.; Penaloza, J.; Perlingeiro, R.; Kyba, M. Skeletal muscle stem cells from PSC-derived teratomas have functional regenerative capacity. *Cell Stem Cell* **2018**, *23*, 74–85. [CrossRef]

231. Costela, M.C.O.; López, M.G.; López, V.C.; Gallardo, M.E. iPSCs: A powerful tool for skeletal muscle tissue engineering. *J. Cell. Mol. Med.* **2019**, *23*. [CrossRef]

232. Hall, M.; Hall, J.; Cadwallader, A.; Pawlikowski, B.; Doles, J.; Elston, T.; Olwin, B. Transplantation of skeletal muscle stem cells. *Methods Mol. Biol.* **2017**, *1556*, 237–244. [PubMed]

233. Quattrocelli, M.; Swinnen, M.; Giacomazzi, G.; Camps, J.; Barthélémy, I.; Ceccarelli, G.; Caluwé, E.; Grosemans, H.; Thorrez, L.; Pelizzo, G.; et al. Mesodermal iPSC–derived progenitor cells functionally regenerate cardiac and skeletal muscle. *J. Clin. Investig.* **2015**, *125*. [CrossRef] [PubMed]

234. Maffioletti, S.; Sarcar, S.; Henderson, A.; Mannhardt, I.; Pinton, L.; Moyle, L.; Steele, H.; Cappellari, O.; Wells, K.; Ferrari, G.; et al. Three-dimensional human iPSC-derived artificial skeletal muscles model muscular dystrophies and enable multilineage tissue engineering. *Cell Rep.* **2018**, *23*, 899–908. [CrossRef] [PubMed]

235. Danišovič, L.; Galambosova, M.; Csobonyeiová, M. Induced pluripotent stem cells for duchenne muscular dystrophy modeling and therapy. *Cells* **2018**, *7*, 253. [CrossRef]

236. Choi, I.; Lim, H.; Estrellas, K.; Mula, J.; Cohen, T.; Zhang, Y.; Donnelly, C.; Richard, J.-P.; Kim, Y.J.; Kim, H.; et al. Concordant but Varied phenotypes among duchenne muscular dystrophy patient-specific myoblasts derived using a human iPSC-based model. *Cell Rep.* **2016**, *15*, 1–12. [CrossRef]

237. Webster, M.; Fan, C. c-MET regulates myoblast motility and myocyte fusion during adult skeletal muscle regeneration. *PLoS ONE* **2013**, *8*, e81757. [CrossRef]

238. Wal, E.; Herrero-Hernandez, P.; Wan, R.; Broeders, M.; Groen, S.; Gestel, T.; Van Ijcken, W.; Cheung, T.; Ploeg, A.; Schaaf, G.; et al. Large-scale expansion of human iPSC-derived skeletal muscle cells for disease modeling and cell-based therapeutic strategies. *Stem Cell Rep.* **2018**, *10*. [CrossRef]

239. Ong, C.S.; Yesantharao, P.; Huang, C.-Y.; Mattson, G.; Boktor, J.; Fukunishi, T.; Zhang, H.; Hibino, N. 3D bioprinting using stem cells. *Pediatr. Res.* **2017**, *83*. [CrossRef]

240. Mandrycky, C.; Wang, D.Z.; Kim, K.; Kim, D.-H. 3D Bioprinting for engineering complex tissues. *Biotechnol. Adv.* **2015**, *34*. [CrossRef] [PubMed]

241. Pollot, B.; Rathbone, C.; Wenke, J.; Guda, T. Natural polymeric hydrogel evaluation for skeletal muscle tissue engineering: Skeletal muscle engineering natural hydrogels. *J. Biomed. Mater. Res. Part. B Appl. Biomater.* **2017**, *106*. [CrossRef] [PubMed]

242. Fuoco, C.; Petrilli, L.L.; Cannata, S.; Gargioli, C. Matrix scaffolding for stem cell guidance toward skeletal muscle tissue engineering. *J. Orthop. Surg. Res.* **2016**, *11*. [CrossRef] [PubMed]

243. Jiao, A.; Moerk, C.; Penland, N.; Perla, M.; Kim, J.; Smith, A.; Murry, C.; Kim, D.-H. Regulation of skeletal myotube formation and alignment by nanotopographically controlled cell-secreted extracellular matrix. *J. Biomed. Mater. Res. Part. A* **2018**, *106*. [CrossRef]

244. Matthews, B.; Vosshall, L. How to turn an organism into a model organism in 10 'easy' steps. *J. Exp. Biol.* **2020**, *223*, jeb218198. [CrossRef]

245. Dickinson, M.; Vosshall, L.; Dow, J. Genome editing in non-model organisms opens new horizons for comparative physiology. *J. Exp. Biol.* **2020**, *223*, jeb221119. [CrossRef]

246. Chargé, S.B.; Rudnicki, M.A. Cellular and molecular regulation of muscle regeneration. *Physiol. Rev.* **2004**, *84*, 209–238. [CrossRef]

247. Hardy, D.; Besnard, A.; Latil, M.; Jouvion, G.; Briand, D.; Thépenier, C.; Pascal, Q.; Guguin, A.; Gayraud-Morel, B.; Cavaillon, J.-M.; et al. Comparative study of injury models for studying muscle regeneration in mice. *PLoS ONE* **2016**, *11*, e0147198. [CrossRef]

248. Hardy, D.; Latil, M.; Gayraud-Morel, B.; Briand, D.; Jouvion, G.; Rocheteau, P.; Chrétien, F. Choosing the appropriate model for studying muscle regeneration in mice: A comparative study of classical protocols. *Morphologie* **2015**, *99*, 168. [CrossRef]

249. Yun, M. Changes in Regenerative Capacity through Lifespan. *Int. J. Mol. Sci.* **2015**, *16*, 25392–25432. [CrossRef]

250. Alvarado, A.S. Regeneration in the metazoans: Why does it happen? *BioEssays* **2000**, *22*, 578–590. [CrossRef]

251. Imperadore, P.; Shah, S.B.; Makarenkova, H.P.; Fiorito, G. Nerve degeneration and regeneration in the cephalopod mollusc Octopus vulgaris: The case of the pallial nerve. *Sci. Rep.* **2017**, *7*, 46564. [CrossRef] [PubMed]

Extracellular Vesicles from Skeletal Muscle Cells Efficiently Promote Myogenesis in Induced Pluripotent Stem Cells

Denisa Baci [1,2], Maila Chirivì [1], Valentina Pace [1], Fabio Maiullari [3], Marika Milan [1], Andrea Rampin [1], Paolo Somma [4], Dario Presutti [1], Silvia Garavelli [5], Antonino Bruno [6], Stefano Cannata [7], Chiara Lanzuolo [8,9], Cesare Gargioli [7], Roberto Rizzi [8,9,*] and Claudia Bearzi [1,9,*]

[1] Institute of Biochemistry and Cell Biology, National Research Council, 00015 Rome, Italy; denisa.baci@uninsubria.it (D.B.); maila.chirivi@yahoo.it (M.C.); va.pace3@gmail.com (V.P.); marika.milan@ibbc.cnr.it (M.M.); rampin88@gmail.com (A.R.); presuttidario@gmail.com (D.P.)
[2] Department of Biotechnology and Life Sciences, University of Insubria, 21100 Varese, Italy
[3] Gemelli Molise Hospital, 86100 Campobasso, Italy; fabio.maiullari3d@gmail.com
[4] Flow Cytometry Core, Humanitas Clinical and Research Center, 20089 Milan, Italy; paolo.somma@humanitasresearch.it
[5] Institute for Endocrinology and Oncology "Gaetano Salvatore", National Research Council, 80131 Naples, Italy; silvia.garavelli@gmail.com
[6] IRCCS MultiMedica, 20138 Milan, Italy; antonino.bruno@multimedica.it
[7] Department of Biology, University of Rome Tor Vergata, 00133 Rome, Italy; cannata@uniroma2.it (S.C.); cesare.gargioli@uniroma2.it (C.G.)
[8] Institute of Biomedical Technologies, National Research Council, 20090 Milan, Italy; chiara.lanzuolo@cnr.it
[9] Fondazione Istituto Nazionale di Genetica Molecolare, 20122 Milan, Italy
[*] Correspondence: roberto.rizzi@cnr.it (R.R.); claudia.bearzi@cnr.it (C.B.);

Abstract: The recent advances, offered by cell therapy in the regenerative medicine field, offer a revolutionary potential for the development of innovative cures to restore compromised physiological functions or organs. Adult myogenic precursors, such as myoblasts or satellite cells, possess a marked regenerative capacity, but the exploitation of this potential still encounters significant challenges in clinical application, due to low rate of proliferation in vitro, as well as a reduced self-renewal capacity. In this scenario, induced pluripotent stem cells (iPSCs) can offer not only an inexhaustible source of cells for regenerative therapeutic approaches, but also a valuable alternative for in vitro modeling of patient-specific diseases. In this study we established a reliable protocol to induce the myogenic differentiation of iPSCs, generated from pericytes and fibroblasts, exploiting skeletal muscle-derived extracellular vesicles (EVs), in combination with chemically defined factors. This genetic integration-free approach generates functional skeletal myotubes maintaining the engraftment ability in vivo. Our results demonstrate evidence that EVs can act as biological "shuttles" to deliver specific bioactive molecules for a successful transgene-free differentiation offering new opportunities for disease modeling and regenerative approaches.

Keywords: iPSC; extracellular vesicles; pericytes; skeletal muscle

1. Introduction

Skeletal muscle is a dynamic tissue with remarkable features for endogenous regeneration provided by muscle progenitors, such as satellite cells. However, in the presence of progressive muscle loss or degeneration, such as muscular dystrophies or aging, satellite cell function is largely affected due to an incorrect asymmetric division or aberrant transcriptional regulation [1–4]. Other adult progenitor cells with myogenic properties, including mesangioblasts [5], pericytes [6,7], muscle side cell population [8], interstitial cells PW1$^+$/PAX7$^-$ [9], or stem cells derived from bone marrow [10] would be considered promising candidates for muscle repair therapy. Despite this, the reduction of proliferative capacity after isolation and the progressive loss of self-renewal potential strongly limit the use of adult progenitor cells for clinical application [11].

On the other hand, induced pluripotent stem cells (iPSCs) represent a valuable source of myogenic progenitors (MPs), essential for cell-based therapy. Indeed, iPSCs not only would allow autologous transplantation but they can also be produced in large quantities, with an unlimited replication ability in vitro. Furthermore, differentiated iPSCs can be used as individual-specific tissue modeling for the validation of innovative therapies, limiting the toxic effects for the patient and providing early indications on the efficacy [12,13].

Many efforts have been made to establish efficient methods for obtaining MPs from iPSCs, mostly relying on the transgenic expression of major myogenesis regulators, such as myoblast determination protein 1 (MyoD) and Pax7 (key myogenic transcription factors) [14–17]. The main disadvantage of these approaches is that forced expression of the MyoD protein leads to cell cycle arrest along with the consequent loss of the in vitro muscle progenitor generation. The risk of unwanted genetic recombination is a widespread limiting issue for future clinical application.

The use of chemical modulators to activate relevant myogenic pathways represents a promising approach to enhance the efficiency of myogenic iPSC differentiation [18–20]. In particular, a myogenic differentiation improvement of human ESC/iPSC through the treatment with a homologous wingless and Int-1 (Wnt) agonist, the glycogen synthase kinase-3 inhibitor (GSK-3, CHIR9902), has been reported [18,19]. Early inhibition of GSK3β is mandatory for the induction of paraxial mesoderm and activation of the myogenic program [21].

In this study we explored the possibility to exploit the content of extracellular vesicles (EVs), released from differentiated myotubes (MTs), in combination with GSK3 inhibitor, in order to synergistically enhance myogenic differentiation.

To date, the scientific interest regarding the role of EVs in cell-to-cell communication, both in physiological and pathological conditions, is rapidly increasing. EVs are similar in composition to their cell of origin, and their cargo can activate signaling pathways in target cells, thus modulating their activities. In particular, the content of EVs derived from skeletal muscle plays a fundamental role for skeletal muscle homeostasis and development [22,23]. Several studies have shown that skeletal muscle cells release protein/nucleic acid complexes within microvesicles, which promote myogenesis and muscle regeneration [24–27]. EVs derived from MTs (MT-derived EVs) were found to be able to promote the differentiation of myoblasts by altering the expression of cyclin-D1 and myogenin [27]. Another study reported that exosomes, a subclass of EVs measuring approximately 100 nm in diameter, secreted during myotube differentiation, contribute significantly to the myogenic differentiation of stem cells derived from human adipose tissue [28].

Previous researches have shown that iPSCs retain molecular characteristics of the cell from which they originate, named 'epigenetic memory', which is able to strengthen the propensity for re-differentiation in the same tissue [29,30]. On the basis of this, in order to enhance muscle differentiation and exploit myogenic predisposition, muscle-derived pericytes (PCs) and skin fibroblasts (FBs) derived from the same donor were employed as cell sources for iPSC generation. PCs surround the endothelial layer of small/medium vessels that reside beneath the microvascular basement membrane. Despite their role in regulating blood flow, angiogenesis, and maintenance of vascular tissue homeostasis [31], not much is known about pericytes as a source of muscle progenitor cells [6,7]. However, several studies have shown that pericytes are strongly predisposed to differentiate into myogenic lineage and repair muscle damage [6,7,32].

In this study, we established a defined transgene-free protocol, which allows iPSCs, derived either from muscular pericytes or skin fibroblasts, to differentiate into MT-like cells when exposed to GSK-3 inhibitor and EV cargo. This combination improved the differentiation yield into muscle cells up to 70% and the fusion index. After 30 days, evidence of an enhanced muscle differentiation was further revealed by an increased expression of myogenic markers. Furthermore, we found a propensity in pericyte-derived iPSCs to re-differentiate toward the skeletal muscular fate compared to fibroblast-derived counterpart.

Finally, in a pilot study, differentiated iPSCs were injected intramuscularly into anterior tibialis (TA) muscle of immunodeficient alpha-sarcoglycan knockout (KO) mice. The differentiated cells were able to integrate into the host regenerating myofibers, revealing a possible application of the proposed method in regenerative medicine.

2. Materials and Methods

2.1. Cell Isolation

Skin and muscle specimens were obtained from 3 healthy donors, aged between 20 and 40, upon informed consent in line with the Declaration of Helsinki. Tissues were digested and muscular cell suspension was cultured in alpha Minimum Essential Medium (αMEM; Thermo Fisher Scientific, Waltham, MA, USA), 20% fetal bovine serum (FBS; Thermo Fisher Scientific), and penicillin (100 U/mL; Thermo Fisher Scientific) and streptomycin (100 μg/mL; Thermo Fisher Scientific). Pericytes were then selected by their ability to grow on plastic at low confluence (0.1–1×10^4 cell/cm^2). Skin cells were plated in Dulbecco's Modified Eagle Medium (DMEM; Thermo Fisher Scientific) supplemented with 10% FBS, 0.5 mM β-mercaptoethanol (Thermo Fisher Scientific), 100 U/mL penicillin, and 100 μg/mL streptomycin (Thermo Fisher Scientific) at a density of 5×10^4 cells/cm^2.

2.2. Tube-Formation Assay

Pericytes and human umbilical vein endothelial cells (HUVEC; Lonza, Basel, Switzerland) were seeded in 8-well Permanox chamber slides coated with Matrigel (Becton Dickinson Franklin Lakes, NJ, USA), either separately (3.75×10^4 cells per well) or co-cultured together at a 1:4 ratio, in Endothelial Cell Growth Basal Medium-2 (EBM-2; Lonza). Cells were incubated for 5 h to allow tube formation. Images of newly formed networks were captured at 10X magnification.

All experiments were performed in duplicates. Analysis was achieved using the Angiogenesis Analyzer tool (ImageJ Software, https://imagej.nih.gov/ij/).

2.3. Pericyte and C2C12 Myogenic Differentiation

Spontaneous skeletal myogenic differentiation of human pericytes and C2C12 cells was induced by plating 10^4cells/cm^2 in αMEM, 20% FBS and penicillin/streptomycin. After the cells reached confluence, we replaced the medium with low-serum medium (2% horse serum, HS, Thermo Fisher Scientific) for about 10 (pericyte differentiation) and 5 (C2C12 differentiation) days.

2.4. Lentiviral Vector Generation

The lentiviral vector employed for the induction of reprogramming was composed of a single excisable polycistronic lentiviral stem cell cassette (STEMCCA), encoding the Yamanaka factors [33]. Low passage 293T cells (Cell Biolabs, San Diego, CA, USA) were used to produce lentiviruses, employing the psPAX2 and vesicular stomatitis virus G protein (VSV-G) packaging constructs and a calcium phosphate transfection protocol. Supernatants containing STEMCCA lentiviruses were collected 48 h later, filtered, and used immediately right after preparation. The lentiviral vector used to introduce a Green Fluorescent Protein (GFP) transgene for the isolation of GFP$^+$-EVs was produced employing the calcium phosphate method into 293FT packaging cells.

2.5. iPSC Generation

To induce reprogramming, we exposed pericytes and fibroblasts, at early passages, to fresh lentiviral medium 3 times at 12 h intervals. Lentiviral medium was then replaced with fresh medium. After a further 5 days, 1×10^3 transduced cells/cm^2 were plated on a feeder layer constituted of inactivated mouse embryonic fibroblast (iMEF). Cells were then cultured in iPSC medium composed of knockout DMEM (Life Technologies, Carlsbad, CA, USA), supplemented with 20% knockout Serum Replacement (Life Technologies), 20 ng/mL of basic fibroblast growth factor (bFGF; Life Technologies), 1% N-2 (Life Technologies), 2% B27 (Life Technologies), 2 mM Glutamax (Life Technologies), 100 µM Eagle's minimum essential medium non-essential amino acid solution (MEM-NEAA, Life Technologies), 100 µM β-mercaptoethanol, 100 U/mL penicillin and 100 µg/mL streptomycin. After iPSC line expansion and characterization was carried out, cells were adapted to feeder-free condition, by seeding them on Geltrex matrix (Thermo Fisher Scientific) in Essential 8 medium (Life Technologies).

2.6. iPSC Multilineage Differentiation

Cardiomyocyte differentiation was performed using STEMdiff Cardiomyocyte Differentiation Kit (StemCell Technologies, Vancouver, BC, Canada) according to the manufacturer's instructions. Briefly, uniform undifferentiated iPSC colonies were harvested and seeded as single cells at 3.5×10^5 cells per well in a 12-well format. After 48 h, the iPSC medium was replaced with Medium A to induce the cells toward a cardiomyocyte fate. On day 2, a full medium change was performed with fresh Medium B. On days 4 and 6, medium B was replaced with fresh Medium C. On day 8, medium was switched to cardiomyocyte Maintenance Medium with full medium changes on days 10, 12 and 14, to promote further differentiation into cardiomyocyte cells.

Neural differentiation was promoted plating 1×10^6 cells/mL in Neural Induction Medium (Thermo Fisher Scientific) for 7 days. On day 8, iPSC-derived neural stem cells were harvested and expanded in Neural Expansion Medium (Thermo Fisher Scientific).

For endothelial differentiation, human iPSC cells were cultured in Roswell Park Memorial Institute medium (RPMI; Sigma-Aldrich, St. Louis, MO, USA) plus B27 medium with 6 µM CHIR99021 (CHIR; Sigma-Aldrich). On day 2, we replaced the medium with fresh RPMI supplemented with B27 and 2 µM CHIR. After 48 h, the medium was changed with EGM-2 medium supplied with vascular endothelial growth factor (VEGF; PeproTech, London, UK), bFGF, and SB431542 (Merck, Darmstadt, Germany). Every other day, the medium was changed with fresh EGM-2 medium supplied with VEGF, bFGF, and SB431542.

2.7. Isolation of MT-derived EVs

EVs were isolated from conditioned medium of C2C12 myoblasts, differentiated into myotubes, using HS, previously centrifuged at $100,000 \times g$ for 16 h at 4 °C for EV depletion. After 48 h of incubation in fresh medium, EVs were harvested and purified by differential centrifugation—cell debris and organelles were eliminated at $500 \times g$ for 20 min followed by another centrifugation at $3500 \times g$ for 15 min at 4 °C. EVs were pelleted by ultracentrifugation at $100,000 \times g$ for 70 min at 4 °C by L-80-XP ultracentrifuge (Beckman-Coulter, Brea, CA, USA). Finally, the pellet was washed with cold PBS (Phosphate Buffered Saline) in order to minimize sticking and trapping of non-vesicular materials. Purified EVs were used immediately after isolation.

2.8. Myogenic Differentiation by MT-Derived EVs

Human iPSCs with no differentiated colonies, expressing pluripotency markers were used for the differentiation process. The iPSCs were cultured under feeder-free conditions using Essential 8 medium on Geltrex matrix. A critical variable for the generation of robust myotube culture was the relative confluence at the onset of differentiation that it should be approximately 30%. After they were seeded for about 48 h, iPSCs were induced toward mesodermal commitment in Essential 6 medium (Life Technologies) and 1% ITS (insulin-transferrin-selenium) supplemented with 10 uM GSK3 inhibitor CHIR (Sigma-Aldrich). After 2 days, we withdrew CHIR from the culture medium. The mesodermal induction medium was replaced with fresh expansion medium composed of Essential 6 medium enriched with 1% ITS, 5 mM LiCl, 10 ng bFGF, 10 ng insulin-like growth factor 1 (IGF-1; Thermo Fisher Scientific) and 50 ug/mL MT-derived EVs. After further 4 days, LiCl was removed from the medium. During this period, cells underwent enhanced proliferation. Between days 8–10, cells reached confluence and were expanded using TryplE (Thermo Fisher Scientific) and Collagen Type I matrix coating (BD Biosciences). The final differentiation and maturation phase into myotubes took additional 2 weeks: by day 20, muscular progenitors were seeded on Collagen type I dishes; after cells reached confluence, growth factors and MT-derived EVs were removed from the medium, and cells were cultured only in Essential 6 medium supplemented with 1% ITS.

2.9. Flow Cytometry and Cell Sorting

Fluorescence-activated cell sorting (FACS) analysis on physical parameters (forward and side light scatter, FSC and SSC, respectively), was first performed in order to exclude small debris, while the LIVE/DEAD Fixable Dead Cell Stain (Invitrogen, Carlsbad, CA, USA) allowed for the discrimination between live and dead cells. Muscle pericytes were labelled with the following conjugated antibodies: anti-alkaline phosphatase-Cy5 (BD Pharmingen), anti-CD45-FITC/CD14-PE (BD Biosciences, San Jose, CA, USA), anti-NG2-PE (BD Pharmingen), anti-CD56-APC (NCAM; BD Biosciences), anti-CD146-Cy5 (MCAM; R&D Systems, Minneapolis, MN, USA), anti-PDGF-R-beta-FITC (R&D Systems), and anti-CD44-APC (BD Pharmingen). Skin fibroblasts were characterized by staining with anti-CD90-FITC (BD Pharmingen). iPSC-derived skeletal muscle progenitor cells were stained with primary antibodies: PAX3 (Thermo Fisher Scientific), MyoD1 (Abcam, Cambridge, UK), PAX7 (DHSB), MyoG (Clone F5D, eBioscience, San Diego, CA, USA), and myosin heavy chain (Clone MF20; R&D Systems) (Abcam), followed by staining with the FITC-conjugated secondary antibody (R&D System). All antibodies were diluted in accordance with the manufacturers' instructions. Fluorescence intensity for surface antigens and intracellular cytokines was detected by flow cytometry using a BD FACS Canto II analyzer. Flow data were analyzed with the FACSDiva 6.1.2 software (Becton Dickinson, Franklin Lakes, NJ, USA) and the FlowLogic software (Miltenyi Biotec, Bergisch Gladbach, Germany).

The ALP$^+$/CD56$^-$ subpopulation was sorted by FACSAria II Cell Sorter (Becton Dickinson) and subsequently characterized by FACS analysis for the expression of pericyte markers (as listed above) following 2 passages in vitro.

To detect and analyze surface EVs markers by FACS analysis, we bound them to 4 μm aldehyde sulphate latex beads (Thermo Fisher Scientific) overnight at 4 °C in rotation. EV-coated beads were then incubated with fluorochrome-conjugated antibodies CD63-APC (eBioscience) and CD81-PE (Invitrogen), and diluted in accordance with the manufacturers' instructions. A "beads only" control sample was used to set gating parameters.

For EV internalization, we labelled the purified vesicles isolated from C2C12 with 5 μg/mL CellMask Deep Red plasma membrane stain (Molecular Probes, Eugene, OR, USA) and 5 mM CellTrace Violet (Invitrogen) at 37 °C for 30 min. The labeled EVs were washed in PBS and ultra-centrifuged at 100,000× g at 4 °C for 90 min, suspended in differentiating medium and used to treat the cells. After 48 h, we detected fluorescence on differentiating cells by flow cytometry.

2.10. Gene Expression Analysis

Total RNA was extracted using small RNA miRNeasy Mini Kit (Qiagen, Hilden, Germany). A total of 1 μg of total RNA was reverse-transcribed to cDNA using SuperScript VILO cDNA synthesis kit (Life Technologies). qRT-PCR were performed using SYBR Green Master Mix (Applied Biosystems, Foster City, CA, USA). Each sample was analyzed in triplicate using QuantStudio 6 Flex Real-Time PCR System Software (Applied Biosystems). The relative gene expression for pluripotency markers was expressed relative to a certified Episomal iPSC lineage (EpiPSC, Thermo Fisher Scientific), and normalized to Glyceraldehyde-3-Phosphate Dehydrogenase (GAPDH) (Table S1).

The expression of the lentiviral vector was assessed by qualitative RT-PCR according to standard procedure. Amplified products were separated by electrophoresis on a 1% agarose gel. Primers were designed to identify cMyc (one of the four human transcription factors included in the polycistronic lentiviral backbone—forward oligonucleotide) and WPRE (woodchuck hepatitis virus post-transcriptional regulatory element, a lentiviral-specific transgene—reverse oligonucleotide) (Table S1).

2.11. Immunohistochemistry and Immunocytochemistry

Cells were fixed in 4% paraformaldehyde for 20 min at room temperature, washed twice in PBS and blocked with 10% donkey serum (Sigma-Aldrich) for 30 min at room temperature. For intracellular immunostaining, we permeabilized cells for 10 min in 0.1% Triton X-100 (Sigma-Aldrich). Immunofluorescence assays were carried out with the following primary antibodies as follows: pericytes were stained with anti-PDGFRβ (1:100 Abcam), anti-α-smooth muscle actin (1:400, SMA; Dako, Santa Clara, CA, USA) and anti-NG2 (1:200, Millipore, Burlington, MA, USA); fibroblasts were labelled with anti-vimentin (1:50, Sigma-Aldrich); HUVEC were incubated with anti-von Willebrand factor (1:100, Abcam); iPSC pluripotency was verified by anti-OCT4, anti-SSEA4, anti-SOX2 and anti-TRA-1-60 (1:100, all from Invitrogen); iPSC-derived MT were identified by anti-myosin heavy chain (MHC; 1:100; R&D).Incubations with the secondary antibodies (1:100, Jackson ImmunoResearch Laboratories, West Grove, PA, USA) were performed for 1 hour at 37 °C. Cells were then counterstained using Vectashield Mounting Medium with DAPI (4′,6-diamidino-2-phenylindole). Fluorescence was detected by microscope (Axio Observer A1, Zeiss, Oberkochen, Germany).

Differentiation evaluation was assessed by immunofluorescence for MHC and fusion index scoring, defined as the ratio between the number of myosin heavy chain expressing myotubes with greater than 2 nuclei with respect to the total number of nuclei.

2.12. Western Blotting Analysis

EVs were also characterized by Western blotting for the expression of specific markers. EVs were lysed in radioimmunoprecipitation assay buffer (RIPA buffer), and supplemented with protease and phosphatase inhibitor cocktails (Roche Diagnostics GmbH, Mannheim, Germany). Proteins (30 μg) were separated on the Nupage Novex on 4–12% Bis-Tris Gel (Life Technologies) and transferred to a Polyvinylidene fluoride (PVDF) membrane Amersham Hybond (GE Healthcare Biosciences, Piscataway, NJ, USA). Membranes were incubated overnight at 4 °C with primary antibodies anti-CD81, anti-CD63, anti-αHSP70 (ExoAb Antibody Kit, System Biosciences, Palo Alto, CA, USA), anti-TSG-101 (Thermo Fisher Scientific), anti-MyoD1 (Abcam), anti-MHC (R&D) followed by peroxidase-linked anti-rabbit IgG or anti-mouse IgG secondary antibodies (GE Healthcare Life science) for 1 h at room temperature. Specific protein bands were detected with Pierce ECL Western Blotting Substrate (Thermo Fisher Scientific).

2.13. In Vivo Studies

Two-month-old male αSGKO/SCIDbg mice (n = 5) were anesthetized with an intramuscular injection of physiologic saline (10 mL/kg) containing ketamine (5 mg/mL) and xylazine (1 mg/mL) and then 5×10^5 PC-derived iPSCs were injected into the Tibialis Anterior muscle (TA), according to standardized procedures [5]. Mice were sacrificed 20 days after implantation for morphological analysis. Experiments on animals were conducted according to the rules of good animal experimentation I.A.C.U.C. no 432 of 12 March 2006 and under Italian Health Ministry approval no. 228/2015-PR. In vivo experiments were conducted in accordance with the principles of the 3Rs (replacement, reduction and refinement).

2.14. Engrafted Human Muscular Cell Identification

Human differentiated iPSCs were identified by immunofluorescence for anti-human lamin A/C (1:100, SIGMA). Anti-laminin (1:100, SIGMA) was used to identify the fibers. The images were obtained by confocal laser scanning microscope.

2.15. Statistical Analysis

Statistical significance of the differences between means was assessed by one-way analysis of variance (ANOVA), followed by the Student-Newman-Keuls test, to determine which groups were significantly different from the others. When only two groups had to be compared, we used the unpaired Student's t-test. $p < 0.05$ was considered significant. Values are expressed as means ± standard deviation (SD). All the analyses were performed using Graph-Pad PRISM 7 and 8.

3. Results

3.1. Pericyte and Fibroblast Isolation and Characterization

Pericytes were isolated from three healthy human skeletal muscle biopsies and characterized by flow cytometry using a specific panel of markers according to previous studies [6]. The harvested cells highly expressed well-known pericyte markers, such as ALP (alkaline phosphatase), PDGFRβ (platelet derived growth factor receptor-beta), CD146 (MCAM, melanoma cell adhesion molecule), NG2 (Neuron/glial antigen 2), and CD44 (HCAM, homing cell adhesion molecule) (Figure 1A) as well as CD56 (NCAM, neural-cell adhesion molecule), a glycoprotein specifically expressed in muscle by human satellite cells [6,34].

Skeletal muscle resident PCs, expressing ALP, represent a myogenic cell compartment, distinct from satellite cells, capable of promoting myofiber regenerating [6]. Therefore, we selected pericytes with myogenic potential by fluorescence-activated cell sorting (FACS), combining the cell surface markers ALP and CD56. We enriched the pericyte population selecting the fraction ALP$^+$CD56$^-$, which represented the 28% of the total population (Figure 1B).

After expansion and before reprogramming, ALP$^+$CD56$^-$ subpopulation was analyzed for the expression of the canonic muscular pericyte markers—almost the totality of the tested cells expressed ALP, PDGFRβ, CD146, NG2, and CD44, while the expression of CD56 was dramatically reduced (Figure 1C), suggesting that ALP$^+$CD56$^-$ fraction retains pericyte features.

These results are in line with previous studies in which pericyte identification was performed through the combination of NG2, PDGFβ, and CD146 markers [35,36]. PC phenotype was further confirmed by the ALP colorimetric assay (Figure 1D) and immunofluorescence positivity for NG2, PDGFRβ, and αSMA (Figure 1E).

We further examined the myogenic potential of ALP$^+$CD56$^-$ cells by measuring myosin heavy chain (MHC) expression, upon skeletal muscle differentiation, induced by cellular confluence and serum depletion [37]. After two weeks, ALP$^+$CD56$^-$ cells spontaneously differentiated into myosin positive multinucleated myotubes, as confirmed by the expression of MHC (Figure 1F). These results indicate that pericytes possess myogenic potential, along with supporting vessel formation and angiogenesis.

PCs are crucial in several phases during angiogenesis and vascular homeostasis, regulating the germination of the capillaries and the stabilization of the vessels. We therefore evaluated the ability of ALP$^+$CD56$^-$ cells to generate networks and to cooperate with endothelial cells (HUVECs) to form capillary-like structures. For this purpose, we transduced cells with a lentivirus expressing GFP, co-cultured with HUVECs (GFP$^+$ ALP$^+$CD56$^-$ cells/HUVECs in a 1:4 ratio), and assembled on Matrigel for 6 h. We found that the ALP$^+$CD56$^-$ cells significantly enhanced capillary-like structure formation of HUVECs. Indeed, PCs co-cultivated with HUVECs displayed higher segment total length, total mesh area and total branch length compared to HUVECs cultured alone (Figure 1G). These results demonstrate that pericytes isolated from skeletal muscle maintain their ability to support vessel formation and myogenic potential after isolation, sorting and expansion procedures.

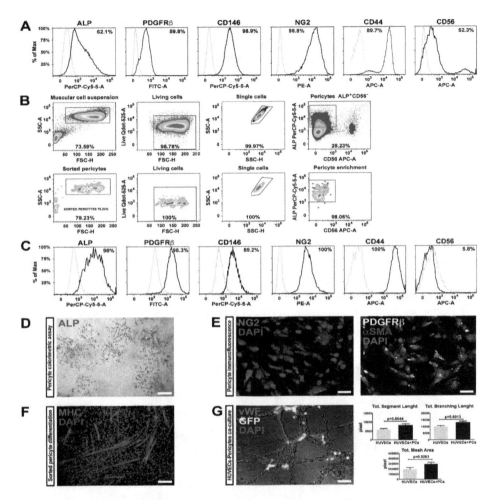

Figure 1. Pericyte characterization. (**A**) Representative histograms indicating the percentage of alkaline phosphatase (ALP$^+$), platelet derived growth factor receptor-beta (PDGFRβ^+), MCAM, melanoma cell adhesion molecule (CD146$^+$), (αSMA$^+$), Neuron/glial antigen 2 (NG2$^+$), HCAM, homing cell adhesion molecule (CD44$^+$) and NCAM, neural-cell adhesion molecule (CD56$^+$) positivity (black peaks) determined by flow cytometry in pre-sorted cells isolated from muscular biopsy (n = 4). Matched isotypes were used as negative controls (grey peaks). (**B**) Representative gating strategy for ALP$^+$ and CD56$^-$ cell sorting (n = 3). Cells were first gated for cell size (side light scatter SSC-A vs. forward light scatter FSC-H) and vitality (Live Qdot-525-A). The muscular cell gate was further analyzed for singlets (SSC-A vs. SSC-H) and their expression for ALP and CD56. Pericytes, ALP$^+$ and CD56$^-$ were then sorted from this gated population. The lower set of four plots confirmed the efficiency of the sorting. (**C**) Representative post-sorting histograms for key pericyte markers after two passages in vitro, indicating an enhanced expression of ALP, NG2, PDGFRβ, CD146, and CD44. (**D**) Sorted pericytes stained for ALP showing fibroblast colony-forming units (CFU-F) when seeded at low confluence. Scale bar represents 300 µm. (**E**) Immunofluorescence labeling for NG2 (red) and the co-staining for PDGFRβ (green) and αSMA (magenta) on sorted ALP$^+$CD56$^-$ cells. Nuclei were stained with DAPI. Scale bar represents 50 µm. (**F**) Representative fluorescence image for myosin heavy chain (MHC) (red), validating the differentiation of sorted pericytes toward skeletal muscle phenotype. Scale bar represents 100 µm. (**G**) Illustrative images of human umbilical vein endothelial cells (HUVEC) in co-culture with pericytes displaying the formation of capillary-like networks with HUVEC labeled for von Willebrand factor (vWF; magenta), and GFP$^+$ pericytes. Nuclei were identified by DAPI (blue). Scale bar represents 100 µm. Tubular structures were photographed at 5× magnification and quantified by the angiogenesis analyzer ImageJ tool. Total segment length, total mesh area and total branching length exhibited significant differences between HUVEC alone and in co-culture with pericytes, as shown in the graphs.

Epigenetic memory inherited from their original tissue have been demonstrated to influence the iPSC differentiation potential [29], suggesting that pericyte myogenic and angiogenic potential could be advantageous in tissue regeneration. Hence, we isolated human adult skin fibroblasts from the same donor of pericytes in order to compare the capability of iPSCs derived from pericytes (PC-derived iPSCs, ALP$^+$CD56$^-$ subpopulation) and fibroblasts (FB-derived iPSCs) to re-differentiate into muscle cells. Skin fibroblasts, isolated by enzymatic digestion, were characterized by immunofluorescence (Figure S1) and FACS analysis (Figure S1) for the expression of vimentin and CD90.

3.2. iPSC Generation and Characterization

We generated human muscular PC-derived iPSCs and skin FB-derived iPSCs from the same donor (n = 3 donors) using a polycistronic vector harboring the four Yamanaka factors (OCT4, Sox2, Klf4, cMyc) [33,38]. Colonies were initially expanded on a feeder layer of inactivated mouse embryonic fibroblasts (iMEF) and then adapted to feeder free conditions replacing iMEF with geltrex matrix (Figure 2A, left panels). iPSC colonies expressed typical pluripotent markers, including OCT4, SSEA4, SOX2, and TRA-1-60, as assessed by immunofluorescence staining (Figure 2A, middle and right panels). These results were confirmed by quantitative real-time PCR (qRT-PCR) for the expression of OCT4, SOX2, NANOG, LIN28, and TERT genes. Certified Episomal iPSC lineage (EpiPSC, Thermo Fisher Scientific) was used as control (Figure 2B).

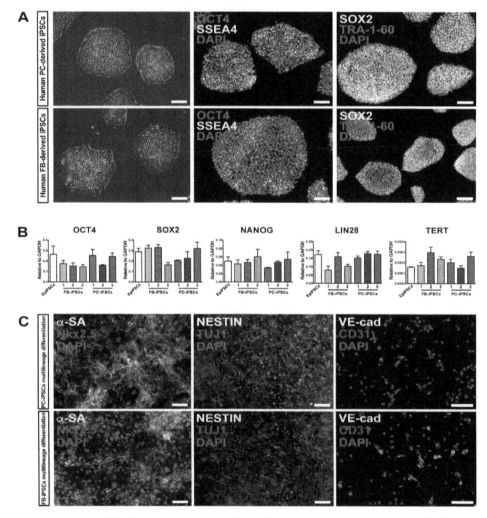

Figure 2. Characterization of human pericyte (PC)- and fibroblast (FB)-derived iPSCs. (**A**) Morphology of PC-derived iPSCs (left upper panel) and FB-derived iPSCs (left lower panel) cultured in feeder-free conditions.

Scale bar represents 100 μm. Immunofluorescence labeling for the expression of the pluripotent markers SSEA4 (yellow), OCT4 (magenta; middle panels), SOX2 (yellow), and TRA-1-60 (magenta; right panels) on PC- and FB-derived iPSCs (PC-iPSCs and FB-iPSCs, upper and lower panels respectively). Nuclei were stained with DAPI. Scale bar represents 100 μm and, for the lower right image, 200 μm. (**B**) Quantitative RT-PCR analysis for the expression of the embryonic genes, OCT4, SOX2, NANOG, LIN28, and TERT—in PC- and FB-derived iPSC lines, derived from three donors (named FB-/PC-derived iPSCs 1, 2, 3), compared to the certified Episomal iPSC lineage (EpiPSC), used as control. Results were normalized to GAPDH. (**C**) Representative fluorescence images demonstrating multilineage differentiation capacity of PC- and FB-derived iPSCs toward cardiomyocyte (alpha-sarcomeric actin–α-SA, Nkx2.5), neuronal (Nestin, TUJ1) and endothelial (CD31, VE-cadherin–VE-cad) lineages. Nuclei were stained with DAPI (blue). Scale bars represent 50 μm (left and middle panels) and 100 μm (right panels).

Qualitative RT-PCR was conducted to verify the silencing of the exogenous transgenes in PC- and FB-derived iPSCs (Figure S2).

In addition, both derived iPSC lines retained the ability to differentiate toward multiple lineages, including cardiomyocytes, neuronal precursors, and endothelial cells (Figure 2C).

3.3. MT-derived EV Characterization

EVs represent an important vector of intercellular communication, acting as vehicles for the transfer of cytosolic factors, proteins, lipids and RNA [39]. EV cargo is cell-type specific, and the molecular composition reflects specific functions of the donor cells.

EV secretion and extracellular signaling occurs during muscle differentiation, repair and regeneration [25,40]. Both myoblasts and myotubes release EVs, but their contribution in muscle physiology and specific biological functions on recipient cells have not been fully elucidated.

Proteomic analysis of muscle-derived EVs revealed that, in addition to proteins involved in their biogenesis, EVs also contain functionally relevant proteins such as myogenic growth factors and contractile proteins [26,40,41].

On the basis of these premises, we have exploited the capacity of EVs, secreted during myotube formation of skeletal myoblasts (C2C12), to promote the differentiation of iPSCs into the myogenic lineage.

EVs were purified from conditioned media of C2C12-derived MTs cultured in 2% EV-depleted horse serum. EV isolation was performed by differential centrifugations according to well-established protocols [42]. EVs were further analyzed by FACS analysis for the expression of CD81 and CD63. We found that MT-derived EVs were enriched in membrane-bound tetraspanins CD63 and CD81, which are common markers for EV subsets released from most cell types (Figure 3A,B). The expression of CD81 is observed on vesicles of various sizes indicating that multivesicular endosomes in muscle cells contain intraluminal vesicles of heterogeneous sizes [27,41]. The expression of proteins associated with EVs, such as tumor susceptibility gene 101 (TSG101), α heat shock 70 kDa protein 4 (HSP70), CD81 and CD63 was further confirmed by Western blot analysis.

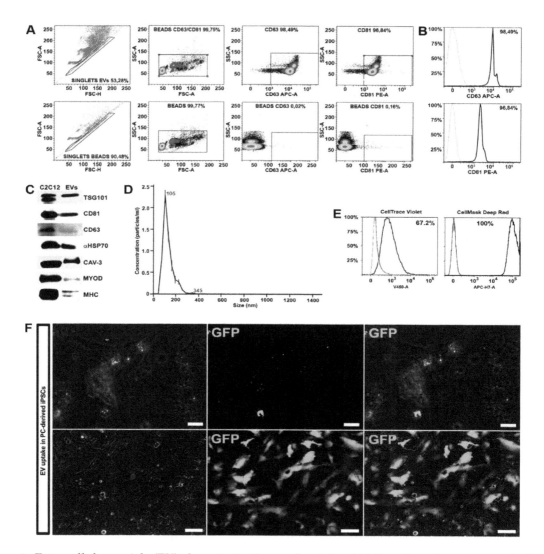

Figure 3. Extracellular vesicle (EV) characterization and uptake. (**A**) Sample gating strategy indicating the percentage of CD63$^+$ and CD81$^+$ in myotube (MT)-derived EVs coated with beads (n = 3). In the upper plots, singlets and subsequently EVs were selected according to physical parameters (FSC-A vs. FSC-H and SSC-A vs. FSC-A, respectively) are shown. Fluorescent intensity signal for CD63 and CD81 was detected on gated EVs (SSC-A vs. APC-A and SSC-A vs. PE-A, respectively). Beads alone were used as control (lower four scatter plots). (**B**) Representative histograms displaying the percentage of EV specific markers, such as CD81 and CD63, determined by flow cytometry in purified MT-derived EVs. Matched isotypes were used as negative controls (grey peaks) (**C**) Western blot for specific the expression of EV markers, such as TSG101, CD81, CD63, aHSP70, and skeletal muscle markers, such as CAV-3, MYOD, MHC, in C2C12-derived myotubes and C2C12 myotube-derived EV lysates. (**D**) Size distribution profile of MT-derived EVs (n = 5). (**E**) Representative histograms, determined by flow cytometry, displaying the percentage of positive cells (black) after the treatment with EVs stained for cell trace violet or cell mask deep red. Non-treated cells (light grey peaks) and cells treated with unstained EVs (dark grey peaks) were used as controls. (**F**) Green spots indicate the presence of fluorescent (GFP$^+$) EVs, derived from GFP transduced myotubes, in the cytoplasm of the recipient differentiating iPSC after 48 h of exposure (upper panels; scale bars represent 20 μm); GFP$^+$ cells 10 days after GFP$^+$ MT-derived EV exposure (lower panels; scale bars represent 100 μm), demonstrating that GFP was transferred through the EVs into the recipient cells.

We found that MT-derived EVs exhibited specific membrane proteins associated with mature muscle tissue, such as caveolin 3 (Cav3), expressed only during the late stage of differentiation, and MHC, a differentiated myotubes marker (Figure 3C). Interestingly, MyoD, a transcription factor implicated in myogenesis, was also detected within the EV cargo.

Finally, the purity, size and concentration of the MT-derived EVs were determined by nanoparticle tracking analysis (NTA), using instrument-optimized analysis settings in NTA 3.1 build 54 software. The results showed a mean size distribution, consistent with what is expected from a sample enriched in microvesicles and exosomes (130.3 ± 0.3 nm), and free from contamination by apoptotic bodies (>1 μm) (Figure 3D).

3.4. Detection of the MT-derived EV Uptake

To exert their functional influence, EV cargo must be internalized within the cell in adequate concentrations. As first step, in order to verify if EVs can transfer their contents to differentiating iPSCs, we performed EV uptake assays. For this experiment, we employed two different methods: FACS analysis and immunofluorescence microscopy. Upon isolation, MT-derived EVs were marked either with cell mask deep red or with cell trace violet. As controls we used untreated cells and cells exposed to unstained EVs. After 48 h, FACS analysis revealed an increased fluorescence of both tracers in recipient cells, indicating a successful uptake (Figure 3E).

In order to demonstrate the EV cargo delivery, we transduced C2C12 cells with a lentivirus expressing the GFP protein, and subsequently differentiated into myotubes. The EVs released by GFP$^+$ myotubes were collected and used to treat the differentiating iPSCs. After 48 h, a fluorescent signal was detected in the cytoplasm of cells undergoing differentiation (Figure 3F, upper panels).

Cells were treated with EVs released by GFP$^+$ myotubes every other day and, after 10 days, approximately 40% of cells expressed GFP in the cytoplasm (Figure 3F, lower panels) indicating a high functional cargo delivery to the recipient cells. EVs may enter into a cell via more than one route, depending on proteins and glycoproteins found on the surface of both the vesicle and the target cell [43]. The mechanisms responsible for MT-derived EVs delivery have not yet been determined highlighting the need for further research [44].

Considering these results, we have shown that EVs target iPSCs via delivery of effector molecules directly affecting their phenotype and functions.

3.5. Myogenic Differentiation by MT-derived EVs

MT-derived EVs express specific cell-adhesion molecules on their surfaces (ITGB1, CD9, CD81, CD44, Myoferlin) that are involved in the recognition and adhesion during the process of myoblast fusion [45–47].

Further, MT-derived EVs contain functionally active proteins of the G-protein family, which are involved in many cellular processes including myogenesis [48].

Wnt signaling and its modulation via GSK3 inhibitors, such as CHIR99021 (CHIR), is essential in the mesoderm induction and to obtain a reliable, reproducible and efficient myogenic differentiation protocol [18,19,49].

On the basis of these findings, we developed a method to induce a robust differentiation of iPSC toward skeletal muscle phenotype combining MT-derived EV cargo and the chemical modulator CHIR for paraxial mesoderm-like muscle progenitor commitment (Figure 4A).

PC- and FB-derived iPSCs, derived from three donors, were divided in four groups and treated as follows: (i) group 1, PC-/FB-derived iPSCs cultured in differentiation medium; (ii) group 2, PC-/FB-derived iPSCs cultured in differentiation medium augmented with EVs; (iii) group 3, PC-/FB-derived iPSCs cultured in differentiation medium enriched with CHIR; and (iv) group 4, PC-/FB-derived iPSCs cultured in differentiation medium supplemented with EVs and CHIR.

Cells were treated with 10 uM CHIR for 48 h to induce the expression of paraxial mesoderm genes. Consistent with other studies [18,19], iPSCs from both sources presented evident morphological changes losing the typical ES-like morphology after 24 h of treatment (Figure 4B). Following replacement of CHIR with FGF2, cells underwent proliferation and reached full confluence approximately at day 8–10.

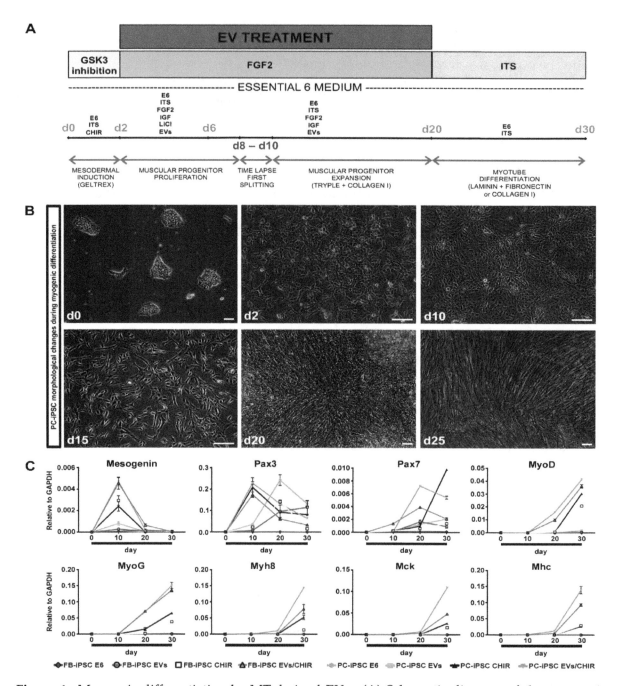

Figure 4. Myogenic differentiation by MT-derived EVs. (**A**) Schematic diagram of the myogenic differentiation procedure: 30% confluent iPSCs were differentiated to early mesoderm using CHIR for 48 h, subsequently proliferation and expansion of muscular progenitors were stimulated utilizing EVs, FGF2, IGF, and the myotube-like cell maturation was induced, removing growth factors from the culture medium. (**B**) Morphological changes of PC-derived iPSC colonies during skeletal muscle differentiation. Scale bars represent 100 μm. (**C**) Representative qRT-PCR for the expression of early (Mesogenin, Pax3, Pax7, MyoD, MyoG) and late (MyH8, MCK, MHC) skeletal muscle genes. The analysis was performed at different time points (d0, d10, d20, d30) in the following conditions: FB- and PC-derived iPSCs not treated with EVs or CHIR (FB-iPSCs E6 and PC-iPSCs E6), exposed to CHIR or EVs only (FB-iPSC EVs, FB-iPSC CHIR, PC-iPSC EVs, PC-iPSC CHIR) and treated with both, EVs and CHIR (FB-iPSC EVs/CHIR and PC-iPSC EVs/CHIR) (n = 3 donors). Results were normalized to GAPDH.

Following 48 h of treatment, CHIR was removed and, in order to enhance the myogenic differentiation, the media were enriched with freshly MT-derived EVs (50 μg/mL) and replenished every 2 days with fresh vesicles until the formation of myoblast-like cells. Between days 15 and

25 paraxial mesoderm-like muscle progenitors can be either expanded or terminally differentiated upon withdrawal of all the growth factors from the medium. The outcome of myotube formation was greater when myoblast-like cells were passaged 2–3 times and consequently exposed longer to MT-derived EVs.

We have analyzed the expression of genes related to mesoderm induction and myogenic differentiation at different time points through qRT-PCR experiments (Figure 4C).

In PC- and FB-derived iPSCs treated with the CHIR/EV combination, pre-myogenic mesoderm genes, such as Mesogenin, Pax3, and Pax7, were upregulated between day 10 and day 20. The myogenic regulatory factor MyoD and MyoG started to be expressed around day 10 and increased up to day 30. Finally, the mature myocyte genes, Myh8 (myosin heavy chain 8), MCK (muscle creatine kinase) and MHC, were detected after day 20 and augmented until the end of the differentiation confirming the increase in differentiation and maturation of the iPSCs treated with both factors.

Cells cultured in differentiation medium were negative for the expression of myogenic genes, while iPSCs treated with EVs exhibited only pre-myogenic genes (Pax3 and Pax7), indicating that the MT-derived EVs are not sufficient, at least within 30 days, to induce myotube differentiation. Lastly, cells exposed to CHIR presented a myogenic inclination similar, but less efficient, to PC-/FB-derived iPSCs treated with the CHIR–EVs mishmash.

Our method proved that the combination CHIR-EVs induces a higher differentiation compared to CHIR treatment (Figure 5A).

To verify whether PC-derived iPSCs, generated from the three donors, possessed a greater propensity to differentiate into myotubes compared to FB-derived iPSCs, we matched the expression of Myh8, MCK, and MHC by qRT-PCR analysis at day 30 of differentiation (Figure 5A). The expression of mature myogenic genes resulted as being higher in differentiated PC-derived iPSCs.

To further determine the role of the EVs/CHIR combination we calculated the fusion index, which was significantly greater compared to the index obtained with the separate exposure of EVs or CHIR (Figure 5B). Consistently, also the cell number expressing MHC was also significantly greater in those generated using the CHIR–EVs cocktail compared to the other treatments (Figure 5C).

The ability of PC-derived iPSCs to generate differentiated cells presenting a characteristic mark of myogenesis, was further confirmed by FACS analysis. Myogenic regulatory factors, Pax3, Pax7, CD56, MYOD, MYOG, and MF20, were used to characterize the expression of myogenic proteins (Figure 5D). At day 30 roughly 80% of the cells were positive for the myocyte mature marker MF20.

Finally, after 25 days of CHIR–EV differentiation, PC-iPSC-derived muscular cells, were implanted in vivo in a limb girdle muscular dystrophy murine model, namely, SCID-Beige α–Sarcoglycan null mice (αSGKO/SCIDbg) [5] in order to evaluate their engraftment capabilities. Three different PC-derived iPSC clones were intramuscularly injected (5×10^5 cells/injection) into the anterior tibialis (TA) muscle of αSGKO/SCIDbg, showing a sufficient engraftment and integration into regenerating muscle fibers revealed by the labelling of human derived cells by immunofluorescence against human specific lamin A/C antibody (Figure 5E).

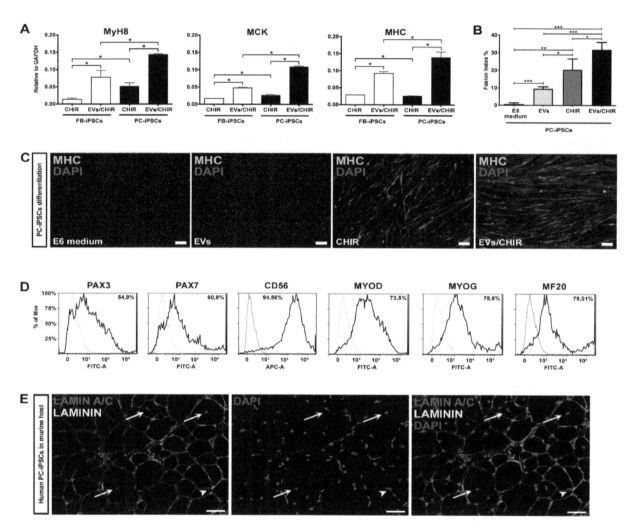

Figure 5. iPSC-derived MT characterization. (**A**) Representative qRT-PCR for the expression of Myh8, MCK and MHC after 30 days of differentiation. The combination CHIR-EVs induced a greater differentiation compared to CHIR treatment and PC-derived iPSCs possessed a greater propensity to differentiate into myotubes compared to FB-derived iPSCs. Results were normalized to GAPDH. (**B**) Fusion index was calculated as the percentage of nuclei within myosin heavy chain–positive myotubes (≥2 nuclei) divided by the total number of nuclei. A minimum of five random fields at 10X magnification were counted. (**C**) Immunofluorescence labeling for MHC (green), validating the differentiation capacity of PC-derived iPSCs toward skeletal muscle phenotype after 30 days of differentiation. The images represent sequentially: PC-derived iPSCs without treatment, exposed to EVs alone, to CHIR only and to the EV–CHIR cocktail. CHIR in combination with MT-derived EVs induced a higher expression of the skeletal marker (n = 3 donors). Nuclei were stained with DAPI. Scale bar represents 100 μm. (**D**) Representative histograms indicating the percentage of PAX3, PAX7, CD56, MYOD, MYOG, and MF20 (black peaks) determined by flow cytometry in PC-iPSC-derived MTs exposed to CHIR and MT-derived EVs after 30 days of differentiation. Matched isotypes were used as negative controls (grey peaks) (n = 3 donors). (**E**) Representative immunofluorescence against human lamin A/C (magenta) and laminin (yellow) on mouse anterior tibialis (TA) injected with human PC-derived iPSC exposed to CHIR-EVs (n = 3 donors). Arrows indicate center-nucleated human derived myofibers, arrowhead labelling integrated human nuclei into mature host muscle fiber. Nuclei were stained with DAPI. Scale bars represent 25 μm.

4. Discussion

In the last few years, there has been a growing interest in the use of iPSCs as a source of myogenic progenitors for cell-based treatment in muscle degenerative diseases. iPSCs overcome several of the limitations related to the use of adult myoblast therapy, such as, non-invasive biopsy for cell isolation, unlimited proliferative capacity in vitro, and a tool for the in vitro correction of genetically mutated somatic cells derived from patients affected by dystrophies [14–16,19,50–52]. Moreover, it is well known that iPSCs maintain the epigenetic memory of the original cell source, influencing the re-differentiation toward the same lineage [30,53]. Pericytes resident in adult skeletal muscle have shown remarkable angiogenic and myogenic differentiation capacities in vitro and in vivo [7]. Hence, in this study, exploiting the advantage of the "epigenetic retention", we proposed the isolation of human derived muscular pericytes to verify whether PC-derived iPSCs are more prone to differentiate into muscular cells compared to FB-derived iPSCs.

To date, the strategies used for iPSC myogenic differentiation are subdivided into two approaches: transgenic (by forced expression of Pax7 or MyoD) or non-transgenic (co-culture, EBs, small molecules) [15,16,51]. The former consists in the differentiation via overexpression of myogenic transcription factors, obtaining efficient iPSC differentiation into myogenic lineage in a relatively short amount of time [15,16,51]. However, forced expression of skeletal master genes drastically reduces the proliferative capacity of skeletal muscle progenitor cells, hindering the molecular mechanisms leading to myogenic differentiation (important for disease modeling in vitro), as well as their in vitro and in vivo self-renewal. Another point to be considered is the potential of insertional mutagenesis events due to the random integration, since these genes are commonly delivered using lentiviral vectors. Integrated virus genomes are frequently associated with chromosomal damage, rearrangements and deletions [54], making these approaches not suitable in terms of clinical applications. On the other hand, the non-transgenic methods use different sequential culture conditions, including cell sorting. These protocols are successful at producing myogenic progenitors capable of engrafting in vivo but lack reproducibility, besides being inefficient and time-consuming [55–57].

First-generation of transgene-free protocols employing different sequential culture conditions were not satisfactory and usually required post-differentiation selection to isolate expandable skeletal muscle progenitor cells [57]. In addition, in some described methods, iPSCs failed to express mature myogenic markers or form myotubes in vitro, underlying the poor efficiency of spontaneous myogenic differentiation method [55,56].

Improvements in muscle differentiation protocols were recently performed by employing a small molecule, CHIR99021, a GSK-3b inhibitor that activates Wnt signaling cascade, which plays a crucial role during early somite induction. These approaches have been proven to be efficient at boosting iPSC towards a myogenic pathway, leading to an ameliorated myotube differentiation in vitro [19,58,59].

Quite recently, considerable attention has been dedicated to extracellular vesicles (EVs) as important mediators of cell-to-cell communication. EVs can influence the behavior of recipient cells and are involved in many processes, including immune signaling, angiogenesis, stress response, proliferation, and cell differentiation [60–62]. Furthermore, EVs, through their paracrine signaling can be used in tissue engineering to modulate cell recruitment, differentiation, and proliferation [63]. Skeletal muscle cells secrete a large number of myokines and EVs that influence the growth, function and development of muscle tissue [26,27,41]. Transcriptome and proteome studies reported that EVs from C2C12 or human myoblasts are enriched in miRNAs and proteins that are implicated in myogenesis [22,27,40,41,64]. EVs isolated from differentiated C2C12 cells express specific cell-adhesion molecules on their surfaces (ITGB1, annexins CD56, CD9, CD81, CD44, Myoferlin), and other myokines (HGF, IGFI/II, FGF2, PDGF, TGFβ, myostatin) involved in myoblast fusion and muscle regeneration. [40,41,45,47,65]. In addition, differentially expressed miRNAs also contained in EVs during C2C12 myotube differentiation, such as miR-1, miR-133a, miR-133b, and miR-206, have been linked with muscle differentiation [64,66]. Interestingly, the Wnt signaling and Sirt 1 that are involved in muscle gene expression and differentiation, were predicted as the most significant targeted pathway by skeletal muscle EVs–miRNAs [64]. In the present study, we found that MT-derived EVs harbored myogenic factors that are crucial in enhancing the iPSC myogenic commitment. Despite several scientific papers reporting transcriptome and proteome profiling of EVs from skeletal muscle, the mechanisms and the key factors playing a major role in promoting skeletal muscle differentiation remain unclear. Evidence suggests that instead of single factors, the diverse EVs myogenic factors such as miRNAs or proteins, synergistically trigger skeletal muscle differentiation in recipient cells [22,26,27,40,41,64]. Further studies are required to define the biological role/function of single myogenic factors in MT-derived EVs.

Here, we have developed an efficient method for iPSC skeletal muscle differentiation combining defined factors with myogenic elements carried by EVs. We were able to generate a consistent number of iPSC-derived positive MHC skeletal muscle cells, evidencing differences in epigenetic signatures between PC-derived iPSCs and their counterpart FB-derived iPSCs. Indeed, quantitative PCR analyses performed at different timepoints and at the end of the differentiation, showed that PC-derived iPSCs are more prone to differentiate in skeletal muscle cells when compared to FB-derived iPSCs. Importantly, the myoblasts obtained with this approach could be expanded, and cryopreserved at all steps during expansion, without losing fusion competence. The obtained MT-like cells were positive for MyoD, MYOG, and MHC, and were able to actively participate in myogenesis in vivo. Transplanted myogenic progenitors demonstrated their ability to successfully engraft and integrate into TA muscle of αSGKO/SCIDbg, identified by the detection of centrally located human lamin A/C positive nuclei, a characteristic perceived only in fusion-competent myoblasts.

In this paper, we explored for the first time EVs as "physiological liposomes" enriched with myogenic factors that were able to trigger skeletal myogenesis in iPSC, raising exciting possibilities for therapeutic use. The use of EVs represent novel tools to deliver signaling molecules for treating muscle-wasting diseases that are better tolerated by the immune system. Additional studies are now required to investigate the role of EVs' skeletal muscle content that may allow the development of better therapeutic approaches to promote skeletal muscle growth, differentiation and regeneration.

Our method may better recapitulate human developmental myogenesis providing inroads for patient-specific drug testing, disease modeling and regenerative approaches.

Author Contributions: Conceptualization, D.B., R.R., and C.B.; data curation, D.B.; formal analysis, D.B., M.C., F.M., S.G., and A.B.; funding acquisition, R.R., and C.B.; investigation, D.B., M.C., V.P., F.M., M.M., A.R., P.S., D.P., S.G., and A.B.; methodology, D.B., M.C., R.R., and C.B.; project administration, D.B., R.R., and C.B.; resources, S.C., C.L., C.G., R.R., and C.B.; supervision, S.C., C.G., R.R., and C.B.; validation, D.B., M.C., V.P., F.M., S.G., and A.B.; writing—original draft preparation, D.B.; writing—review and editing, C.L., C.G., R.R., and C.B. All authors have read and agreed to the published version of the manuscript.

Acknowledgments: We acknowledge Gustavo Mostoslavsky from Boston University School of Medicine, for providing the STEMCCA plasmid. We thank Massimiliano Gubello for the English editing and proofreading. We want also to thank the reviewers for their insightful comments in previous version of the manuscript.

References

1. Bianchi, A.; Mozzetta, C.; Pegoli, G.; Lucini, F.; Valsoni, S.; Rosti, V.; Petrini, C.; Cortesi, A.; Gregoretti, F.; Antonelli, L.; et al. Dysfunctional polycomb transcriptional repression contributes to lamin A/C-dependent muscular dystrophy. *J. Clin. Investig.* **2020**, *130*, 2408–2421. [CrossRef] [PubMed]

2. Cossu, G.; Tajbakhsh, S. Oriented cell divisions and muscle satellite cell heterogeneity. *Cell* **2007**, *129*, 859–861. [CrossRef] [PubMed]

3. Kuang, S.; Kuroda, K.; Le Grand, F.; Rudnicki, M.A. Asymmetric self-renewal and commitment of satellite stem cells in muscle. *Cell* **2007**, *129*, 999–1010. [CrossRef]

4. Lanzuolo, C. Epigenetic alterations in muscular disorders. *Comp. Funct. Genom.* **2012**, *2012*, 256892. [CrossRef]

5. Fuoco, C.; Salvatori, M.L.; Biondo, A.; Shapira-Schweitzer, K.; Santoleri, S.; Antonini, S.; Bernardini, S.; Tedesco, F.S.; Cannata, S.; Seliktar, D.; et al. Injectable polyethylene glycol-fibrinogen hydrogel adjuvant improves survival and differentiation of transplanted mesoangioblasts in acute and chronic skeletal-muscle degeneration. *Skelet. Muscle* **2012**, *2*, 24. [CrossRef]

6. Dellavalle, A.; Sampaolesi, M.; Tonlorenzi, R.; Tagliafico, E.; Sacchetti, B.; Perani, L.; Innocenzi, A.; Galvez, B.G.; Messina, G.; Morosetti, R.; et al. Pericytes of human skeletal muscle are myogenic precursors distinct from satellite cells. *Nat. Cell Biol.* **2007**, *9*, 255–267. [CrossRef]

7. Fuoco, C.; Sangalli, E.; Vono, R.; Testa, S.; Sacchetti, B.; Latronico, M.V.; Bernardini, S.; Madeddu, P.; Cesareni, G.; Seliktar, D.; et al. 3D hydrogel environment rejuvenates aged pericytes for skeletal muscle tissue engineering. *Front. Physiol.* **2014**, *5*, 203. [CrossRef]

8. Asakura, A.; Seale, P.; Girgis-Gabardo, A.; Rudnicki, M.A. Myogenic specification of side population cells in skeletal muscle. *J. Cell Biol.* **2002**, *159*, 123–134. [CrossRef]

9. Mitchell, K.J.; Pannerec, A.; Cadot, B.; Parlakian, A.; Besson, V.; Gomes, E.R.; Marazzi, G.; Sassoon, D.A. Identification and characterization of a non-satellite cell muscle resident progenitor during postnatal development. *Nat. Cell Biol.* **2010**, *12*, 257–266. [CrossRef]

10. Ferrari, G. Muscle regeneration by bone marrow-derived myogenic progenitors. *Science* **1998**, *279*, 1528–1530. [CrossRef]

11. Negroni, E.; Bigot, A.; Butler-Browne, G.S.; Trollet, C.; Mouly, V. Cellular Therapies for Muscular Dystrophies: Frustrations and Clinical Successes. *Hum. Gene Ther.* **2016**, *27*, 117–126. [CrossRef] [PubMed]

12. Shi, Y.; Inoue, H.; Wu, J.C.; Yamanaka, S. Induced pluripotent stem cell technology: A decade of progress. *Nat. Rev. Drug Discov.* **2017**, *16*, 115–130. [CrossRef] [PubMed]

13. Bearzi, C.; Gargioli, C.; Baci, D.; Fortunato, O.; Shapira-Schweitzer, K.; Kossover, O.; Latronico, M.V.; Seliktar, D.; Condorelli, G.; Rizzi, R. PlGF-MMP9-engineered iPS cells supported on a PEG-fibrinogen hydrogel scaffold possess an enhanced capacity to repair damaged myocardium. *Cell Death Dis.* **2014**, *5*, e1053. [CrossRef] [PubMed]

14. Darabi, R.; Arpke, R.W.; Irion, S.; Dimos, J.T.; Grskovic, M.; Kyba, M.; Perlingeiro, R.C. Human ES- and iPS-derived myogenic progenitors restore DYSTROPHIN and improve contractility upon transplantation in dystrophic mice. *Cell Stem Cell* **2012**, *10*, 610–619. [CrossRef]

15. Goudenege, S.; Lebel, C.; Huot, N.B.; Dufour, C.; Fujii, I.; Gekas, J.; Rousseau, J.; Tremblay, J.P. Myoblasts derived from normal hESCs and dystrophic hiPSCs efficiently fuse with existing muscle fibers following transplantation. *Mol. Ther. J. Am. Soc. Gene Ther.* **2012**, *20*, 2153–2167. [CrossRef] [PubMed]

16. Tedesco, F.S.; Gerli, M.F.; Perani, L.; Benedetti, S.; Ungaro, F.; Cassano, M.; Antonini, S.; Tagliafico, E.; Artusi, V.; Longa, E.; et al. Transplantation of genetically corrected human iPSC-derived progenitors in mice with limb-girdle muscular dystrophy. *Sci. Transl. Med.* **2012**, *4*, 140ra189. [CrossRef]

17. Uchimura, T.; Otomo, J.; Sato, M.; Sakurai, H. A human iPS cell myogenic differentiation system permitting high-throughput drug screening. *Stem Cell Res.* **2017**, *25*, 98–106. [CrossRef]

18. Borchin, B.; Chen, J.; Barberi, T. Derivation and FACS-mediated purification of PAX3+/PAX7+ skeletal muscle precursors from human pluripotent stem cells. *Stem Cell Rep.* **2013**, *1*, 620–631. [CrossRef]

19. Shelton, M.; Metz, J.; Liu, J.; Carpenedo, R.L.; Demers, S.P.; Stanford, W.L.; Skerjanc, I.S. Derivation and expansion of PAX7-positive muscle progenitors from human and mouse embryonic stem cells. *Stem Cell Rep.* **2014**, *3*, 516–529. [CrossRef]

20. Xu, C.; Tabebordbar, M.; Iovino, S.; Ciarlo, C.; Liu, J.; Castiglioni, A.; Price, E.; Liu, M.; Barton, E.R.; Kahn, C.R.; et al. A zebrafish embryo culture system defines factors that promote vertebrate myogenesis across species. *Cell* **2013**, *155*, 909–921. [CrossRef]

21. von Maltzahn, J.; Chang, N.C.; Bentzinger, C.F.; Rudnicki, M.A. Wnt signaling in myogenesis. *Trends Cell Biol.* **2012**, *22*, 602–609. [CrossRef] [PubMed]

22. Rome, S.; Forterre, A.; Mizgier, M.L.; Bouzakri, K. Skeletal Muscle-Released Extracellular Vesicles: State of the Art. *Front. Physiol.* **2019**, *10*, 929. [CrossRef] [PubMed]

23. Trovato, E.; Di Felice, V.; Barone, R. Extracellular Vesicles: Delivery Vehicles of Myokines. *Front. Physiol.* **2019**, *10*, 522. [CrossRef] [PubMed]

24. Guescini, M.; Maggio, S.; Ceccaroli, P.; Battistelli, M.; Annibalini, G.; Piccoli, G.; Sestili, P.; Stocchi, V. Extracellular Vesicles Released by Oxidatively Injured or Intact C_2C1_2 Myotubes Promote Distinct Responses Converging toward Myogenesis. *Int. J. Mol. Sci.* **2017**, *18*, 2488. [CrossRef] [PubMed]

25. Murphy, C.; Withrow, J.; Hunter, M.; Liu, Y.; Tang, Y.L.; Fulzele, S.; Hamrick, M.W. Emerging role of extracellular vesicles in musculoskeletal diseases. *Mol. Asp. Med.* **2018**, *60*, 123–128. [CrossRef] [PubMed]

26. Romancino, D.P.; Paterniti, G.; Campos, Y.; De Luca, A.; Di Felice, V.; d'Azzo, A.; Bongiovanni, A. Identification and characterization of the nano-sized vesicles released by muscle cells. *FEBS Lett.* **2013**, *587*, 1379–1384. [CrossRef]

27. Forterre, A.; Jalabert, A.; Berger, E.; Baudet, M.; Chikh, K.; Errazuriz, E.; De Larichaudy, J.; Chanon, S.; Weiss-Gayet, M.; Hesse, A.M.; et al. Proteomic analysis of C_2C1_2 myoblast and myotube exosome-like vesicles: A new paradigm for myoblast-myotube cross talk? *PLoS ONE* **2014**, *9*, e84153. [CrossRef]

28. Choi, J.S.; Yoon, H.I.; Lee, K.S.; Choi, Y.C.; Yang, S.H.; Kim, I.S.; Cho, Y.W. Exosomes from differentiating human skeletal muscle cells trigger myogenesis of stem cells and provide biochemical cues for skeletal muscle regeneration. *J. Control. Release* **2016**, *222*, 107–115. [CrossRef]

29. Polo, J.M.; Liu, S.; Figueroa, M.E.; Kulalert, W.; Eminli, S.; Tan, K.Y.; Apostolou, E.; Stadtfeld, M.; Li, Y.; Shioda, T.; et al. Cell type of origin influences the molecular and functional properties of mouse induced pluripotent stem cells. *Nat. Biotechnol.* **2010**, *28*, 848–855. [CrossRef]

30. Rizzi, R.; Di Pasquale, E.; Portararo, P.; Papait, R.; Cattaneo, P.; Latronico, M.V.; Altomare, C.; Sala, L.; Zaza, A.; Hirsch, E.; et al. Post-natal cardiomyocytes can generate iPS cells with an enhanced capacity toward cardiomyogenic re-differentation. *Cell Death Differ.* **2012**, *19*, 1162–1174. [CrossRef]

31. Chappell, J.C.; Bautch, V.L. Vascular development: Genetic mechanisms and links to vascular disease. *Curr. Top. Dev. Biol.* **2010**, *90*, 43–72. [CrossRef] [PubMed]

32. Birbrair, A.; Zhang, T.; Wang, Z.M.; Messi, M.L.; Enikolopov, G.N.; Mintz, A.; Delbono, O. Skeletal muscle pericyte subtypes differ in their differentiation potential. *Stem Cell Res.* **2013**, *10*, 67–84. [CrossRef]

33. Somers, A.; Jean, J.C.; Sommer, C.A.; Omari, A.; Ford, C.C.; Mills, J.A.; Ying, L.; Sommer, A.G.; Jean, J.M.; Smith, B.W.; et al. Generation of transgene-free lung disease-specific human induced pluripotent stem cells using a single excisable lentiviral stem cell cassette. *Stem Cells (Dayt. Ohio)* **2010**, *28*, 1728–1740. [CrossRef] [PubMed]

34. Cappellari, O.; Cossu, G. Pericytes in development and pathology of skeletal muscle. *Circ. Res.* **2013**, *113*, 341–347. [CrossRef] [PubMed]

35. Winkler, E.A.; Bell, R.D.; Zlokovic, B.V. Pericyte-specific expression of PDGF beta receptor in mouse models with normal and deficient PDGF beta receptor signaling. *Mol. Neurodegener.* **2010**, *5*, 32. [CrossRef]

36. Huang, F.J.; You, W.K.; Bonaldo, P.; Seyfried, T.N.; Pasquale, E.B.; Stallcup, W.B. Pericyte deficiencies lead to aberrant tumor vascularizaton in the brain of the NG2 null mouse. *Dev. Biol.* **2010**, *344*, 1035–1046. [CrossRef]

37. Peault, B.; Rudnicki, M.; Torrente, Y.; Cossu, G.; Tremblay, J.P.; Partridge, T.; Gussoni, E.; Kunkel, L.M.; Huard, J. Stem and Progenitor Cells in Skeletal Muscle Development, Maintenance, and Therapy. *Mol. Ther. J. Am. Soc. Gene Ther.* **2007**, *15*, 867–877. [CrossRef]

38. Sommer, A.G.; Rozelle, S.S.; Sullivan, S.; Mills, J.A.; Park, S.M.; Smith, B.W.; Iyer, A.M.; French, D.L.; Kotton, D.N.; Gadue, P.; et al. Generation of human induced pluripotent stem cells from peripheral blood using the STEMCCA lentiviral vector. *J. Vis. Exp. JoVE* **2012**, *68*, e4327. [CrossRef]

39. Raposo, G.; Stoorvogel, W. Extracellular vesicles: Exosomes, microvesicles, and friends. *J. Cell Biol.* **2013**, *200*, 373–383. [CrossRef]

40. Demonbreun, A.R.; McNally, E.M. Muscle cell communication in development and repair. *Curr. Opin. Pharm.* **2017**, *34*, 7–14. [CrossRef]

41. Le Bihan, M.-C.; Bigot, A.; Jensen, S.S.; Dennis, J.L.; Rogowska-Wrzesinska, A.; Lainé, J.; Gache, V.; Furling, D.; Jensen, O.N.; Voit, T.; et al. In-depth analysis of the secretome identifies three major independent secretory pathways in differentiating human myoblasts. *J. Proteom.* **2012**, *77*, 344–356. [CrossRef] [PubMed]

42. Thery, C.; Amigorena, S.; Raposo, G.; Clayton, A. Isolation and characterization of exosomes from cell culture supernatants and biological fluids. *Curr. Protoc. Cell Biol.* **2006**, *30*, 3–22. [CrossRef]

43. Mulcahy, L.A.; Pink, R.C.; Carter, D.R. Routes and mechanisms of extracellular vesicle uptake. *J. Extracell. Vesicles* **2014**, *3*, 24641. [CrossRef] [PubMed]

44. Murphy, D.E.; de Jong, O.G.; Brouwer, M.; Wood, M.J.; Lavieu, G.; Schiffelers, R.M.; Vader, P. Extracellular vesicle-based therapeutics: Natural versus engineered targeting and trafficking. *Exp. Mol. Med.* **2019**, *51*, 32. [CrossRef] [PubMed]

45. Grabowska, I.; Szeliga, A.; Moraczewski, J.; Czaplicka, I.; Brzoska, E. Comparison of satellite cell-derived myoblasts and C_2C1_2 differentiation in two- and three-dimensional cultures: Changes in adhesion protein expression. *Cell Biol. Int.* **2011**, *35*, 125–133. [CrossRef] [PubMed]

46. Guescini, M.; Guidolin, D.; Vallorani, L.; Casadei, L.; Gioacchini, A.M.; Tibollo, P.; Battistelli, M.; Falcieri, E.; Battistin, L.; Agnati, L.F.; et al. C_2C1_2 myoblasts release micro-vesicles containing mtDNA and proteins involved in signal transduction. *Exp. Cell Res.* **2010**, *316*, 1977–1984. [CrossRef] [PubMed]

47. Mylona, E.; Jones, K.A.; Mills, S.T.; Pavlath, G.K. CD44 regulates myoblast migration and differentiation. *J. Cell. Physiol.* **2006**, *209*, 314–321. [CrossRef]

48. Estelles, A.; Sperinde, J.; Roulon, T.; Aguilar, B.; Bonner, C.; LePecq, J.B.; Delcayre, A. Exosome nanovesicles displaying G protein-coupled receptors for drug discovery. *Int. J. Nanomed.* **2007**, *2*, 751–760.

49. Tan, J.Y.; Sriram, G.; Rufaihah, A.J.; Neoh, K.G.; Cao, T. Efficient derivation of lateral plate and paraxial mesoderm subtypes from human embryonic stem cells through GSKi-mediated differentiation. *Stem Cells Dev.* **2013**, *22*, 1893–1906. [CrossRef]

50. Roca, I.; Requena, J.; Edel, M.; Alvarez-Palomo, A. Myogenic Precursors from iPS Cells for Skeletal Muscle Cell Replacement Therapy. *J. Clin. Med.* **2015**, *4*, 243–259. [CrossRef]

51. Shoji, E.; Woltjen, K.; Sakurai, H. Directed Myogenic Differentiation of Human Induced Pluripotent Stem Cells. *Methods Mol. Biol.* **2016**, *1353*, 89–99. [CrossRef] [PubMed]

52. Tanaka, A.; Woltjen, K.; Miyake, K.; Hotta, A.; Ikeya, M.; Yamamoto, T.; Nishino, T.; Shoji, E.; Sehara-Fujisawa, A.; Manabe, Y.; et al. Efficient and reproducible myogenic differentiation from human iPS cells: Prospects for modeling Miyoshi Myopathy in vitro. *PLoS ONE* **2013**, *8*, e61540. [CrossRef]

53. Kim, K.; Zhao, R.; Doi, A.; Ng, K.; Unternaehrer, J.; Cahan, P.; Huo, H.; Loh, Y.H.; Aryee, M.J.; Lensch, M.W.; et al. Donor cell type can influence the epigenome and differentiation potential of human induced pluripotent stem cells. *Nat. Biotechnol.* **2011**, *29*, 1117–1119. [CrossRef] [PubMed]

54. Thomas, C.E.; Ehrhardt, A.; Kay, M.A. Progress and problems with the use of viral vectors for gene therapy. *Nat. Rev. Genet.* **2003**, *4*, 346–358. [CrossRef]

55. Zheng, J.K.; Wang, Y.; Karandikar, A.; Wang, Q.; Gai, H.; Liu, A.L.; Peng, C.; Sheng, H.Z. Skeletal myogenesis by human embryonic stem cells. *Cell Res.* **2006**, *16*, 713–722. [CrossRef]

56. Awaya, T.; Kato, T.; Mizuno, Y.; Chang, H.; Niwa, A.; Umeda, K.; Nakahata, T.; Heike, T. Selective development of myogenic mesenchymal cells from human embryonic and induced pluripotent stem cells. *PLoS ONE* **2012**, *7*, e51638. [CrossRef] [PubMed]

57. Zhu, S.; Wurdak, H.; Wang, J.; Lyssiotis, C.A.; Peters, E.C.; Cho, C.Y.; Wu, X.; Schultz, P.G. A small molecule primes embryonic stem cells for differentiation. *Cell Stem Cell* **2009**, *4*, 416–426. [CrossRef]

58. Choi, I.Y.; Lim, H.; Estrellas, K.; Mula, J.; Cohen, T.V.; Zhang, Y.; Donnelly, C.J.; Richard, J.P.; Kim, Y.J.; Kim, H.; et al. Concordant but Varied Phenotypes among Duchenne Muscular Dystrophy Patient-Specific Myoblasts Derived using a Human iPSC-Based Model. *Cell Rep.* **2016**, *15*, 2301–2312. [CrossRef]

59. Chal, J.; Oginuma, M.; Al Tanoury, Z.; Gobert, B.; Sumara, O.; Hick, A.; Bousson, F.; Zidouni, Y.; Mursch, C.; Moncuquet, P.; et al. Differentiation of pluripotent stem cells to muscle fiber to model Duchenne muscular dystrophy. *Nat. Biotechnol.* **2015**, *33*, 962–969. [CrossRef]

60. Valadi, H.; Ekstrom, K.; Bossios, A.; Sjostrand, M.; Lee, J.J.; Lotvall, J.O. Exosome-mediated transfer of mRNAs and microRNAs is a novel mechanism of genetic exchange between cells. *Nat. Cell Biol.* **2007**, *9*, 654–659. [CrossRef] [PubMed]

61. Xu, D.; Tahara, H. The role of exosomes and microRNAs in senescence and aging. *Adv. Drug Deliv. Rev.* **2013**, *65*, 368–375. [CrossRef] [PubMed]

62. Gutzeit, C.; Nagy, N.; Gentile, M.; Lyberg, K.; Gumz, J.; Vallhov, H.; Puga, I.; Klein, E.; Gabrielsson, S.; Cerutti, A.; et al. Exosomes Derived from Burkitt's Lymphoma Cell Lines Induce Proliferation, Differentiation, and Class-Switch Recombination in B Cells. *J. Immunol. (Baltim. Md. 1950)* **2014**, *192*, 5852–5862. [CrossRef] [PubMed]

63. Muylaert, D.E.; Fledderus, J.O.; Bouten, C.V.; Dankers, P.Y.; Verhaar, M.C. Combining tissue repair and tissue engineering; bioactivating implantable cell-free vascular scaffolds. *Heart (Br. Card. Soc.)* **2014**, *100*, 1825–1830. [CrossRef] [PubMed]

64. Forterre, A.; Jalabert, A.; Chikh, K.; Pesenti, S.; Euthine, V.; Granjon, A.; Errazuriz, E.; Lefai, E.; Vidal, H.; Rome, S. Myotube-derived exosomal miRNAs downregulate Sirtuin1 in myoblasts during muscle cell differentiation. *Cell Cycle* **2014**, *13*, 78–89. [CrossRef]

65. Charlton, C.A.; Mohler, W.A.; Blau, H.M. Neural cell adhesion molecule (NCAM) and myoblast fusion. *Dev. Biol.* **2000**, *221*, 112–119. [CrossRef]

6

Genetic Control of Muscle Diversification and Homeostasis: Insights from *Drosophila*

Preethi Poovathumkadavil * and Krzysztof Jagla

Institute of Genetics Reproduction and Development, iGReD, INSERM U1103, CNRS UMR6293, University of Clermont Auvergne, 28 Place Henri Dunant, 63000 Clermont-Ferrand, France; christophe.jagla@uca.fr
* Correspondence: preethi.poovathumkadavil@uca.fr

Abstract: In the fruit fly, *Drosophila melanogaster*, the larval somatic muscles or the adult thoracic flight and leg muscles are the major voluntary locomotory organs. They share several developmental and structural similarities with vertebrate skeletal muscles. To ensure appropriate activity levels for their functions such as hatching in the embryo, crawling in the larva, and jumping and flying in adult flies all muscle components need to be maintained in a functionally stable or homeostatic state despite constant strain. This requires that the muscles develop in a coordinated manner with appropriate connections to other cell types they communicate with. Various signaling pathways as well as extrinsic and intrinsic factors are known to play a role during *Drosophila* muscle development, diversification, and homeostasis. In this review, we discuss genetic control mechanisms of muscle contraction, development, and homeostasis with particular emphasis on the contractile unit of the muscle, the sarcomere.

Keywords: *Drosophila*; muscle; genetic control; muscle diversification; muscle homeostasis

1. Introduction

1.1. General Overview

Drosophila melanogaster, a holometabolic insect with a short lifespan, has served as a simple model to study myogenesis [1,2] and contractile proteins [3] for decades. Myogenesis in *Drosophila* occurs in two waves, one during the embryonic stage that gives rise to the larval body wall or somatic muscles and the second during pupal development that gives rise to adult flight, leg, and abdominal muscles [4]. All these muscles are voluntary, syncytial (multinucleate), and striated making them similar to vertebrate skeletal muscles [5]. Multiple signaling pathways, genes, and processes are conserved from *Drosophila* to vertebrates [6,7]. Muscles provide force to ensure various locomotory behaviors such as crawling, walking, jumping, and flying in *Drosophila*. Thus, they need to carry high levels of a mechanical load and are subject to constant strains, which can potentially disrupt homeostasis. Muscle movements need to be precise and coordinated, where communication with other tissues such as the nervous system provides critical inputs [8]. Muscles are the major reservoir for amino acids in the body that contribute to muscle mass and protein homeostasis [9]. All muscle functionalities require that they are correctly formed in the first place to attain a homeostatic state in which they are physiologically active and stable. Muscle intrinsic signaling as well as signaling from external organs contribute to muscle homeostasis. Muscles display a high degree of plasticity or flexibility at the signaling, metabolic, myonuclear, mitochondrial, and stem cell levels.

This review is divided into three parts. The first part presents an overview of the mechanisms of muscle contraction in *Drosophila*. The second part focuses on the development of the larval and adult muscles. In the third part, we discuss the maintenance of muscle homeostasis in normal conditions and the adverse effects of the loss of this homeostasis in pathological conditions. Throughout the review, the focus is on sarcomeres, which are the basic contractile units of the muscle.

1.2. Major Structural Components of the Drosophila Muscle and Their Vertebrate Counterparts

In *Drosophila*, muscle function is coordinated by sensory, excitatory, and mechanical inputs by its connection to the nervous system via neuromuscular junctions and to the epidermis via myotendinous junctions akin to vertebrate systems though they present differences, some of which are outlined below.

1.2.1. Sarcomeres

Sarcomeres are the basic contractile units of the muscle and provide the force for contraction during movements (Figure 1). They are repetitively arranged in a regular pattern that gives a striated appearance under the microscope to vertebrate skeletal muscles as well as *Drosophila* somatic, flight, and leg muscles [10,11]. Sarcomeric length, functional domains, and many component proteins are conserved between invertebrates and vertebrates, although studies also point to interesting differences among species, which appear to be adaptations to individual muscle function [12–15]. Despite structural differences in *Drosophila* sarcomeric proteins in comparison to vertebrate counterparts, they have similar functional interactions and possess conserved functional domains; for example, the PEVK domain of the *Drosophila* titin, Sallimus (Sls) confers elasticity similar to vertebrates [16]. Thus, the sarcomere provides an example of nature reusing and repurposing components across evolution.

1.2.2. Myotendinous Junctions (MTJs)

In *Drosophila*, the MTJ is an attachment formed between the muscle and specialized groups of tendon-like cells of ectodermal origin called tendon cells, also known as apodemes (Figure 1a). Unlike vertebrates, *Drosophila* does not have an internal skeleton and tendon cells help anchor the muscles firmly to the cuticular exoskeleton instead, which helps transmit the contractile forces to the body to generate motion. This makes them functionally similar to vertebrate tendons despite their distinct embryological origins, mesodermal for vertebrates and ectodermal for *Drosophila* [17,18]. The formation and maintenance of the MTJ is mediated through the ECM by specific integrin heterodimers on the muscle and tendon ends in *Drosophila* similar to vertebrates [19–22].

1.2.3. Neuromuscular Junctions (NMJs)

The NMJ is the point of contact between the motor neurons of the nervous system and the muscle, which enables environmental inputs to be transmitted via synapses to the muscle (Figure 1a). The *Drosophila* larval NMJ is an established model for NMJ formation and function. This NMJ is glutamatergic and responds to the neurotransmitter glutamate unlike vertebrate NMJs that are cholinergic and respond to acetylcholine. However, they are of particular interest owing to their similarity to mammalian brain glutamatergic synapses that express multiple genes orthologous to *Drosophila* genes and the ease with which NMJ assembly can be studied in this model [23–25]. It continues to be an active field of study with focus equally shifting to adult motor neurons formed after metamorphosis [26,27].

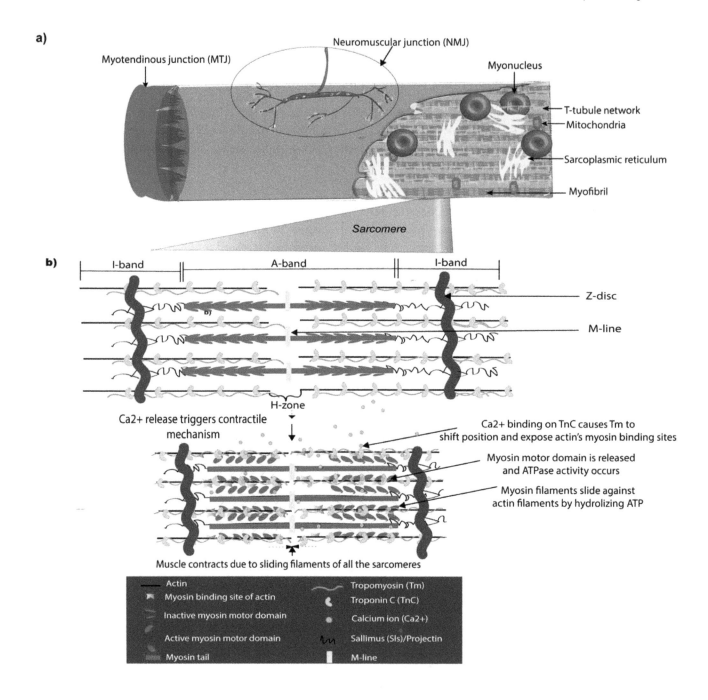

Figure 1. Schematic representation of the larval body wall or somatic muscle structure and the sliding filament theory of muscle contraction. (**a**) Muscle structure with myofibrils and the network of myonuclei, sarcoplasmic reticulum (SR), T-tubules, and mitochondria. The muscle is connected to the nervous system via the neuromuscular junction (NMJ) and to the epidermis via the myotendinous junction (MTJ). Myofibrils are formed of repetitive contractile units, the sarcomeres. (**b**) The structure of a sarcomere and the mechanism of contraction proposed by the sliding filament theory. Ca^{2+} ions released upon neurotransmitter signaling from the NMJ launch a cascade by binding to TroponinC (TnC) on the thin filaments of sarcomeres. This Ca^{2+} binding causes a conformation change in Tropomyosin (Tm) bound to actin, exposing actin's myosin binding sites. This permits the activated myosin motor domain to bind to actin and slide against it by utilizing the energy stored in Adenosine Triphosphate (ATP).

2. The Sarcomere and Molecular Mechanisms of Muscle Contraction

Voluntary muscle contraction is a highly coordinated process that depends on cooperative signaling from sensory neurons via interneurons and motor neurons to the NMJ of the muscle [28–30]. Given that the principal muscle function is to generate movements by contracting, the sarcomeric contractile units are indispensable for muscle function and their maintenance is crucial. The *Drosophila* adult indirect flight muscle (IFM) is established as a model to study sarcomere assembly and the functions of its components [31]. IFMs are built of multiple myofibers and have a stereotypic pattern of sarcomeric proteins forming highly ordered myofibrils similar to human skeletal muscles allowing the study of sarcomere malformations under mutant conditions. The IFM is also a model to study stretch activation (SA) [32]. During SA, there is a high frequency of contraction although the nervous system input frequency is much lower. This is possible due to the delayed increase in tension following muscle stretching. SA is a mechanism found in all muscles though it has particular significance in certain muscle types with rhythmic activity such as human cardiac muscles and the fruit fly flight muscles. In contrast to the multi-fiber IFM muscles of the adult, the somatic muscles in the *Drosophila* embryo and larvae are built of only one muscle fiber per muscle and present a much simpler model to study myofibers.

A sarcomere is a specialized structure adapted for muscle contraction (Figure 1). During myofibrillogenesis, newly formed sarcomeres align in repeating units along the length of a muscle to form a myofibril and multiple myofibrils covered by the plasma membrane form a myofiber. A sarcomere is built of thin-actin and thick-myosin filaments with associated proteins facilitating contraction-relaxation cycles. The thick filaments consist of myosin polymers with each myosin consisting of a myosin tail and two myosin heads, which are capable of attaching to actin during muscle contraction. The two ends of a sarcomere are demarcated by a Z-disc, a huge protein complex that anchors the thin filaments that form I-bands on either side of a sarcomere, while the thick filaments form an A-band in the center (Figure 1). In between the two I-bands is an H-zone lacking myosin heads and in the center of the H-zone is an M-line that corresponds to another large protein complex that anchors the thick filaments [33].

Sarcomere function is intricately linked to other organelles such as the mitochondria [34], myonuclei [35], sarcoplasmic reticulum (SR), and T-tubules [10,36]. The efficient function of sarcomeres is closely coupled with the periodic arrangement of the SR and T-tubules around them [10,36–38]. T-tubules are regular tubular invaginations of the plasma membrane at each sarcomere. The membrane organelle SR is linked to the myonuclei and T-tubules to facilitate the exchange of proteins and ions. The SR is the major intracellular reservoir of calcium (Ca^{2+}) ions in the muscle, which are essential for muscle contraction. The T-tubule and SR form a specialized triad/dyad structure, which is indispensable for correct muscle functioning by excitation-contraction (EC) coupling. This EC coupling enables the transmission of excitation potentials from the NMJ to the SR, which triggers Ca^{2+} release from the SR that in turn initiates sarcomeric sliding movements leading to muscle contraction. Apart from Ca^{2+}, other ions contribute to muscle contraction [39]. The Na^+K^+-ATPase is a Na^+-K^+ pump that can pump Na^+ out of and K^+ into the cells against their normal concentration gradients. In muscles, the concentration of these ions fine-tunes the force of contraction [40]. In *Drosophila*, muscles are one of the major organs that express the Na^+K^+-ATPase α subunit [41]. One form of the Na^+K^+-ATPase β subunit, Nrv1 interacts with Dystroglycan (Dg), which is part of a complex that helps transmit forces into the muscle cell [42].

The mechanism of muscle contraction is explained by the sliding filament theory [43,44], reviewed by Hugh Huxley [33]. This theory proposes that the myosin head domain acts as a motor and slides against the actin filament powered by the energy stored in ATP. This sliding of the central myosin along the thin filaments causes the two I bands on either side to come closer to each other. During contraction, environmental inputs are transmitted by the nervous system to the NMJ leading to Ca^{2+} binding to the Troponin C (TnC) subunit of the Troponin (Tn) complex. This leads to the Troponin T (TnT) subunit that binds to the actin binding protein Tropomyosin (Tm) triggering a conformational change in Tm, thus shifting its position on actin and exposing the myosin binding site of actin [45–47]. Myosin that is turned 'on' by a myosin regulatory light chain (Rlc) phosphorylation [48] liberates the motor domains in the myosin head that were folded onto the myosin tail, thus facilitating its binding to actin. Subsequent ATP hydrolysis and energy release, thanks to its ATPase activity, permits it to move along the thin filament to contract the muscle. For the muscle to relax, the Troponin I (TnI) troponin subunit inhibits the actomyosin interaction [49] so that Tm covers the myosin binding site of actin and the myosin is switched 'off' and folded back onto the myosin tail [50,51]. This coordinated key muscle function highlights the importance of ionic and sarcomeric component homeostasis in muscles, which implies the supply and maintenance of the right quantities of the right ions and sarcomeric components at the right time to ensure muscle functionality.

During contraction, the MTJ helps anchor the myofibrils and transmits forces [19,52]. Tight interactions between sarcomeric components ensure myofibrillar integrity and prevent disintegration due to contractile forces. CapZ binds to the actin barbed end and links it to the Z-disc [13] while Z-disc proteins such as the filamin Cher [53], Zasp, and α-actinin anchor the thin filaments [54]. Similarly, the M-line protein Obscurin that associates with the thick filament [55], Muscle LIM protein at 84B (Mlp84B) that cooperates with Sallimus (Sls) known as the *Drosophila* titin [56], integrins [57], and other proteins ensure muscle integrity. Sarcomeres are subject to constant mechanical strain due to the thin and thick filament friction and need to be consistently replenished to ensure their function over a lifetime. Since these muscles are voluntary, they also need to be able to stop contracting at will and go back to their natural state. Defective sarcomeric formation, maintenance, and homeostasis are associated with muscular diseases [15,58].

3. Muscle Diversification—On the Road to Muscle Homeostasis

Muscle development is a finely orchestrated, synchronized process that occurs in spatial and temporal coordination with the development of other communicating tissues to finally form a homeostatic muscle. There are similarities as well as differences between *Drosophila* and vertebrate myogenesis [59]. During development, each muscle diversifies to attain an identity tailored to its specific functional requirements. The study of muscle diversification during development is of interest in the context of homeostasis for two primary reasons:

(a)   Events similar to those occurring during development need to be reinitiated to repair and regenerate an injured muscle and reestablish muscle homeostasis [60]. This is a new field of study in *Drosophila* stemming from the recent discovery of muscle satellite cells in adult flies [61].

(b)   The two waves of myogenesis in *Drosophila* result in two homeostatic states, one in the larva and one in the adult. The larval homeostatic states are highly dynamic given the large growth spurt that occurs over the three larval instars. This might provide insights into mechanisms of muscle atrophy and hypertrophy. Forkhead box sub-group O (Foxo), for example, has been shown to inhibit larval muscle growth by repressing *diminutive* (*myc*) [62]. In mice, excess c-Myc has been shown to induce cardiac hypertrophy [63].

3.1. Embryonic Myogenesis of Larval Muscles

Embryonic myogenesis gives rise to monofiber larval somatic muscles whose main function is to aid in hatching and the peristaltic, crawling movements of the larvae. The embryonic and larval somatic musculature consists of a stereotypical pattern of muscles in each segment, with 30 muscles in most abdominal hemisegments (A2–A6) (figure in Table 1). There are fewer muscles in the posterior and first abdominal hemisegment and a slightly different set of muscles in the three thoracic hemisegments (T1–T3). Embryonic muscles arise from the mesoderm germ layer and their development requires intrinsic mesodermal cues and extrinsic cues from the adjacent epidermal and neural cells. Thus, they develop in synchrony with the development of muscle-interactors such as tendon cells and motor neurons and need to 'speak a common language' to communicate for coordinated development and maintenance.

Somatic muscle specification and differentiation have been reviewed extensively in the past [1,2,7,60–62] and this review presents complementary as well as new information that emphasizes the role of developmental factors in future muscle homeostasis.

3.1.1. Muscle Diversification by the Specification of Muscle Founder Cells Expressing Identity Transcription Factors (iTFs)

The embryo undergoes gastrulation by invagination [64], which brings the three germ layers, the ectoderm, the somatic muscle forming mesoderm, and endoderm in juxtaposition with each other. This helps provide extrinsic signals to the developing mesoderm. Following this juxtaposition, the mesoderm is divided into domains by morphogenic signaling [65] giving rise to a somatic muscle domain in which the transcription factor (TF) Twist (Twi) provides a myogenic switch [66]. Subsequently, equivalence or promuscular cell clusters expressing the neurogenic gene *lethal of scute* (*l'sc*) form and one muscle progenitor cell is singled out from each cluster by lateral inhibition involving Notch and Ras/MAPK signaling [67,68]. The remaining Notch activated cells in the equivalence groups become fusion competent myoblasts (FCMs). This process is reminiscent and coincides temporally with the specification of neural lineages from the neurectoderm [69,70], which occurs during embryonic stages 8–11, while muscle cell identity specification occurs during stages 9–11.

The singled-out muscle progenitors divide asymmetrically to give rise to founder cells (FCs), which are believed to carry all the information necessary to give rise to the diversity of muscle types. Asymmetric divisions of progenitors can give rise to two FCs, an FC and a Numb negative adult muscle precursor (AMP) or an FC and a cardiac progenitor, which subsequently migrate away from each other [67,71,72]. Each FC contains the information to establish one muscle's identity since it can form correct attachments and be correctly innervated even in the absence of myoblast fusion with surrounding FCMs [73,74]. It expresses its characteristic code of TFs known as muscle identity transcription factors (iTFs) (Figure 2). The expression of a combinatorial code of iTFs in distinct progenitors is the result of their spatial positioning as well as tissue specific convergence of multiple signaling cascades [75]. For example, Wg signaling from the adjacent developing central nervous system (CNS) is implicated in the specification of Slouch (Slou) positive FCs [76] highlighting the importance of coordinated tissue development.

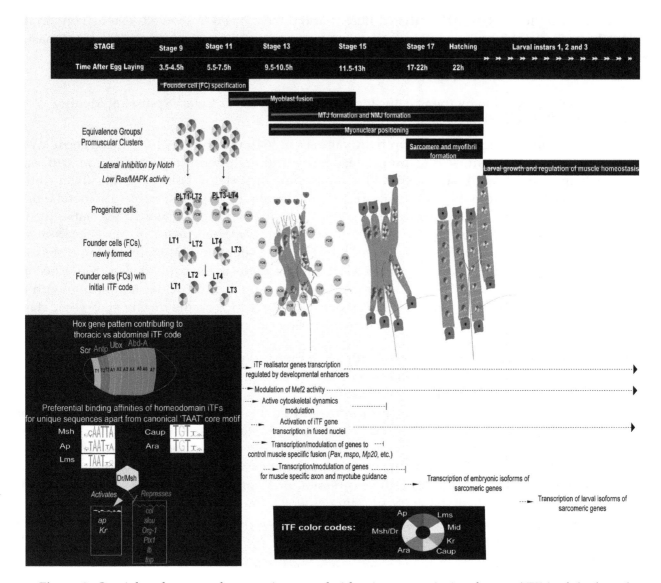

Figure 2. Spatial and temporal expression muscle identity transcription factors (iTFs) of the larval lateral transverse (LT) muscles. Sizes are not up to scale. Following the specification of progenitor cells by a lateral inhibition by Notch and low Ras/MAPK activity, founder cells (FCs) expressing muscle specific iTFs are specified for each LT muscle, LT1, LT2, LT3, and LT4 with a contribution from homeobox (Hox) genes to specify thoracic versus abdominal identities. Each iTF has preferential binding abilities to certain enhancers. The iTF expression is followed by the regulation of transcription and modulation of expression of their realisator genes which establish muscle identity over the course of development. The spatial and temporal expression of iTFs coupled with their modulation of realisator genes, which include generic muscle genes, in collaboration with Mef2 begs the question about their contribution to muscle homeostasis. Abbreviations: FCM: Fusion competent myoblasts; FC: Founder cells; LT: Lateral transverse muscles; iTF: Identity transcription factor.

3.1.2. The Role of iTFs

After the initial discovery of distinct Slou expressing FCs [77], many other TFs expressed in discrete subsets of FCs were subsequently identified and collectively named muscle identity transcription factors or iTFs (Table 1). A loss or gain of iTF function can cause muscle loss [78,79] or transformation of one muscle to another muscle fate [80,81] and impede muscle development [82] thus disrupting muscle patterns. The iTFs such as Ap, Slou, Eve, Kr, Lb, and Lms are also expressed in the CNS [78]. Many identified iTFs such as Dr/Msh, Lms, Ap, Ara, Caup, Lb, Slou, Eve, Ptx1, and Tup are homeodomain TFs that are known to recognize similar canonical TAAT containing binding motifs, but they could have preferential high affinity binding motifs (Figure 2), as has been shown for Slou [83] and Caup [84]. The iTFs from other TF families are Twi, Nau, Kr, Kn/Col, Mid, Six4, Poxm, Org-1, and Vg. Newly identified iTFs for a subset of dorsal muscles are Sine occulis (So), No ocelli (Noc), and the cofactor ETS-domain lacking (Edl) [85], which act sequentially with their cofactors. The iTF Vg also acts with a cofactor, Sd [86].

Table 1. The iTF expression patterns in embryonic somatic muscle founder cells.

iTF	Human Orthologs	FCs Expressing iTF [1]	References	Embryonic Somatic Muscle Pattern
Apterous (Ap)	LHX	LT1, LT2, LT3, LT4, VA2, VA3	[78]	
Araucan (Ara)	IRX	LT1, LT2, LT3, LT4, SBM, DT1-*DO3*	[87]	
Caupolican (Caup)	IRX	LT1, LT2, LT3, LT4, SBM, DT1-*DO3*	[87]	
Collier (Col)/Knot (Kn)	EBF	*DA2*, DA3-*DO5*, *DT1-DO3*, *LL1-DO4*	[82,85,88]	
Drop (Dr)/Muscle segment homeobox (Msh)	MSX	DO1, DO2, LT1-LT2, LT3-LT4, VA2, VA3	[89,90]	
Even-skipped (Eve)	EVX	DA1, *DO2*	[91,92]	External muscles are represented in dark brown, intermediate muscles in a medium shade of brown, and internal muscles in fuchsia.
Krüppel (Kr)	KLF	DA1, DO1, *LT1-LT2*, *LT3*-LT4, LL1, *VA1*-VA2, *DO2*, VL3, VO2, VO5	[87,92,93]	
Ladybird (Lb)	LBX	SBM	[94]	
Lateral muscles scarcer (Lms)	-	LT1-LT2, LT3-LT4	[95]	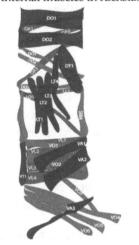
Midline (Mid)	TBX20	*LT3*-LT4, LO1, *VA1*-VA2	[96]	
Nautilus (Nau)	MYOD	DO1, DA2, DA3-DO5, DO3, LL1- DO4, LO1, VA1	[79,85,88,97]	
Optomotor-blind-related-1 (Org-1)	TBX1	LO1, VT1, SBM	[98]	
Pox meso (Poxm)	PAX	DT1-*DO3*, VA1-VA2, VA3	[99]	
Ptx1	PITX	Ventral muscles	[100]	
Runt		DO2, VA3, VO4	[92,101]	
Slouch (Slou)/S59	NKX1	DT1-*DO3*, *VA1*-VA2, VA3, VT1, *LO1*	[77,80,87]	
Scalloped (Sd)	TEF-1	*All FCs transiently*, maintained in VL1, VL2, VL3, VL4	[86]	
Vestigial (Vg)	VGLL	DA1-DA2, DA3, LL1, VL1, VL2, VL3, VL4	[86]	
Tailup (Tup)	ISL	DA1, DA2, DO1, DO2	[81]	
Eyes absent (Eya)		Differential temporal expression in multiple FCs	[85,102]	
Six4	SIX	Differential temporal expression in multiple FCs	[102,103]	
Sine occulis (So)	SIX	*DA2*, DA3-*DO5*, *LL1-DO4*	[85]	
No ocelli (Noc)	ZNF	DA3-DO5	[85]	
ETS-domain lacking (Edl)	-	*DA2, DA3*	[85]	

[1] In the 'FCs Expressing iTF' column, each FC name is shown in the colour corresponding to the muscle it generates as depicted in the figure in the column on the extreme right. FCs known to be generated from an asymmetric division of the same progenitor cell are hyphenated. FCs with transient expression are shown in italics.

The iTF code can be hierarchic and activate other iTFs as has been shown for Org-1 that activates Slou and Lb [98]. In addition to hierarchy, there seems to be isoform specificity in iTF expression [85]. Certain iTFs confer identity by repressing other iTFs. Dr, for example, represses Lb that is normally active only in the SBM muscle and Eve that is normally continually expressed in only the DA1 muscle [104], while Tup represses Col in DA2 [81]. The expression levels of one isoform of the chromatin remodeling factor Sin3A is implicated in modulating the response to iTFs by acting on the *slou* enhancer [105].

The same iTFs can be expressed in different muscles, but with different co-iTFs. The identity code for one specific muscle subset, the lateral transverse or LT muscles, which comprises the four muscles LT1-4, for example, is known to be set up by a combinatorial expression of Dr [89], Ap [78], Kr [93], Lms [95], and the Ara/Caup complex [87] (Figure 2). Dr appears to directly or indirectly activate the transcription of many LT iTFs such as *Kr*, *ap*, and itself while repressing non-LT iTFs such as *col*, *slou*, *Org-1*, *Ptx1*, *lb*, and *tup* [83] and its expression is lost by mid embryonic stages. Only Lms is specific to all four LT muscles while others are also expressed in other muscle subsets, although not in combination with the same co-iTFs. This seems to be the way the iTF code is set up, where they are repurposed in different combinations to define the identity of different muscles [81,85,88]. Even amongst the LT muscles, each muscle has a specific combination of these iTFs (Figure 2). Some iTFs such as Lms are persistently expressed while others such as Ap and Kr are transient. A characteristic feature of Kr is that it is transiently expressed and subsequently lost from one of the two sibling FCs that arise from the progenitor that expresses it [87,93].

The thoracic LT muscles have slightly different characteristics such as a different number of myonuclei, which might depend on the iTF code along with individual iTF dynamics in conjunction with other TFs [106]. Homeotic or Hox genes such as *Antennapedia* (*Antp*), *Abdominal-A* (*Abd-A*), *Abdominal-B* (*Abd-B*), and *Ultrabithorax* (*Ubx*) control the muscle pattern along the anterior-posterior axis and are thus part of the iTF code [106–108] (Figure 2). The mechanism of Hox gene regulation in muscles could be by repressing genes specifying alternative fates by altering the epigenetic landscape in a tissue specific manner [109]. Hox genes could also be involved in the coordination of the proper innervation of muscles [110].

Once an FC initiates its diversification with a specific identity determined by an iTF code, it starts differentiating by activating realisator genes acting downstream of iTFs. Some muscle identity realisator genes have been identified. They include several muscular differentiation genes such as *sallimus* (*sls*), *Paxillin* (*Pax*), *Muscle protein 20* (*Mp20*), and *M-spondin* (*mspo*), which are differentially expressed in muscle subsets to control the acquisition of specific muscle properties such as the number of myoblast fusion events or the specific attachment to tendon cells. [111,112]. Thus, an iTF code and a downstream realisator gene code are both essential to generate a diversity of muscle types with specific functions and to set the foundation for muscle homeostasis.

3.1.3. Mef2, a Key Muscle Differentiation Factor and Its Interactions with iTFs

The *Drosophila* Myocyte enhancer factor 2 (Mef2) acts along with iTFs and their realisator genes to cause the muscle to differentiate. Mef2, similar to its vertebrate ortholog MEF2, is indispensable for muscle differentiation [113–115]. It has an equally important role in fully differentiated muscles and the control of its expression and activity is dynamic. Though it is expressed in the mesoderm during all stages, its loss of function does not prevent initial muscle specification and FC generation, but completely blocks subsequent differentiation so that muscle cells undergo apoptosis in later embryonic stages [116,117]. Mef2 activity levels change over time and appear to be adapted to varying target gene expression requirements during different developmental stages [86,118]. It regulates a vast array of muscle specific genes [119,120], sometimes in cooperation with other TFs such as Cf2 [121,122]. It is itself regulated by various mechanisms including autoregulation [123], signal and TF integration at its specific cis regulatory modules (CRMs) [124], or post transcriptionally by highly conserved miRNAs such as miR-92b [125]. TFs such as Twi and Lameduck (Lmd) [119,126] acting on muscle specific CRMs and Akirin-bearing chromatin remodeling complexes [127] are known regulators of Mef2 transcriptional activity. The RNA modifying enzyme Ten-eleven-translocation family protein (Tet) shows a strong overlap with Mef2 expression in somatic muscles and its depletion in muscle precursors leads to larval locomotion defects [128] though the relationship between the two factors is unclear.

The iTFs Vg and Sd physically interact with each other and with Mef2 either alone or in combination [129]. Each of them has a spatially and temporally controlled expression pattern and altering their expression levels severely affects the development of specific ventral muscles during late stages by affecting the levels of realisator genes. Thus, iTFs could play a key role in the modulation of Mef2 interactions. Given the central role of Mef2 in muscle development, disrupted Mef2 expression can have deleterious consequences at all stages of muscle development and maintenance.

3.1.4. Myoblast Fusion and Myonuclear Positioning

In order to form a differentiated muscle, in the mid-stage embryo, a specific number of neighboring FCMs fuse with the FC to form a syncytium (Figure 2). The formation of syncytial fibers by myoblast fusion is complete by the end of stage 15 [130–132]. As fusion proceeds, the round-shaped FC becomes a myotube that elongates, becomes polarized, and locally sends out filopodia in the presumptive area of MTJ and NMJ formation. Fusion involves complementary cell adhesion molecules (CAMs) such as Dumbfounded (Duf) or its paralogue Roughest (Rst) expressed on FCs [133,134] and Stick and Stones (Sns) or its paralogue Hibris (Hbs) expressed on FCMs [135,136], respectively. They trigger a signaling cascade, thereby modulating cytoskeleton dynamics to form a fusogenic synapse that helps integrate the FCM nucleus into the FC/myotube. In *Drosophila*, the iTF code dictates the number of fusion events by controlling the expression level of fusion genes encoding actin cytoskeleton modulators such as *Muscle Protein 20* (*Mp20*) and *Paxillin* (*Pax*) or the ECM component *m-spondin* (*mspo*) [112]. A recent study provides insights into the FCM-FC transcription dynamics in a syncytial myotube [137]. FCMs appear to be naïve and respond to the local environment that recruits them for fusion. Upon fusion, the FCM adopts an FC transcriptional program triggered by the transcription of certain muscle specific iTFs. However, once fusion is complete, differences in gene transcription among myonuclei within the same muscle are observed. For example, not all myonuclei transcribe the iTFs at a given timepoint, which could help maintain an mRNA-protein balance. Evidence from this study suggests that even after fusion is complete the FC nucleus that seeded the muscle retains a transcriptional program that is distinct from other myonuclei.

As fusion proceeds, at around stage 14, the nuclei of newly fused FCMs start exhibiting characteristic movements until they are positioned peripherally to maximize the internuclear distances. This process, also observed in vertebrate muscles [138,139], has been extensively studied in the LT muscles in the *Drosophila* embryo. In these muscles the new myonuclei initially cluster into two groups, unlike in vertebrates where nuclei cluster in the center of the myotube [140], then disperse and are finally arranged along the periphery of the myotube. Correct myonuclear positioning is dependent on the LINC complex [141] that links the inner nuclear membrane (INM) to the outer nuclear membrane (ONM) and the ONM to the microtubules (MT) and the actin cytoskeleton. Mispositioned myonuclei in *Drosophila* larvae cause locomotion defects, and in humans, are associated with various diseases [142]. This is not surprising considering the close association of myonuclei with muscle structural components such as the NMJ, MTJ, actin cytoskeleton, microtubule, SR, Golgi complex, and T-tubules. During the larval growth spurt following hatching, myonuclei increase in size along with the increasing muscle size by Myc dependent endoreplication to adapt transcription to muscle functionality requirements [62].

3.1.5. Myotendinous Junction (MTJ) Formation

MTJ formation has been previously reviewed [17,143–145]. Once FCs are specified, they migrate towards the ectoderm while tendon precursor cells are specified in the ectoderm in parallel in a muscle independent fashion by the induction of expression of the early growth response factor (Egr)-like zinc finger TF, Stripe (Sr). Interestingly, tendon progenitor cells in mice express the Sr orthologs, the early growth response TFs EGR1 and EGR2 [146]. The StripeB (SrB) isoform is induced during the precursor stage to maintain the tendon cells in a non-differentiated state until later when they differentiate following signals from the approaching muscles. These signals lead to an increase in the expression of the StripeA (SrA) isoform in an integrin dependent manner by promoting *stripe* splicing by the short isoform How(S) of the splice factor interactor How [147]. SrA induces the expression of tendon differentiation markers such as *short stop (shot)*, *delilah (dei)*, and *β1-tubulin (β1-tub)*. At stage 14, tendon cells guide myotubes to their final attachment sites. The targeting of muscles to tendon cells at stage 15 is facilitated by muscle type dependent and generic CAMs as well as signaling molecules. These include Slit-Robo [148] in some ventral muscles, Derailed (Drl) [149] in LT muscles, Kon-tiki (Kon), Glutamate receptor interacting protein (Grip), and Echinoid (Ed), probably involving integrin complexes [149–152]. Once muscles target their tendon cells, integrin complexes assemble on the muscle and tendon cells facilitated by the αPS2-βPS integrin heterodimer on the muscle end and αPS1-βPS on the tendon cell end to stabilize the attachments [153]. Each attachment site is muscle type specific and the iTF code could potentially modulate the expression of genes such as *kon* [137].

MTJ formation is complete by the end of stage 16 and is then further refined to withstand contractile forces. Talin phosphorylation contributes to MTJ refinement [154]. This is followed by myofibril maturation and attachment to the MTJ. Once muscles start contraction, mechanical forces stabilize the MTJ by reducing integrin turnover [155]. The MTJ grows along with the massive larval growth spurt following hatching.

3.1.6. Sarcomere Assembly and Myofibrillogenesis

Sarcomere assembly has been extensively studied in the *Drosophila* indirect flight muscles (IFM) [31] and other invertebrate models as well as in vertebrate models and cultured human cells [156,157]. These studies point to similarities as well as differences in vertebrate and insect muscles. The premyofibril theory that is widely accepted for vertebrate sarcomere assembly proposes the formation of premyofibrils along the cell periphery containing non muscle myosin, which then incorporate muscle myosin to form nascent myofibrils that subsequently form mature myofibrils [158,159]. In the early stages, distinct Mhc positive fibrils and I-Z-I complexes containing thin filaments protruding from α-actinin positive central Z bodies are seen in invertebrates as well as vertebrates [160,161]. In *Drosophila*, it has been proposed that the individual components of the sarcomere are assembled separately as latent complexes and are then assembled into sarcomeres without assembling into premyofibrils [162–164]. Most studies on *Drosophila* sarcomere assembly have been using the IFM as a model and not much attention has been given to embryonic sarcomere development.

In the *Drosophila* embryo, sarcomere assembly is initiated at stage 17. Individual sarcomere constituents are first assembled and then integrated into a mature sarcomere by integrin dependent interdigitation [162]. The precise stage at which each sarcomere component is added is currently not known. Certain sarcomeric proteins such as actin [165] and myosin [166] express sarcomere specific as well as generic cytoplasmic isoforms with roles in other muscle components such as the MTJ. TFs such as Mef2, Chorion factor 2 (Cf2), and E2F transcription factor 1 (E2f1) have been shown to regulate the expression of sarcomeric genes [122,167]. *Drosophila* has six actin isoforms including Act57B and Act87E that are muscle specific and incorporate into larval sarcomeres [165]. Thin filament formation and elongation requires actin binding factors such as the *Drosophila* formin Dishevelled Associated Activator of Morphogenesis (DAAM) [168] and Sarcomere length short (Sals) [169], which localize to the growing thin filament pointed ends. Once the thin actin filament attains its final length, it is capped by a short embryonic isoform of Tmod [169,170]. While non-muscle myosin is a component of premyofibrils in vertebrates, this does not seem to be the case in *Drosophila*, which has only one non-muscle myosin, Zipper (Zip). During stage 16, it colocalizes with PS2 integrin at muscle attachment sites and at stage 17 when sarcomeres form, it also colocalizes to Z-discs and is essential for myofibril formation [162,171]. PS2 integrin follows a similar expression pattern in culture with initial occurrence at contact sites, then at Z-discs [172]. The observation of Zip association with PS2 before sarcomere assembly is significant because myofibrils attach to the MTJ via integrin complexes with Zip acting downstream of PS2 signaling [52]. Therefore, it would appear that the embryo is getting individual components ready for future integration into myofibrils.

By stage 17 of embryogenesis, several sarcomere proteins localize to Z-discs and thin and thick filament organization and myofibril structures are seen. A knockdown of Z-disc proteins Zip, Zasp, and α-actinin at this stage disrupts sarcomerogenesis [162], though Zasp mutant sarcomeres disintegrate after initial correct formation. The myoblast fusion protein Rolling pebbles (Rols7) also colocalizes to the Z-discs during sarcomerogenesis [173], but its function remains to be elucidated. Integrins are distributed along the width of the muscle and align with Z-discs during embryonic sarcomerogenesis. Their loss results in clumping, where I-Z-I body components stay distinct from Mhc containing components. In addition, integrins associate with the ECM and mutant larvae for the ECM type IV collagen Col4a1 present abnormalities in thin-thick filament interdigitation and the degeneration of body wall muscles [162,172,174]. They are also present at epidermal muscle attachment sites along with several Z-disc proteins. Mature sarcomeres align themselves to form myofibrils that attach to the MTJ via the terminal Z-disc to be able to sustain muscle contractions [162,173].

Auld and Folker showed that myonuclear movements are intricately linked to sarcomere and myofibril formation [35]. Their study showed that the Z-disc protein Zasp66, one of the *Drosophila* Zasp family of proteins, localizes as puncta to the cytoplasmic face of the nuclei along with F-actin during initial stages of sarcomerogenesis. At later stages, puncta were observed throughout the muscle. They showed that LINC complex components such as Klarsicht (Klar) and Klaroid (Koi) coordinate initial colocalization of puncta around the nucleus. However, Z-disc-like structures still formed and aligned into myofibrils in LINC component depleted muscles, although they had altered morphology suggesting a specialized role for myonuclei-associated Zasp66 puncta. *sals* mutants display clustered myonuclei at muscle ends as well as myofibrils with numerous shorter sarcomeres suggesting a role for correct myonuclear positioning in myofibril organization [169].

Embryonic myofibrillogenesis within the egg is complete by late stage 17. Asynchronous, episodic contractions occur during the process of myofibril assembly, but coordinated contractions only occur later after mature NMJ formation results in adequate motor inputs [175,176]. Following hatching, during larval stages when the muscles rapidly grow in size, new sarcomeres are generated and organized into myofibrils during an approximately five-day period [62]. In fully mature larval muscles, T-tubules and the SR organize themselves around each sarcomere for excitation-contraction coupling and this organization is Amphiphysin (Amph) dependent [37]. The iTF code could play a role in modulating the muscle specific expression of sarcomeric genes, as has been shown for Vg and Sd that form a complex with Mef2 to modulate Mef2 targets involved in sarcomerogenesis including *Act57B* and *Mhc* [129].

3.1.7. Innervation and Neuromuscular Junction (NMJ) Formation

The development of the NMJ of larval somatic muscles has been previously reviewed [24,25,177–179] and represents another example of intricate communication between two different tissues. After neuroblasts differentiate into motor neurons (MNs) in parallel with FC specification [180–182], their dendrites in the CNS are organized in a 'myotopic map' reflecting the innervation pattern of their target muscles and MNs can reach target locations even in the absence of muscles [182]. Each neuroblast expresses a characteristic code of TFs that defines its identity as is the case for muscle FCs expressing iTFs [26]. By stage 12, MN axons fasciculate in each hemisegment within three peripheral nerves, the intersegmental nerve (ISN), segmental nerve (SN), and transverse nerve (TN) that extend towards specific target muscles from the ventral nerve chord (VNC). The ISN, SN, and TN branch stereotypically as they extend growth cones towards muscles to form MN nerve branches that further defasciculate into axons to innervate muscles. The SN nerve, for example, branches into SNa, SNb, SNc, and SNd with a subset of MNs from the SNa innervating a muscle subset including LT muscles [181].

At around stage 14, each MN extends numerous filopodia from axon growth cones towards muscles to explore their target muscles. Muscles in turn extend myopodia that cluster together on axon growth cone arrival and intermingle with growth cone filopodia. Muscles also form lamellipodia during innervation [183]. Target muscle recognition and contact are facilitated by muscle and MN specific CAMs, Cell Surface and Secreted (CSS) proteins, and other proteins [184]. Certain guidance molecules such as the homophilic Connectin (Con) are expressed in the SNa MN as well as the LT muscles it innervates [185]. Con is also expressed in the DT1 muscle and its expression is potentially modulated by the iTF code [137]. Some MNs and the muscles they innervate express the same iTF, as is the case for the Eve expressing DA1 muscle and its innervating aCC MN in the ISNb [91,181,182,186]. Eve indirectly modulates the MN expression of the Netrin repulsive presynaptic receptor Unc-5 in the ISNb [187] to guide MN axons. Upon MN contact, muscles start to accumulate Glutamate Receptor (GluR) at synaptic zones mediated by Disks large (Dlg) to form primitive synapses in an innervation dependent fashion [188,189]. By the end of stage 17, non-target synapses are pruned and mature synapses form, which exhibit a stereotyped morphology of boutons with active zones for vesicle release on the presynaptic end and novel synthesis and clustering of more GluR on the postsynaptic end [190]. Once NMJ formation is complete, muscles are ready to contract in a coordinated manner.

During larval stages, some MNs are remodeled and this is reflected in the larval CNS myotopic map [191]. Until the third larval instar, the NMJ grows by arborization and addition of boutons, a process that requires the gene *miles to go* (*mtgo*), which is an ortholog of mammalian *FNDC3* genes [192], and integrins [193]. There is also an activity dependent refinement of the synapse mediated by Ca^{2+} [194]. Tenurins, a conserved family of transmembrane proteins enriched in the vertebrate brain that possesses glutamatergic synapses are implicated in *Drosophila* axon guidance as well as synaptic organization and signaling with muscle specific expression [195].

As muscles form, abdominal adult muscle precursors (AMPs) arrange themselves in niches between specific peripheral nerves and muscles. They form an interconnected network connecting to each other and to the peripheral nerves by extending filopodia [196–198]. All embryonic muscle development processes finally lead to the formation of functional larval body wall muscles that closely communicate with the epidermis via the MTJ and with the nervous system via the NMJ to ensure larval locomotion.

3.2. Pupal Myogenesis of Adult Muscles

Adult muscles are generated during a second wave of myogenesis during pupal metamorphosis where most larval muscles are histolyzed. Metamorphosis marks the end of larval muscle homeostatic states. Adult flies have a pair of wings in the thoracic segment T2 and three pairs of legs in thoracic segments T1–T3, which are powered by specialized thoracic flight and appendicular muscles, respectively (figure in Table 2). Adult myogenesis has been reviewed recently in [199,200]. All adult thoracic muscles including the indirect flight muscles (IFMs), direct flight muscles (DFMs), and leg muscles possess a multi-fiber structure similar to vertebrate skeletal muscles. However, unlike heterogenous mammalian skeletal muscles with one muscle composed of slow and fast fiber types, each *Drosophila* muscle appears to have a single fiber type. IFMs are constituted of the dorsoventral muscles (DVMs) and the dorsal longitudinal muscles (DLMs), which facilitate upward and downward wing strokes respectively during flight. The muscle fibers that build the IFM and leg muscles differ in organization and morphology to adapt to different functionalities. The IFMs are fibrillar, asynchronous muscles while the tergal depressor of the trochanter (TDT) or leg jump muscles and DFM are tubular, synchronous muscles [201–203]. Similar to mammals, individual fiber types in the adult fly differ in component constitution such as expressing specific myosin heavy chain isoforms [203,204]. The generation of adult muscles is initiated by a series of coordinated processes again requiring close communication between tissues.

3.2.1. Myoblast Pool Generation by Adult Muscle Precursors (AMPs) during Larval Stages

Embryonic myogenesis sets the foundation for adult muscle development since the asymmetric divisions of embryonic muscle progenitor cells give rise to adult muscle precursors (AMPs) in addition to the embryonic muscle FCs. AMPs are Notch positive, Numb negative cells that remain quiescent with persistent Twist (Twi) expression until initial pupal stages when they get reactivated [205] and contribute to adult muscle development. Abdominal AMPs are closely associated with the larval muscles and with the peripheral nervous system (PNS) enabling crosstalk and providing positional cues to the AMPs that give rise to adult abdominal muscles [196–198]. In the thoracic segments, AMPs associate with wing and leg imaginal discs, which are epidermal cell clusters set aside in the embryo and larva and act as precursors for the future generation of adult wings and legs, respectively [206]. During the first and second instar larval stages, these AMPs undergo symmetric divisions giving rise to an imaginal disc associated monolayer of Twi and Notch positive adepithelial cells. In the abdominal segments, they proliferate while remaining associated with their muscle fibers similar to vertebrate satellite cells [207,208]. During the third larval instar, due to the activation of Wg signaling from the imaginal discs, AMPs undergo asymmetric divisions forming one stem cell and one Numb positive post-mitotic myoblast where Notch signaling is inhibited [209,210]. Thus, a large pool of myoblasts is primed for metamorphosis.

The myoblasts primed to form IFM express high levels of Vestigial (Vg), which represses Notch and promotes IFM differentiation [211], and low levels of the TF Cut (Ct) while DFM myoblasts express high Ct levels, with the levels being governed extrinsically by the ectoderm [212]. DFM myoblasts also express Lms [95]. The myoblasts associated with the leg imaginal disc on the other hand express Ladybird (Lb) similar to vertebrate limb bud myoblasts that express the Lb orthologue LBX1 [213,214], which represses Vg. Mutant *vg*, *ct*, *lms*, and *lb* flies have severely disrupted muscle pattern or function and they thus contribute to the adult muscle iTF code (Table 2). Vg, Lms, and Lb also act as embryonic somatic muscle iTFs expressed in a subset of embryonic muscles [86,94,95] (Table 1). Among embryonic myogenic factors, it was noticed that Apterous (Ap) expression defines all prospective flight muscle epidermal muscle attachment sites in the wing disc [215]. Similar to embryonic stages, Duf positive adult FC specification takes place by the third larval instar, but in contrast to embryos it is driven by Heartless (Htl) mediated Fibroblast growth factor (Fgf) signaling and Hox genes [212,214,216,217].

Table 2. The iTF expression patterns in myoblasts of adult muscles.

Adult iTF	Human Orthologs	Adult Myoblast Expression	Embryonic iTF Function [1]	References	Adult Flight and Leg Muscle Pattern
Vestigial (Vg)	VGLL	IFM	DA1-DA2, DA3, LL1, VL1, VL2, VL3, VL4	[211]	Indirect flight muscles (IFM) are shown in shades of red and the direct flight muscles (DFM) in dark brown. Among the leg muscles, only the tergal depressor of trochanter (TDT) muscles are highlighted in olive green. Other leg muscles are in a light shade of green.
Extradenticle (Exd)	PBX	IFM		[218]	
Homeothorax (Hth)	MEIS	IFM		[218]	
Spalt major (Salm)	SALL	IFM		[219]	
Erect wing (Ewg)	NRF1	IFM		[220]	
Cut (Ct)		DFM		[213,214]	
Lateral muscles scarcer (Lms)	–	DFM	LT1-LT2, LT3-LT4	[95]	
Apterous (Ap)	LHX	DFM	LT1, LT2, LT3, LT4, VA2, VA3	[215]	
Ladybird (Lb)	LBX	Leg muscles	SBM	[214]	

[1] In the 'Adult myoblast expression' column, names are shown in the colour corresponding to the muscles they generate as depicted in the figure in the column on the extreme right. Embryonic FCs known to be generated from an asymmetric division of the same progenitor cell are hyphenated.

3.2.2. Histolysis of Larval Muscles, Adult iTF Code Refinement, and the Contribution of AMPs

During pupal stages, most of the larval muscles are histolyzed in the thoracic as well as abdominal hemisegments [221,222]. Myoblasts generated from AMPs either fuse with non-histolyzed larval muscle scaffolds to which they associate or give rise to adult muscles de novo [221]. In the T2 mesothoracic segment, three larval dorsal oblique muscles, DO1, DO2, and DO3 escape histolysis and serve as templates for the formation of the DLMs while the DVMs and leg muscles are generated de novo. At the end of the third larval instar, the myoblasts start expressing the muscle differentiation factor Mef2 in an ecdysone dependent manner [123]. As with embryonic myogenesis, adult muscle formation is seeded by FCs, with the number of FCs generated corresponding to the number of muscles they will seed [217]. The DLMs are an exception where the three remnant larval muscles serve as FCs and express the marker Duf. Nevertheless, if the larval muscles giving rise to adult DLMs are ablated they still form muscles de novo by an innervation dependent process, although with aberrations [223].

During early pupal stages myoblasts start migrating. MNs play a significant role in initial adult myogenesis by regulating myoblast proliferation during the second larval instar and subsequent myoblast migration during pupal stages. In denervated flies, DVM muscle formation is severely compromised and it leads to the reduction in DLM size when using larval muscles as templates whereas if larval templates are ablated, their de novo formation is abolished [223]. In the abdominal segments, myoblasts migrate and associate with nerves to form adult muscles [224]. In the thoracic segments, the wing and leg discs evaginate and myoblasts migrate along them to reach their destinations where adult muscles are generated. The myoblasts either fuse with FCs or with larval templates using a similar machinery to embryonic myoblast fusion to form fully differentiated adult muscles by 36 h after puparium formation (APF). Muscles extend as they fuse and attach to the MTJ on either end [221,225,226].

Apart from Vg, Ct, and Lb that act as adult muscle iTFs (Table 2) to confer myoblast identity in the imaginal discs during larval stages, the expression of the embryonic iTF Ap is initiated during pupal stages in myoblasts that will give rise to the DFM but not IFM in addition to epidermal attachment sites [215]. Unlike the embryonic FCs, it is expressed in adult FCMs instead of adult FCs, but similar to the embryonic FCs they contribute to the same muscle's iTF code along with Lms. This hints at specific muscle patterning information derived from these iTFs. Ap is necessary for the correct formation of DFMs and continues to be expressed in fully formed DFMs. It is also necessary for IFM attachment by regulating Stripe (Sr) expression which, similar to the embryo, is essential for adult muscle attachment. In *lms* mutants, the wing disc Vg domain is expanded and although muscles seem normal, the adult wings exhibit a held-out phenotype suggesting contraction abnormalities [95]. As fusion begins, the IFM FCs also express the adult iTFs Extradenticle (Exd), Homeothorax (Hth), and Spalt major (Salm), which genetically interact to specify a fibrillar versus tubular fate by regulating fiber specific gene expression and splicing regulated by Arrest (Aret) [201,218,219]. The iTF Erect wing (Ewg) also significantly contributes to IFM identity [220].

3.2.3. MTJ Formation

The wing and leg imaginal discs generate Sr positive tendon-like precursor cell clusters starting from the third larval instar until the beginning of pupation. Sr expression is initiated by Notch signaling [227,228]. Leg muscles attach to the internal tendons on one end and the tendon cells in the exoskeleton on the other end. At about 3 h APF, the leg disc Sr positive tendon precursor cells invaginate into an evaginating leg disc and are closely associated with myoblasts that give rise to leg muscles [18]. Disrupting tendon precursors also disrupts myoblast localization. The epidermal tendon precursor cells' shape changes to form tubular structures during invagination giving rise to internal tendons to which each leg muscle attaches on one end with tendon specificity. DLM muscles that form by the splitting of remnant larval muscles extend filopodia on either end as they grow and split. Still in the process of splitting, their filopodia interdigitate with those of their target tendon cells and initiate MTJ formation that requires Kon, integrins, Tsp, and Talin similar to embryos. DLM filopodia disappear after a mature MTJ forms by 30 h APF and tendon cells elongate due to tension [163]. In the abdomen, MTJ maturation follows a similar process but is complete only by 40 h APF [229].

3.2.4. Sarcomere Assembly

Similar to embryos, premyofibrils are absent in DLM muscles. Mhc positive complexes are observed throughout the muscle by 26 h APF and assemble rapidly and synchronously across the entire muscle into myofibrils at 30 h APF immediately following tension generated by MTJ maturation [163,230]. This myofibril assembly fails in the absence of muscle attachment. The terminal Z-disc attaches to the MTJ mediated by integrins and IAPs [52]. Myofibrils are refined to regular arrays of sarcomeres over the next several hours where more sarcomeres are added. DLM myofibrils are flanked by MT arrays during initial stages of assembly that are dissembled by the end of pupation. The myofibril length then increases without other structural changes to reach its final length shortly after eclosion [231]. In the IFM, distinct transcriptional dynamics are associated with different stages of myofibrillogenesis, with the iTF Salm contributing to the transition after 30 h APF and its expression is maintained to establish IFM fate [230,232]. A similar sequence of myofibrillogenesis occurs in abdominal muscles that form mature MTJ by 50 h APF when myofibril assembly synchronously starts and is refined further to form the transversely aligned sarcomeres seen in abdominal muscles. Thin and thick filament complexes appear separately, then start interdigitating to form immature myofibrils by 46 h when muscles have stably attached to MTJ and exhibit spontaneous contractions. They subsequently assemble into ordered myofibrils by 50 h APF and are refined over the next several hours to begin coordinated contraction [229].

During IFM sarcomere assembly, thin filaments elongate from their pointed ends as is the case during embryonic myogenesis [170]. They initially form a dispersed pattern by the polymerization of actin into nascent thin filaments which become regularly patterned after 30 h APF. At this time, active incorporation of actin at both ends of the thin filament and further refinement and growth occurs by new actin monomer incorporation at the pointed ends of thin filaments and the formation of new thin filaments at the sarcomere periphery. Tmod and Sals that are located to pointed ends are necessary for thin filament length control [170,233]. The nebulin repeat containing protein Lasp regulates thin filament length by regulating its stability [234]. The *Drosophila* formin Fhos mediates thin filament assembly by initially regulating actin monomer incorporation into thin filaments during mid pupal stages and then localizes near Z-discs to facilitate radial growth of thin filament arrays to increase myofibril diameter [233]. In *Drosophila*, IFM thick filaments are associated with many insect-specific proteins such as myofilin [235], arthrin which is a ubiquitinated actin [236], paramyosin [237], minipramyosin [238], and flightin [239,240] not found in vertebrates, which could represent proteins adapted for flight [241]. The insect and IFM specific protein flightin is implicated in regulating the thick filament length by associating with myosin filaments as they grow [242,243]. Z-disc formation fails in the IFM if actin lacks its α-actinin binding domain showing the importance of sarcomere component interdigitation [244]. A downregulation of Sls results in smaller Z-discs around which a normal thick filament assembly occurs with abnormally long thick filaments at the periphery lacking the Z-disc [164,245]. As myofibrils grow, the Z-disc protein Zasp controls the final myofibril diameter by switching to growth restricting isoforms [246]. After complete myofibril growth, coordinated contractions can be initiated after mature NMJ formation.

3.2.5. Innervation and NMJ Formation

Embryonic neuroblast lineages undergo a second larval wave of neurogenesis where embryonic neuroblasts are re-specified to give rise to adult MN lineages whose dendrites are organized in a 'myotopic map' within the CNS that reflects the innervation pattern of their target adult muscles similar to embryonic/larval stages [247–250]. MNs innervate adult muscles in a stereotypical pattern. For DLMs generated from larval templates, the primary larval ISN branch remains while secondary branches are initially retracted, and extensive new branching is generated as the muscles fuse with adult myoblasts and then split. Initial nerve arrival is muscle independent, but subsequent nerve branching occurs only in the presence of the target muscle [251]. Among DVMs, DVM I and DVM II are innervated by new branches arising from the larval ISN while the larval SN innervates DVM III [251,252]. The 14 leg muscles are innervated by around 50 MNs arising from specific neuroblasts in the CNS in a stereotypical pattern [250]. Following initial innervation, the NMJ is formed by extensive branching and synapse formation. The glial cells at the IFM NMJ express the glutamate *Drosophila* Excitatory Amino Acid Transporter 1 (dEAAT1) unlike during other stages for efficient neurotransmission [253]. Muscle iTFs contribute to correct innervation since malformed muscles cause MN branching aberrations as has been shown for Ewg [220].

In the end, a stereotypical muscle pattern along with stereotypical innervation generates fully functional adult muscles.

3.2.6. Programmed Cell Death Following Eclosion of New Adults

Some larval abdominal muscles persist through metamorphosis and are used for the eclosion of new adults. These muscles degenerate after eclosion along with associated nerves [254].

4. The Maintenance of Muscle Homeostasis

4.1. Muscle Homeostasis under Normal Conditions

Functional larval somatic muscles and adult muscles represent two different homeostatic states during the fly lifetime. The embryonic wave of myogenesis takes only one day leading to the formation of functional larval muscles, which undergo continuous growth and refinement during the larval stages spanning five days. Larval muscle homeostasis needs to be coordinated with larval growth during the three larval instars until metamorphosis to ensure functional stability. Following metamorphosis and the pupal wave of myogenesis over a period of five days, adult flies eclose from their pupae and adult muscle homeostasis needs to be maintained during the fly lifespan of several weeks.

The stereotypical muscle pattern is associated with iTFs and their realisator genes that also exhibit tightly controlled spatial and temporal expression patterns in larval and adult muscles. Therefore, some of the iTFs can play a key role in the maintenance of muscle specific homeostasis by regulating the levels of key myogenic factors such as Mef2 as well as the expression of realisator genes [111,112,129,137] (Figure 2). The control of the level of activity of the key differentiation TF Mef2 is quintessential throughout the fly lifetime since this in turn controls the muscle specific levels of its vast array of target genes [118,129]. In the embryo, various genes were shown to require different Mef2 activity, with early expressing genes such as *Act57B* requiring lower levels compared to late expressing genes such as *Mhc* [118]. In the adult, the development and maintenance of the adult DLM muscles have been observed to be sensitive to the levels of Mef2 as well as its antagonist Holes in muscles (Him). Tubular adult muscles such as the TDT and DVM muscles seem to require lower Mef2 activity than the fibrillar DLM muscles since RNAi lines affect these muscles differently [255,256]. TFs such as Cf2 and E2f1 acting along with Mef2 could also contribute to setting the muscle homeostatic state [122,167]. A study identified putative Cf2 and Mef2 binding site clusters for multiple sarcomeric genes including *Mhc, Tm1, Tm2, up, wupA* (or *TnI*), and *paramyosin* (*Prm*) [122]. On Cf2 depletion, the stoichiometry of proteins such as TnT, TnI, and Prm was found to be altered and this imbalance worsened over the course of development. Another study detected E2f binding site enrichment upstream of myogenic genes such as *how, sals, Tm1, Mef2,* etc. This study also showed that E2f1 depletion altered the gene expression levels of *Tm2, Act88F, Mlc2, how,* and *Mef2* [167].

One hallmark of muscle homeostasis in *Drosophila* larval and adult muscles is the expression of fiber specific protein isoforms. Many sarcomeric genes switch between embryonic, larval, and/or adult isoforms during development, with different muscle types also exhibiting isoform specificity. Isoform switching usually occurs by switching to a predominant isoform. Embryonic *Mhc* transcripts contain exon 19, which is spliced out of adult versions and results in a different carboxy terminal [242,257]. Embryonic isoforms lack the functionality for the high ATPase rate and sliding velocity required for adult muscles [258]. The IFM muscles initially express an Mhc isoform containing exon 19 and switch to the adult exon 18 containing isoform during late stages of myofibril assembly [242]. A shorter embryonic/larval isoform of the pointed end capping protein Tmod is associated with actin during pupal sarcomere assembly and there is a switch to a longer Tmod isoform in eclosed adults [170]. Adult *Drosophila* muscles express fiber specific actins, with Act88F being expressed in the IFM and Act79B in the TDT, for example [202]. Two IFM specific Tm1 isoforms are expressed in adult flies [259,260]. Kettin is the predominant *Drosophila* titin isoform in embryos and the IFM muscles switch to the IFM specific predominant long Sls(700) isoform [245]. Zasp52 and other Zasp proteins also switch to adult isoforms [246,261], with Zasp52 expressing an exon 8 containing isoform absent in embryos, but present in the IFM and TDT. Obscurin expresses a single larval isoform and two IFM isoforms [262].

Isoform switches are potentially associated with cis regulatory modules (CRMs) that seem to be arranged in sequential modules mirroring developmental expression and regulation by different TFs and cofactors. Marin et al. identified an upstream regulatory element (URE) and an intronic regulatory element (IRE) in intron 1 of the *wupA* (or *TnI*) gene that acted synergistically and was capable of driving LacZ tagged TnI expression. Mas et al. identified similar elements in the *up* (or *TnT*) gene [263]. They showed that these elements synergistically interact in larval muscles, whereas the contribution of the IRE is higher in adult muscles. In addition, they showed that there was decreasing IRE contribution from the IFM to the jump muscles to the visceral muscles [264]. Garcia-Zaragoza et al. followed up on this study and identified the URE and potential IRE elements of *Tm1*, *Tm2*, and *Mhc*. *Tm1* was previously shown to be coordinately regulated by two intronic enhancers in cooperation with Mef2 and its interactor PAR domain protein 1 (Pdp1) [265–267]. Mature muscles need to ensure the activation and maintenance of the correct protein isoforms [268] since aberrant isoform expression impedes muscle function. For example, transient overexpression of a shorter Tmod isoform during mid-to late IFM assembly leads to normal length thin filaments at the periphery of the myofibrils that are correctly capped by the long Tmod isoform. However, they exhibit shorter core thin filaments within the myofibril caused by the permanent association of the shorter Tmod at their pointed ends, which cannot be dynamically uncapped to permit thin filament elongation. Therefore, this prevents its elongation causing defective sarcomeres that interfere with flight during adult stages [170]. The embryonic Mhc isoform fails to substitute for the IFM isoform due to different physiological properties [258,269].

Post transcriptional mechanisms such as phosphorylation could potentially contribute to muscle homeostasis. Thin and thick filament disruptions, for example, are associated with concomitant flightin phosphorylation deregulations [239]. Tm1 IFM isoforms are phosphorylated only in adult flies, which could have functional implications [260]. Impaired Talin phosphorylation leads to severe muscle detachment at late embryonic stages [154]. This means the right CRM regulatory mechanisms as well as post translational mechanisms such as phosphorylation [48,270] need to be dynamically maintained since specific protein domains are necessary for muscle specific functionality [269,271,272].

The accumulation of insoluble protein aggregates in the muscle is associated with protein aggregate myopathies (PAM) and in *Drosophila*, p38b deficiency leads to the deposition of polyubiquitinated protein aggregates in adult thoracic muscles and to locomotor defects [273]. Loss of components of the proteasome, which mediate protein turnover were shown to cause protein aggregates and progressive muscle atrophy in larval muscles [274]. Ubiquitin protein ligases such as Mind bomb 2 (Mib2) and Ubiquitin protein ligase E3A (Ube3A), which tag proteins for proteasomal degradation, have been associated with muscle defects. The loss of function of *mib2* was shown to trigger embryonic muscle apoptosis [275] and the over or under expression of *Ube3a* alters larval NMJ neurotransmission with associated altered number of active zones [276]. Proteostasis is thus integral to muscle maintenance.

Muscle contraction is associated with multiple biochemical and morphological changes as well as large mechanical strains. This necessitates efficient mechanisms to withstand these forces to prevent muscle disintegration during contraction and to reinstate the stable muscle state (Figure 3). Protein stoichiometry is integral to sarcomere integrity since varying the expression levels of one protein has a cascading effect on the levels of other sarcomeric proteins leading to altered muscle functionality [277,278]. Sarcomeric integrity during contractions is maintained by components such as Mlp84B, Cher, small heat shock proteins (sHsps) such as dCryAB and Hsp67Bc and integrin-mediated adhesions. Mlp84B localizes to the Z-disc and genetically interacts with Sls. Mlp84B-Sls transheterozygotes exacerbate individual mutant phenotypes disrupting myofibrillar integrity [56]. Cher also interacts with Sls in addition to actin stably anchoring them to each other [53]. In addition, Cher interacts physically with dCryAB and a disruption of this interaction affects sarcomeric integrity [279]. The chaperone Hsp67Bc also colocalizes to the Z-disc although its function is unknown [280]. Integrin mediated adhesions maintain sarcomeric integrity and reduced adhesion results in the progressive age-dependent loss of sarcomeric cytoarchitecture [57]. Integrin and IAP stoichiometries at the MTJ are important to respond to different types of forces [166]. The myonuclear LINC complex and associated components such as Msp300 and Spectraplakin, which regulate MT organization, play a role in myonuclear maintenance by providing elasticity to resist contractile forces with the help of the MT network that surrounds it [281–283]. In addition, Msp300 associates with the Z-disc and keeps the mitochondria and SR anchored to the Z-disc during contractions [284]. Its presence around myonuclei near the larval NMJ also regulates glutamate receptor density to control locomotion [285].

NMJ activity perturbations lead to homeostatic synaptic plasticity, which enables compensatory modulations of the NMJ synaptic strength to resist these perturbations and stabilize synaptic activity. Lifelong synaptic plasticity ensures efficient neurotransmission of signals at the NMJ. The NMJ adapts various homeostatic mechanisms to maintain appropriate muscle function levels [286–289]. Mutants for *endophilin* (*endo*) exhibit tremendous synaptic overgrowth, but the overall synaptic strength is stabilized by reducing the active zone number in synaptic buttons, which modulates neurotransmitter release [286]. The NMJ adapts a homeostatic scaling mechanism called presynaptic homeostatic potentiation (PHP), where there is a compensatory increase in neurotransmitter release to maintain muscle excitation in response to abnormally reduced GluR on the postsynaptic end. This compensation appears to be associated with an uncharacteristic multilayer ring of electron dense T-bars in active zones to increase the neurotransmitter release [289]. The PHP maintenance has been shown to require inositol triphosphate (IP$_3$) directed signaling [290]. During the larval growth spurt, NMJ homeostasis needs to be maintained even though the presynaptic end grows slower than the muscle surface that tends to accumulate GluRs. Ziegler et al. showed that the amino acid transporter, Juvenile hormone Inducible-21 (JhI-21) is a gene that coevolved with GluRs, is expressed at presynaptic ends and plays a role in suppressing excess GluR accumulation [288].

The close association of the mesoderm with other germ layers right from the embryonic stage and the continued association with epidermal and nervous tissues over the fly lifetime highlights the importance of coordinated intrinsic and extrinsic signaling for homeostasis.

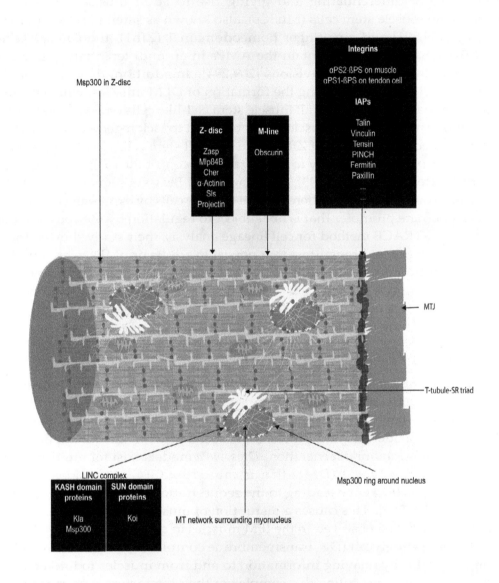

Figure 3. Maintenance of myofibril integrity and homeostasis. The integrin complex links the myofibrils to the MTJ via the extracellular matrix (ECM) and senses the forces transmitted by the MTJ. Integrins and Integrin Associated Proteins (IAPs) constitute the integrin complex. Integrin complex turnover and constitution are adapted to the forces sensed during contraction. The dense microtubule (MT) network anchored to the myonuclei by the Msp300 ring associated with the LINC complex on the nuclear envelope provides myonuclear elasticity during contractions to prevent disintegration of myonuclei and dissociation of the myofibril network. Msp300 in the Z-disc ensure regular spacing of organelles such as mitochondria and the SR for contractions. Z-disc and M-line components provide anchorage and elasticity to ensure sarcomeric integrity.

4.2. Re-Establishment of Muscle Homeostasis Following Muscle Injury

Muscle regeneration has not been described in the larva. However, the larval stem cell-like AMPs that are capable of differentiating and giving rise to adult muscles were noted to have similarities to vertebrate muscle stem cells (MuSCs), also known as satellite cells. Similar to MuSCs, the Notch pathway [209,291] and zinc-finger homeodomain 1 (Zfh1), the *Drosophila* homolog of the vertebrate ZEB1/ZEB2 [292,293], maintain the AMPs in an undifferentiated state and they are capable of self-renewal by asymmetric divisions [209,294]. In addition, they are capable of fusion with existing larval muscle remnants during the formation of DLM muscles, which is reminiscent of muscle repair. It was initially thought that all muscle stem cell-like cells or AMPs are depleted during adult muscle formation and thus adult muscles were believed to lack regenerative capacity. Recently, Chaturvedi et al. identified a population of Zfh1 positive adult stem cells closely apposed to the adult muscle, which appear to possess the ability to proliferate and contribute to muscle regeneration upon injury [61] similar to vertebrate MuSCs [293]. Boukhatmi and Bray subsequently showed that Notch directly regulates Zfh1 to antagonize the differentiation of these cells by expressing a short Zfh1 isoform transcribed from an alternate promoter that is not subject to regulation by the conserved micro RNA, miR-8 [292]. Using the G-TRACE method for cell lineage analysis, their study showed that these cells, which they termed population of progenitors that persist in adults or pMPs, were mitotically active and incorporated into adult muscles even under normal conditions. Thus, they reiterated that these cells contributed to adult muscle homeostasis. Since this is a recent discovery, further studies could provide insights into the extent of repair in *Drosophila* adult muscles and the mechanisms involved in re-establishing and maintaining muscle identity and homeostasis.

4.3. Muscle Homeostasis under Pathological Conditions

Multiple studies in *Drosophila* models have reproduced defects observed in human pathological conditions and could provide important insights into disruptions of muscle homeostasis under pathological conditions. Many myopathies and neuromuscular disorders are associated with or even caused by myonuclear defects and others are associated with sarcomeric defects leading to muscle dysfunction, wasting, and/or degeneration. *Drosophila* models exist for multisystemic disorders such as Myotonic Dystrophy Type 1 (DM1) that is caused by CTG expansions in the *Dystrophia Myotonica Protein Kinase (DMPK)* gene leading to the sequestration of RNA binding proteins such as MBNL1 in nuclear foci [295,296]. This causes a disruption of muscle homeostasis as indicated by the progressive muscle degeneration observed in the IFM muscles in a model expressing 480 CTG repeats. The Dystrophin (Dys)-Dystroglycan (Dg) transmembrane complex at the plasma membrane acts as a crucial signaling mediator by relaying information to and from muscles to interacting tissues via the ECM. Mutations in genes constituting this complex or their interactors thus cause a disruption of homeostasis, thereby causing diseases such as Duchenne Muscular Dystrophy (DMD) where there is muscle wasting. In *Drosophila*, *Dg* was shown to be under miRNA regulation by miR-9a to ensure correct MTJ formation [297]. Large scale genetic and interactome screens in *Drosophila* have identified factors affecting muscle integrity such as stress response components [298] and components of the Hippo signaling pathway [42].

Laminopathies are disorders caused by mutations in the human *LMNA* genes which code for lamins present in the INM providing structural support and regulating gene expression. One *Drosophila* model revealed increased reductive stress due to the nuclear translocation of Nrf2, which is normally sequestered in the cytoplasm and released only during oxidative stress [299]. Chandran et al. observed a loss of muscle proteostasis in a *Drosophila* model of laminopathies and corroborated this by RNA-seq analyses of human muscle biopsy tissues. Interestingly, they were able to rescue the muscular phenotypes by the modulation of the AMPK pathway which could present future therapeutic directions [300]. Apart from laminopathies, other myopathies such as Centronuclear Myopathies (CNM) are associated with myonuclear positioning defects [301]. Muscle development studies in

Drosophila are beginning to unveil mechanisms for myonuclear positioning and factors that disrupt this [141,284,302,303].

Other studies in *Drosophila* are providing insights into pathological features caused by disruptions in sarcomeric components. Muscular phenotypes caused by a mutation in the *Tm2* gene was found to be rescued by a suppressor mutation in the *wupA* gene coding for TnI [304]. *Drosophila* models exist for myosin myopathies such as Inclusion Body Myopathy Type 3 and Laing Distal Myopathy (LDM). A study has shown that the formation of large aggregates in muscles similar to those seen in human patients with *ZASP* mutations is caused by an imbalance in the levels of Zasp isoforms [246]. Dahl-Halvarsson et al. showed that the overexpression of the Thin protein, a homolog of the human TRIM family of proteins that is implicated in maintaining sarcomeric integrity, could alleviate LDM-like phenotypes [305].

5. Discussion

In vertebrates, the loss of skeletal muscle homeostasis is the cause of various muscular disorders. Studies in vertebrate systems are complicated by the presence of large gene families for multiple genes. *Drosophila* is a simple model organism with various conserved pathways and genes to study muscle homeostasis while at the same time mostly having one to a few genes orthologous to large vertebrate gene families that perform functions similar to vertebrate genes. Thus, it appears that genes are reused/repurposed over the course of evolution instead of 'reinventing the wheel'. *Drosophila* muscle development has been studied for decades. The embryonic somatic muscles being uni-fiber muscles present a simple model to study development since all muscles have been well characterized along with their specific attachment sites and innervating MNs [143,180]. The IFM muscles have been equally well characterized [31,221,252]. In addition, a large number of tools are available in *Drosophila* to study in vivo mechanisms [306].

A better understanding of developmental and post developmental processes would help us gain a better understanding of the mechanisms of maintenance and disruption of homeostasis. The short life cycle of the fruit fly facilitates the quick and detailed study of processes making it a valuable model for the study of factors that initiate, maintain, and disrupt muscle homeostasis. The study of muscle regeneration following muscle injury, where developmental processes need to be re-initiated, represents an example of how the *Drosophila* model could help understand the mechanisms of muscle homeostasis. Some potential therapeutic targets have been unveiled by studies in *Drosophila* models of myopathies [300,305]. The recent discovery of stem cell-like cells associated with adult muscles is an exciting new direction of research to study muscle regeneration and homeostasis [61]. In vertebrates, aging is related to a depletion of the MuSC population leading to sarcopenia or age-related gradual loss of muscle mass and function [307] that is also characteristic of pathological conditions such as DMD [308]. The short life span of the *Drosophila* model presents a huge advantage to study homeostatic disruptions during aging.

Large gaps exist in our understanding of pathological mechanisms and simpler models could provide valuable insights and therapeutic directions. In *Drosophila*, although a lot of attention has been given to the major muscle components including the sarcomeres, MTJ and NMJ, muscle organelles that play an equally central role such as the SR, T-tubules, golgi complex, and transport vesicles have received lesser attention, although myonuclei are beginning to be studied in detail. Given the detailed characterization and tools available for this established model system that has already helped advance research [309,310], it would continue to serve as an important backbone for research into various physiological processes including muscle development and homeostasis.

Author Contributions: Conceptualization, P.P.; writing—original draft preparation, P.P.; writing—review and editing, P.P. and K.J.; visualization, P.P.; supervision, K.J. All authors have read and agreed to the published version of the manuscript.

References

1. Bate, M. The embryonic development of larval muscles in Drosophila. *Development* **1990**, *110*, 791. [PubMed]
2. Abmayr, S.M.; Erickson, M.S.; Bour, B.A. Embryonic development of the larval body wall musculature of Drosophila melanogaster. *Trends Genet.* **1995**, *11*, 153–159. [CrossRef]
3. Fyrberg, E. Study of contractile and cytoskeletal proteins using Drosophila genetics. *Cell Motil. Cytoskelet.* **1989**, *14*, 118–127. [CrossRef]
4. Dobi, K.C.; Schulman, V.K.; Baylies, M.K. Specification of the somatic musculature in Drosophila. *Wiley Interdiscip. Rev. Dev. Biol.* **2015**, *4*, 357–375. [CrossRef]
5. Mukund, K.; Subramaniam, S. Skeletal muscle: A review of molecular structure and function, in health and disease. *Wiley Interdiscip. Rev. Syst. Biol. Med.* **2020**, *12*, e1462. [CrossRef] [PubMed]
6. Taylor, M. Comparison of muscle development in Drosophila and vertebrates. In *Muscle development in Drosophila*; Sink, H., Ed.; Landes Bioscience/Springer: Georgetown, TX, USA; New York, NY, USA, 2006; pp. 169–203.
7. Piccirillo, R.; Demontis, F.; Perrimon, N.; Goldberg, A.L. Mechanisms of muscle growth and atrophy in mammals and Drosophila. *Dev. Dyn. Off. Publ. Am. Assoc. Anat.* **2014**, *243*, 201–215. [CrossRef]
8. Kohsaka, H.; Guertin, P.A.; Nose, A. Neural Circuits Underlying Fly Larval Locomotion. *Curr. Pharm. Des.* **2017**, *23*, 1722–1733. [CrossRef]
9. Wolfe, R.R. The underappreciated role of muscle in health and disease. *Am. J. Clin. Nutr.* **2006**, *84*, 475–482. [CrossRef]
10. Veratti, E. Investigations on the fine structure of striated muscle fiber read before the Reale Istituto Lombardo, 13 March 1902. *J. Biophys. Biochem. Cytol.* **1961**, *10*, 1–59. [CrossRef]
11. Hanson, J.; Huxley, H.E. Structural Basis of the Cross-Striations in Muscle. *Nature* **1953**, *172*, 530–532. [CrossRef]
12. Royuela, M.; Fraile, B.; Arenas, M.I.; Paniagua, R. Characterization of several invertebrate muscle cell types: A comparison with vertebrate muscles. *Microsc. Res. Tech.* **2000**, *48*, 107–115. [CrossRef]
13. Littlefield, R.S.; Fowler, V.M. Thin filament length regulation in striated muscle sarcomeres: Pointed-end dynamics go beyond a nebulin ruler. *Semin. Cell Dev. Biol.* **2008**, *19*, 511–519. [CrossRef] [PubMed]
14. Lemke, S.B.; Schnorrer, F. Mechanical forces during muscle development. *Mech. Dev.* **2017**, *144*, 92–101. [CrossRef] [PubMed]
15. Wang, L.; Geist, J.; Grogan, A.; Hu, L.-Y.R.; Kontrogianni-Konstantopoulos, A. Thick Filament Protein Network, Functions, and Disease Association. *Compr. Physiol.* **2018**, *8*, 631–709. [CrossRef] [PubMed]
16. Hooper, S.L.; Thuma, J.B. Invertebrate Muscles: Muscle Specific Genes and Proteins. *Physiol. Rev.* **2005**, *85*, 1001–1060. [CrossRef] [PubMed]
17. Schweitzer, R.; Zelzer, E.; Volk, T. Connecting muscles to tendons: Tendons and musculoskeletal development in flies and vertebrates. *Dev. Camb. Engl.* **2010**, *137*, 2807–2817. [CrossRef]
18. Soler, C.; Laddada, L.; Jagla, K. Coordinated Development of Muscles and Tendon-Like Structures: Early Interactions in the Drosophila Leg. *Front. Physiol.* **2016**, *7*, 22. [CrossRef]
19. Lemke, S.B.; Weidemann, T.; Cost, A.-L.; Grashoff, C.; Schnorrer, F. A small proportion of Talin molecules transmit forces at developing muscle attachments in vivo. *PLoS Biol.* **2019**, *17*, e3000057. [CrossRef]
20. Richier, B.; Inoue, Y.; Dobramysl, U.; Friedlander, J.; Brown, N.H.; Gallop, J.L. Integrin signaling downregulates filopodia during muscle-tendon attachment. *J. Cell Sci.* **2018**, *131*, jcs217133. [CrossRef]
21. Nawrotzki, R.; Willem, M.; Miosge, N.; Brinkmeier, H.; Mayer, U. Defective integrin switch and matrix composition at alpha 7-deficient myotendinous junctions precede the onset of muscular dystrophy in mice. *Hum. Mol. Genet.* **2003**, *12*, 483–495. [CrossRef]
22. Marshall, J.L.; Chou, E.; Oh, J.; Kwok, A.; Burkin, D.J.; Crosbie-Watson, R.H. Dystrophin and utrophin expression require sarcospan: Loss of α7 integrin exacerbates a newly discovered muscle phenotype in sarcospan-null mice. *Hum. Mol. Genet.* **2012**, *21*, 4378–4393. [CrossRef] [PubMed]
23. Broadie, K.; Bate, M. The Drosophila NMJ: A genetic model system for synapse formation and function. *Semin. Dev. Biol.* **1995**, *6*, 221–231. [CrossRef]
24. Menon, K.P.; Carrillo, R.A.; Zinn, K. Development and plasticity of the Drosophila larval neuromuscular junction. *WIREs Dev. Biol.* **2013**, *2*, 647–670. [CrossRef] [PubMed]

25. Harris, K.P.; Littleton, J.T. Transmission, Development, and Plasticity of Synapses. *Genetics* **2015**, *201*, 345–375. [CrossRef]

26. Lacin, H.; Truman, J.W. Lineage mapping identifies molecular and architectural similarities between the larval and adult Drosophila central nervous system. *eLife* **2016**, *5*, e13399. [CrossRef]

27. Pérez-Moreno, J.J.; O'Kane, C.J. GAL4 Drivers Specific for Type Ib and Type Is Motor Neurons in Drosophila. *G3 Genes Genomes Genet.* **2019**, *9*, 453. [CrossRef]

28. Dasari, S.; Cooper, R.L. Modulation of sensory–CNS–motor circuits by serotonin, octopamine, and dopamine in semi-intact Drosophila larva. *Neurosci. Res.* **2004**, *48*, 221–227. [CrossRef]

29. Kohsaka, H.; Takasu, E.; Morimoto, T.; Nose, A. A Group of Segmental Premotor Interneurons Regulates the Speed of Axial Locomotion in Drosophila Larvae. *Curr. Biol.* **2014**, *24*, 2632–2642. [CrossRef]

30. Babski, H.; Jovanic, T.; Surel, C.; Yoshikawa, S.; Zwart, M.F.; Valmier, J.; Thomas, J.B.; Enriquez, J.; Carroll, P.; Garcès, A. A GABAergic Maf-expressing interneuron subset regulates the speed of locomotion in Drosophila. *Nat. Commun.* **2019**, *10*, 4796. [CrossRef]

31. Vigoreaux, J.O. Genetics of the Drosophila flight muscle myofibril: A window into the biology of complex systems. *BioEssays* **2001**, *23*, 1047–1063. [CrossRef]

32. Campbell, K.B.; Chandra, M. Functions of stretch activation in heart muscle. *J. Gen. Physiol.* **2006**, *127*, 89–94. [CrossRef] [PubMed]

33. Huxley, H.E. Fifty years of muscle and the sliding filament hypothesis. *Eur. J. Biochem.* **2004**, *271*, 1403–1415. [CrossRef] [PubMed]

34. Wang, Z.-H.; Clark, C.; Geisbrecht, E.R. Analysis of mitochondrial structure and function in the Drosophila larval musculature. *Mitochondrion* **2016**, *26*, 33–42. [CrossRef] [PubMed]

35. Auld, A.L.; Folker, E.S. Nucleus-dependent sarcomere assembly is mediated by the LINC complex. *Mol. Biol. Cell* **2016**, *27*, 2351–2359. [CrossRef] [PubMed]

36. Al-Qusairi, L.; Laporte, J. T-tubule biogenesis and triad formation in skeletal muscle and implication in human diseases. *Skelet. Muscle* **2011**, *1*, 26. [CrossRef]

37. Razzaq, A.; Robinson, I.M.; McMahon, H.T.; Skepper, J.N.; Su, Y.; Zelhof, A.C.; Jackson, A.P.; Gay, N.J.; O'Kane, C.J. Amphiphysin is necessary for organization of the excitation-contraction coupling machinery of muscles, but not for synaptic vesicle endocytosis in Drosophila. *Genes Dev.* **2001**, *15*, 2967–2979. [CrossRef]

38. Ackermann, M.A.; Ziman, A.P.; Strong, J.; Zhang, Y.; Hartford, A.K.; Ward, C.W.; Randall, W.R.; Kontrogianni-Konstantopoulos, A.; Bloch, R.J. Integrity of the network sarcoplasmic reticulum in skeletal muscle requires small ankyrin 1. *J. Cell Sci.* **2011**, *124*, 3619–3630. [CrossRef]

39. Maughan, D.W.; Godt, R.E. Equilibrium distribution of ions in a muscle fiber. *Biophys. J.* **1989**, *56*, 717–722. [CrossRef]

40. Clausen, T. Na$^+$-K$^+$ Pump Stimulation Improves Contractility in Damaged Muscle Fibers. *Ann. N. Y. Acad. Sci.* **2006**, *1066*, 286–294. [CrossRef]

41. Lebovitz, R.M.; Takeyasu, K.; Fambrough, D.M. Molecular characterization and expression of the (Na$^+$ + K$^+$)-ATPase alpha-subunit in Drosophila melanogaster. *EMBO J.* **1989**, *8*, 193–202. [CrossRef]

42. Yatsenko, A.S.; Kucherenko, M.M.; Xie, Y.; Aweida, D.; Urlaub, H.; Scheibe, R.J.; Cohen, S.; Shcherbata, H.R. Profiling of the muscle-specific dystroglycan interactome reveals the role of Hippo signaling in muscular dystrophy and age-dependent muscle atrophy. *BMC Med.* **2020**, *18*, 8. [CrossRef] [PubMed]

43. Huxley, H.; Hanson, J. Changes in the Cross-Striations of Muscle during Contraction and Stretch and their Structural Interpretation. *Nature* **1954**, *173*, 973–976. [CrossRef]

44. Huxley, A.F.; Niedergerke, R. Structural Changes in Muscle During Contraction: Interference Microscopy of Living Muscle Fibres. *Nature* **1954**, *173*, 971–973. [CrossRef] [PubMed]

45. Potter, J.D.; Sheng, Z.; Pan, B.-S.; Zhao, J. A Direct Regulatory Role for Troponin T and a Dual Role for Troponin C in the Ca^{2+} Regulation of Muscle Contraction. *J. Biol. Chem.* **1995**, *270*, 2557–2562. [CrossRef] [PubMed]

46. Qiu, F.; Lakey, A.; Agianian, B.; Hutchings, A.; Butcher, G.W.; Labeit, S.; Leonard, K.; Bullard, B. Troponin C in different insect muscle types: Identification of two isoforms in Lethocerus, Drosophila and Anopheles that are specific to asynchronous flight muscle in the adult insect. *Biochem. J.* **2003**, *371*, 811–821. [CrossRef] [PubMed]

47. Vibert, P.; Craig, R.; Lehman, W. Steric-model for activation of muscle thin filaments 1 1 Edited by P.E. Wright. *J. Mol. Biol.* **1997**, *266*, 8–14. [CrossRef]

48. Farman, G.P.; Miller, M.S.; Reedy, M.C.; Soto-Adames, F.N.; Vigoreaux, J.O.; Maughan, D.W.; Irving, T.C. Phosphorylation and the N-terminal extension of the regulatory light chain help orient and align the myosin heads in Drosophila flight muscle. *J. Struct. Biol.* **2009**, *168*, 240–249. [CrossRef]

49. Beall, C.J.; Fyrberg, E. Muscle abnormalities in Drosophila melanogaster heldup mutants are caused by missing or aberrant troponin-I isoforms. *J. Cell Biol.* **1991**, *114*, 941–951. [CrossRef]

50. Lee, K.H.; Sulbarán, G.; Yang, S.; Mun, J.Y.; Alamo, L.; Pinto, A.; Sato, O.; Ikebe, M.; Liu, X.; Korn, E.D.; et al. Interacting-heads motif has been conserved as a mechanism of myosin II inhibition since before the origin of animals. *Proc. Natl. Acad. Sci. USA* **2018**, *115*, E1991–E2000. [CrossRef]

51. Jung, H.S.; Komatsu, S.; Ikebe, M.; Craig, R. Head-head and head-tail interaction: A general mechanism for switching off myosin II activity in cells. *Mol. Biol. Cell* **2008**, *19*, 3234–3242. [CrossRef]

52. Green, H.J.; Griffiths, A.G.; Ylänne, J.; Brown, N.H. Novel functions for integrin-associated proteins revealed by analysis of myofibril attachment in Drosophila. *eLife* **2018**, *7*, e35783. [CrossRef] [PubMed]

53. González-Morales, N.; Holenka, T.K.; Schöck, F. Filamin actin-binding and titin-binding fulfill distinct functions in Z-disc cohesion. *PLoS Genet.* **2017**, *13*, e1006880. [CrossRef] [PubMed]

54. Liao, K.A.; González-Morales, N.; Schöck, F. Zasp52, a Core Z-disc Protein in Drosophila Indirect Flight Muscles, Interacts with α-Actinin via an Extended PDZ Domain. *PLoS Genet.* **2016**, *12*, e1006400. [CrossRef] [PubMed]

55. Katzemich, A.; West, R.J.H.; Fukuzawa, A.; Sweeney, S.T.; Gautel, M.; Sparrow, J.; Bullard, B. Binding partners of the kinase domains in Drosophila obscurin and their effect on the structure of the flight muscle. *J. Cell Sci.* **2015**, *128*, 3386–3397. [CrossRef] [PubMed]

56. Clark, K.A.; Bland, J.M.; Beckerle, M.C. The Drosophila muscle LIM protein, Mlp84B, cooperates with D-titin to maintain muscle structural integrity. *J. Cell Sci.* **2007**, *120*, 2066. [CrossRef] [PubMed]

57. Perkins, A.D.; Ellis, S.J.; Asghari, P.; Shamsian, A.; Moore, E.D.W.; Tanentzapf, G. Integrin-mediated adhesion maintains sarcomeric integrity. *Dev. Biol.* **2010**, *338*, 15–27. [CrossRef]

58. Prill, K.; Dawson, J.F. Assembly and Maintenance of Sarcomere Thin Filaments and Associated Diseases. *Int. J. Mol. Sci.* **2020**, *21*, 542. [CrossRef]

59. Ciglar, L.; Furlong, E.E. Conservation and divergence in developmental networks: A view from Drosophila myogenesis. *Cell Differ. Cell Div. Growth Death* **2009**, *21*, 754–760. [CrossRef]

60. Karalaki, M.; Fili, S.; Philippou, A.; Koutsilieris, M. Muscle regeneration: Cellular and molecular events. *Vivo Athens Greece* **2009**, *23*, 779–796.

61. Chaturvedi, D.; Reichert, H.; Gunage, R.D.; VijayRaghavan, K. Identification and functional characterization of muscle satellite cells in Drosophila. *eLife* **2017**, *6*, e30107. [CrossRef]

62. Demontis, F.; Perrimon, N. Integration of Insulin receptor/Foxo signaling and dMyc activity during muscle growth regulates body size in Drosophila. *Dev. Camb. Engl.* **2009**, *136*, 983–993. [CrossRef] [PubMed]

63. Xiao, G.; Mao, S.; Baumgarten, G.; Serrano, J.; Jordan, M.C.; Roos, K.P.; Fishbein, M.C.; MacLellan, W.R. Inducible activation of c-Myc in adult myocardium in vivo provokes cardiac myocyte hypertrophy and reactivation of DNA synthesis. *Circ. Res.* **2001**, *89*, 1122–1129. [CrossRef] [PubMed]

64. Martin, A.C. The Physical Mechanisms of Drosophila Gastrulation: Mesoderm and Endoderm Invagination. *Genetics* **2020**, *214*, 543. [CrossRef] [PubMed]

65. Azpiazu, N.; Lawrence, P.A.; Vincent, J.P.; Frasch, M. Segmentation and specification of the Drosophila mesoderm. *Genes Dev.* **1996**, *10*, 3183–3194. [CrossRef]

66. Baylies, M.K.; Bate, M. twist: A Myogenic Switch in Drosophila. *Science* **1996**, *272*, 1481. [CrossRef] [PubMed]

67. Carmena, A.; Bate, M.; Jiménez, F. Lethal of scute, a proneural gene, participates in the specification of muscle progenitors during Drosophila embryogenesis. *Genes Dev.* **1995**, *9*, 2373–2383. [CrossRef]

68. Carmena, A.; Buff, E.; Halfon, M.S.; Gisselbrecht, S.; Jiménez, F.; Baylies, M.K.; Michelson, A.M. Reciprocal Regulatory Interactions between the Notch and Ras Signaling Pathways in the Drosophila Embryonic Mesoderm. *Dev. Biol.* **2002**, *244*, 226–242. [CrossRef]

69. Doe, C.Q.; Skeath, J.B. Neurogenesis in the insect central nervous system. *Curr. Opin. Neurobiol.* **1996**, *6*, 18–24. [CrossRef]

70. Crews, S.T. Drosophila Embryonic CNS Development: Neurogenesis, Gliogenesis, Cell Fate, and Differentiation. *Genetics* **2019**, *213*, 1111. [CrossRef]

71. Gomez Ruiz, M.; Bate, M. Segregation of myogenic lineages in Drosophila requires numb. *Development* **1997**, *124*, 4857.

72. Liu, J.; Qian, L.; Wessells, R.J.; Bidet, Y.; Jagla, K.; Bodmer, R. Hedgehog and RAS pathways cooperate in the anterior–posterior specification and positioning of cardiac progenitor cells. *Dev. Biol.* **2006**, *290*, 373–385. [CrossRef] [PubMed]

73. Rushton, E.; Drysdale, R.; Abmayr, S.M.; Michelson, A.M.; Bate, M. Mutations in a novel gene, myoblast city, provide evidence in support of the founder cell hypothesis for Drosophila muscle development. *Development* **1995**, *121*, 1979. [PubMed]

74. Prokop, A.; Landgraf, M.; Rushton, E.; Broadie, K.; Bate, M. Presynaptic Development at the Drosophila Neuromuscular Junction: Assembly and Localization of Presynaptic Active Zones. *Neuron* **1996**, *17*, 617–626. [CrossRef]

75. Halfon, M.S.; Carmena, A.; Gisselbrecht, S.; Sackerson, C.M.; Jiménez, F.; Baylies, M.K.; Michelson, A.M. Ras Pathway Specificity Is Determined by the Integration of Multiple Signal-Activated and Tissue-Restricted Transcription Factors. *Cell* **2000**, *103*, 63–74. [CrossRef]

76. Cox, V.T.; Beckett, K.; Baylies, M.K. Delivery of wingless to the ventral mesoderm by the developing central nervous system ensures proper patterning of individual slouch-positive muscle progenitors. *Dev. Biol.* **2005**, *287*, 403–415. [CrossRef] [PubMed]

77. Dohrmann, C.; Azpiazu, N.; Frasch, M. A new Drosophila homeo box gene is expressed in mesodermal precursor cells of distinct muscles during embryogenesis. *Genes Dev.* **1990**, *4*, 2098–2111. [CrossRef]

78. Bourgouin, C.; Lundgren, S.E.; Thomas, J.B. Apterous is a drosophila LIM domain gene required for the development of a subset of embryonic muscles. *Neuron* **1992**, *9*, 549–561. [CrossRef]

79. Keller, C.A.; Grill, M.A.; Abmayr, S.M. A Role for nautilus in the Differentiation of Muscle Precursors. *Dev. Biol.* **1998**, *202*, 157–171. [CrossRef]

80. Knirr, S.; Azpiazu, N.; Frasch, M. The role of the NK-homeobox gene slouch (S59) in somatic muscle patterning. *Development* **1999**, *126*, 4525.

81. Boukhatmi, H.; Frendo, J.L.; Enriquez, J.; Crozatier, M.; Dubois, L.; Vincent, A. Tup/Islet1 integrates time and position to specify muscle identity in Drosophila. *Development* **2012**, *139*, 3572. [CrossRef]

82. Crozatier, M.; Vincent, A. Requirement for the Drosophila COE transcription factor Collier in formation of an embryonic muscle: Transcriptional response to notch signalling. *Development* **1999**, *126*, 1495. [PubMed]

83. Busser, B.W.; Shokri, L.; Jaeger, S.A.; Gisselbrecht, S.S.; Singhania, A.; Berger, M.F.; Zhou, B.; Bulyk, M.L.; Michelson, A.M. Molecular mechanism underlying the regulatory specificity of a Drosophila homeodomain protein that specifies myoblast identity. *Dev. Camb. Engl.* **2012**, *139*, 1164–1174. [CrossRef] [PubMed]

84. Busser, B.W.; Gisselbrecht, S.S.; Shokri, L.; Tansey, T.R.; Gamble, C.E.; Bulyk, M.L.; Michelson, A.M. Contribution of distinct homeodomain DNA binding specificities to Drosophila embryonic mesodermal cell-specific gene expression programs. *PLoS ONE* **2013**, *8*, e69385. [CrossRef] [PubMed]

85. Dubois, L.; Frendo, J.-L.; Chanut-Delalande, H.; Crozatier, M.; Vincent, A. Genetic dissection of the Transcription Factor code controlling serial specification of muscle identities in Drosophila. *eLife* **2016**, *5*, e14979. [CrossRef] [PubMed]

86. Deng, H.; Bell, J.B.; Simmonds, A.J. Vestigial is required during late-stage muscle differentiation in Drosophila melanogaster embryos. *Mol. Biol. Cell* **2010**, *21*, 3304–3316. [CrossRef]

87. Carrasco-Rando, M.; Tutor, A.S.; Prieto-Sánchez, S.; González-Pérez, E.; Barrios, N.; Letizia, A.; Martín, P.; Campuzano, S.; Ruiz-Gómez, M. Drosophila araucan and caupolican integrate intrinsic and signalling inputs for the acquisition by muscle progenitors of the lateral transverse fate. *PLoS Genet.* **2011**, *7*, e1002186. [CrossRef]

88. Enriquez, J.; de Taffin, M.; Crozatier, M.; Vincent, A.; Dubois, L. Combinatorial coding of Drosophila muscle shape by Collier and Nautilus. *Dev. Biol.* **2012**, *363*, 27–39. [CrossRef]

89. Nose, A.; Isshiki, T.; Takeichi, M. Regional specification of muscle progenitors in Drosophila: The role of the msh homeobox gene. *Development* **1998**, *125*, 215.

90. Lord, P.C.W.; Lin, M.-H.; Hales, K.H.; Storti, R.V. Normal Expression and the Effects of Ectopic Expression of the Drosophila muscle segment homeobox (msh) Gene Suggest a Role in Differentiation and Patterning of Embryonic Muscles. *Dev. Biol.* **1995**, *171*, 627–640. [CrossRef]

91. Knirr, S.; Frasch, M. Molecular Integration of Inductive and Mesoderm-Intrinsic Inputs Governs even-skipped Enhancer Activity in a Subset of Pericardial and Dorsal Muscle Progenitors. *Dev. Biol.* **2001**, *238*, 13–26. [CrossRef]

92. Fujioka, M.; Wessells, R.J.; Han, Z.; Liu, J.; Fitzgerald, K.; Yusibova, G.L.; Zamora, M.; Ruiz-Lozano, P.; Bodmer, R.; Jaynes, J.B. Embryonic even skipped-dependent muscle and heart cell fates are required for normal adult activity, heart function, and lifespan. *Circ. Res.* **2005**, *97*, 1108–1114. [CrossRef] [PubMed]

93. Ruiz-Gomez, M.; Romani, S.; Hartmann, C.; Jackle, H.; Bate, M. Specific muscle identities are regulated by Kruppel during Drosophila embryogenesis. *Development* **1997**, *124*, 3407. [PubMed]

94. Jagla, T.; Bellard, F.; Lutz, Y.; Dretzen, G.; Bellard, M.; Jagla, K. ladybird determines cell fate decisions during diversification of Drosophila somatic muscles. *Development* **1998**, *125*, 3699. [PubMed]

95. Müller, D.; Jagla, T.; Bodart, L.M.; Jährling, N.; Dodt, H.-U.; Jagla, K.; Frasch, M. Regulation and functions of the lms homeobox gene during development of embryonic lateral transverse muscles and direct flight muscles in Drosophila. *PLoS ONE* **2010**, *5*, e14323. [CrossRef]

96. Kumar, R.P.; Dobi, K.C.; Baylies, M.K.; Abmayr, S.M. Muscle cell fate choice requires the T-box transcription factor midline in Drosophila. *Genetics* **2015**, *199*, 777–791. [CrossRef]

97. Corbin, V.; Michelson, A.M.; Abmayr, S.M.; Neel, V.; Alcamo, E.; Maniatis, T.; Young, M.W. A role for the Drosophila neurogenic genes in mesoderm differentiation. *Cell* **1991**, *67*, 311–323. [CrossRef]

98. Schaub, C.; Nagaso, H.; Jin, H.; Frasch, M. Org-1, the Drosophila ortholog of Tbx1, is a direct activator of known identity genes during muscle specification. *Development* **2012**, *139*, 1001. [CrossRef]

99. Duan, H.; Zhang, C.; Chen, J.; Sink, H.; Frei, E.; Noll, M. A key role of Pox meso in somatic myogenesis of Drosophila. *Development* **2007**, *134*, 3985. [CrossRef]

100. Vorbrüggen, G.; Constien, R.; Zilian, O.; Wimmer, E.A.; Dowe, G.; Taubert, H.; Noll, M.; Jäckle, H. Embryonic expression and characterization of a Ptx1 homolog in Drosophila. *Mech. Dev.* **1997**, *68*, 139–147. [CrossRef]

101. Drysdale, R.; Rushton, E.; Bate, M. Genes required for embryonic muscle development in Drosophila melanogaster A survey of the X chromosome. *Rouxs Arch. Dev. Biol. Off. Organ EDBO* **1993**, *202*, 276–295. [CrossRef]

102. Liu, Y.-H.; Jakobsen, J.S.; Valentin, G.; Amarantos, I.; Gilmour, D.T.; Furlong, E.E.M. A Systematic Analysis of Tinman Function Reveals Eya and JAK-STAT Signaling as Essential Regulators of Muscle Development. *Dev. Cell* **2009**, *16*, 280–291. [CrossRef] [PubMed]

103. Clark, I.B.N.; Boyd, J.; Hamilton, G.; Finnegan, D.J.; Jarman, A.P. D-six4 plays a key role in patterning cell identities deriving from the Drosophila mesoderm. *Dev. Biol.* **2006**, *294*, 220–231. [CrossRef] [PubMed]

104. Jagla, T.; Bidet, Y.; Da Ponte, J.P.; Dastugue, B.; Jagla, K. Cross-repressive interactions of identity genes are essential for proper specification of cardiac and muscular fates in Drosophila. *Development* **2002**, *129*, 1037. [PubMed]

105. Dobi, K.C.; Halfon, M.S.; Baylies, M.K. Whole-Genome Analysis of Muscle Founder Cells Implicates the Chromatin Regulator Sin3A in Muscle Identity. *Cell Rep.* **2014**, *8*, 858–870. [CrossRef] [PubMed]

106. Capovilla, M.; Kambris, Z.; Botas, J. Direct regulation of the muscle-identity gene apterous by a Hox protein in the somatic mesoderm. *Development* **2001**, *128*, 1221. [PubMed]

107. Michelson, A.M. Muscle pattern diversification in Drosophila is determined by the autonomous function of homeotic genes in the embryonic mesoderm. *Development* **1994**, *120*, 755.

108. Enriquez, J.; Boukhatmi, H.; Dubois, L.; Philippakis, A.A.; Bulyk, M.L.; Michelson, A.M.; Crozatier, M.; Vincent, A. Multi-step control of muscle diversity by Hox proteins in the Drosophila embryo. *Dev. Camb. Engl.* **2010**, *137*, 457–466. [CrossRef]

109. Domsch, K.; Carnesecchi, J.; Disela, V.; Friedrich, J.; Trost, N.; Ermakova, O.; Polychronidou, M.; Lohmann, I. The Hox transcription factor Ubx stabilizes lineage commitment by suppressing cellular plasticity in Drosophila. *eLife* **2019**, *8*, e42675. [CrossRef]

110. Hessinger, C.; Technau, G.M.; Rogulja-Ortmann, A. The Drosophila Hox gene Ultrabithorax acts in both muscles and motoneurons to orchestrate formation of specific neuromuscular connections. *Development* **2017**, *144*, 139. [CrossRef]

111. Junion, G.; Bataillé, L.; Jagla, T.; Da Ponte, J.P.; Tapin, R.; Jagla, K. Genome-wide view of cell fate specification: Ladybird acts at multiple levels during diversification of muscle and heart precursors. *Genes Dev.* **2007**, *21*, 3163–3180. [CrossRef]

112. Bataillé, L.; Delon, I.; Da Ponte, J.P.; Brown, N.H.; Jagla, K. Downstream of Identity Genes: Muscle-Type-Specific Regulation of the Fusion Process. *Dev. Cell* **2010**, *19*, 317–328. [CrossRef] [PubMed]

113. Black, B.L.; Olson, E.N. Transcriptional control of muscle development by myocyte enhancer factor-2 (Mef2) proteins. *Annu. Rev. Cell Dev. Biol.* **1998**, *14*, 167–196. [CrossRef] [PubMed]

114. Pon, J.R.; Marra, M.A. MEF2 transcription factors: Developmental regulators and emerging cancer genes. *Oncotarget* **2016**, *7*, 2297–2312. [CrossRef]

115. Taylor, M.V.; Hughes, S.M. Mef2 and the skeletal muscle differentiation program. *Skelet. Muscle Dev. 30th Anniv. MyoD* **2017**, *72*, 33–44. [CrossRef]

116. Bour, B.A.; O'Brien, M.A.; Lockwood, W.L.; Goldstein, E.S.; Bodmer, R.; Taghert, P.H.; Abmayr, S.M.; Nguyen, H.T. Drosophila MEF2, a transcription factor that is essential for myogenesis. *Genes Dev.* **1995**, *9*, 730–741. [CrossRef] [PubMed]

117. Ranganayakulu, G.; Zhao, B.; Dokidis, A.; Molkentin, J.D.; Olson, E.N.; Schulz, R.A. A Series of Mutations in the D-MEF2 Transcription Factor Reveal Multiple Functions in Larval and Adult Myogenesis in Drosophila. *Dev. Biol.* **1995**, *171*, 169–181. [CrossRef] [PubMed]

118. Elgar, S.J.; Han, J.; Taylor, M.V. mef2 activity levels differentially affect gene expression during Drosophila muscle development. *Proc. Natl. Acad. Sci. USA* **2008**, *105*, 918–923. [CrossRef]

119. Cunha, P.M.F.; Sandmann, T.; Gustafson, E.H.; Ciglar, L.; Eichenlaub, M.P.; Furlong, E.E.M. Combinatorial binding leads to diverse regulatory responses: Lmd is a tissue-specific modulator of Mef2 activity. *PLoS Genet.* **2010**, *6*, e1001014. [CrossRef]

120. Junion, G.; Jagla, T.; Duplant, S.; Tapin, R.; Da Ponte, J.-P.; Jagla, K. Mapping Dmef2-binding regulatory modules by using a ChIP-enriched in silico targets approach. *Proc. Natl. Acad. Sci. USA* **2005**, *102*, 18479. [CrossRef]

121. Tanaka, K.K.K.; Bryantsev, A.L.; Cripps, R.M. Myocyte Enhancer Factor 2 and Chorion Factor 2 Collaborate in Activation of the Myogenic Program in Drosophila. *Mol. Cell. Biol.* **2008**, *28*, 1616. [CrossRef]

122. García-Zaragoza, E.; Mas, J.A.; Vivar, J.; Arredondo, J.J.; Cervera, M. CF2 activity and enhancer integration are required for proper muscle gene expression in Drosophila. *Mech. Dev.* **2008**, *125*, 617–630. [CrossRef] [PubMed]

123. Cripps, R.M.; Lovato, T.L.; Olson, E.N. Positive autoregulation of the Myocyte enhancer factor-2 myogenic control gene during somatic muscle development in Drosophila. *Dev. Biol.* **2004**, *267*, 536–547. [CrossRef] [PubMed]

124. Nguyen, H.T.; Xu, X. Drosophila mef2 Expression during Mesoderm Development Is Controlled by a Complex Array of cis-Acting Regulatory Modules. *Dev. Biol.* **1998**, *204*, 550–566. [CrossRef] [PubMed]

125. Chen, Z.; Liang, S.; Zhao, Y.; Han, Z. miR-92b regulates Mef2 levels through a negative-feedback circuit during Drosophila muscle development. *Dev. Camb. Engl.* **2012**, *139*, 3543–3552. [CrossRef] [PubMed]

126. Cripps, R.M.; Black, B.L.; Zhao, B.; Lien, C.L.; Schulz, R.A.; Olson, E.N. The myogenic regulatory gene Mef2 is a direct target for transcriptional activation by Twist during Drosophila myogenesis. *Genes Dev.* **1998**, *12*, 422–434. [CrossRef] [PubMed]

127. Nowak, S.J.; Aihara, H.; Gonzalez, K.; Nibu, Y.; Baylies, M.K. Akirin links twist-regulated transcription with the Brahma chromatin remodeling complex during embryogenesis. *PLoS Genet.* **2012**, *8*, e1002547. [CrossRef]

128. Wang, F.; Minakhina, S.; Tran, H.; Changela, N.; Kramer, J.; Steward, R. Tet protein function during Drosophila development. *PLoS ONE* **2018**, *13*, e0190367. [CrossRef]

129. Deng, H.; Hughes, S.C.; Bell, J.B.; Simmonds, A.J. Alternative requirements for Vestigial, Scalloped, and Dmef2 during muscle differentiation in Drosophila melanogaster. *Mol. Biol. Cell* **2009**, *20*, 256–269. [CrossRef]

130. Haralalka, S.; Abmayr, S.M. Myoblast fusion in Drosophila. *Exp. Cell Res.* **2010**, *316*, 3007–3013. [CrossRef]

131. Deng, S.; Azevedo, M.; Baylies, M. Acting on identity: Myoblast fusion and the formation of the syncytial muscle fiber. *Semin. Cell Dev. Biol.* **2017**, *72*, 45–55. [CrossRef]

132. Lee, D.M.; Chen, E.H. Drosophila Myoblast Fusion: Invasion and Resistance for the Ultimate Union. *Annu. Rev. Genet.* **2019**, *53*, 67–91. [CrossRef] [PubMed]

133. Ruiz-Gómez, M.; Coutts, N.; Price, A.; Taylor, M.V.; Bate, M. Drosophila Dumbfounded: A Myoblast Attractant Essential for Fusion. *Cell* **2000**, *102*, 189–198. [CrossRef]

134. Strünkelnberg, M.; Bonengel, B.; Moda, L.M.; Hertenstein, A.; de Couet, H.G.; Ramos, R.G.P.; Fischbach, K.-F. rst and its paralogue kirre act redundantly during embryonic muscle development in Drosophila. *Development* **2001**, *128*, 4229.

135. Bour, B.A.; Chakravarti, M.; West, J.M.; Abmayr, S.M. Drosophila SNS, a member of the immunoglobulin superfamily that is essential for myoblast fusion. *Genes Dev.* **2000**, *14*, 1498–1511. [PubMed]

136. Artero, R.D.; Castanon, I.; Baylies, M.K. The immunoglobulin-like protein Hibris functions as a dose-dependent regulator of myoblast fusion and is differentially controlled by Ras and Notch signaling. *Development* **2001**, *128*, 4251.

137. Bataillé, L.; Boukhatmi, H.; Frendo, J.-L.; Vincent, A. Dynamics of transcriptional (re)-programming of syncytial nuclei in developing muscles. *BMC Biol.* **2017**, *15*. [CrossRef]

138. Azevedo, M.; Baylies, M.K. Getting into Position: Nuclear Movement in Muscle Cells. *Trends Cell Biol.* **2020**, *30*, 303–316. [CrossRef]

139. Roman, W.; Gomes, E.R. Nuclear positioning in skeletal muscle. *SI Nucl. Position.* **2018**, *82*, 51–56. [CrossRef]

140. Cadot, B.; Gache, V.; Gomes, E.R. Moving and positioning the nucleus in skeletal muscle - one step at a time. *Nucl. Austin Tex* **2015**, *6*, 373–381. [CrossRef]

141. Starr, D.A.; Fridolfsson, H.N. Interactions Between Nuclei and the Cytoskeleton Are Mediated by SUN-KASH Nuclear-Envelope Bridges. *Annu. Rev. Cell Dev. Biol.* **2010**, *26*, 421–444. [CrossRef]

142. Folker, E.S.; Baylies, M.K. Nuclear positioning in muscle development and disease. *Front. Physiol.* **2013**, *4*, 363. [CrossRef] [PubMed]

143. Volk, T. Singling out Drosophila tendon cells: A dialogue between two distinct cell types. *Trends Genet.* **1999**, *15*, 448–453. [CrossRef]

144. Schnorrer, F.; Dickson, B.J. Muscle Building: Mechanisms of Myotube Guidance and Attachment Site Selection. *Dev. Cell* **2004**, *7*, 9–20. [CrossRef] [PubMed]

145. Subramanian, A.; Schilling, T.F. Tendon development and musculoskeletal assembly: Emerging roles for the extracellular matrix. *Dev. Camb. Engl.* **2015**, *142*, 4191–4204. [CrossRef]

146. Lejard, V.; Blais, F.; Guerquin, M.-J.; Bonnet, A.; Bonnin, M.-A.; Havis, E.; Malbouyres, M.; Bidaud, C.B.; Maro, G.; Gilardi-Hebenstreit, P.; et al. EGR1 and EGR2 involvement in vertebrate tendon differentiation. *J. Biol. Chem.* **2011**, *286*, 5855–5867. [CrossRef]

147. Volohonsky, G.; Edenfeld, G.; Klämbt, C.; Volk, T. Muscle-dependent maturation of tendon cells is induced by post-transcriptional regulation of stripeA. *Development* **2007**, *134*, 347. [CrossRef]

148. Kramer, S.G.; Kidd, T.; Simpson, J.H.; Goodman, C.S. Switching Repulsion to Attraction: Changing Responses to Slit During Transition in Mesoderm Migration. *Science* **2001**, *292*, 737. [CrossRef]

149. Callahan, C.A.; Bonkovsky, J.L.; Scully, A.L.; Thomas, J.B. derailed is required for muscle attachment site selection in Drosophila. *Development* **1996**, *122*, 2761.

150. Schnorrer, F.; Kalchhauser, I.; Dickson, B.J. The Transmembrane Protein Kon-tiki Couples to Dgrip to Mediate Myotube Targeting in Drosophila. *Dev. Cell* **2007**, *12*, 751–766. [CrossRef]

151. Estrada, B.; Gisselbrecht, S.S.; Michelson, A.M. The transmembrane protein Perdido interacts with Grip and integrins to mediate myotube projection and attachment in the Drosophila embryo. *Development* **2007**, *134*, 4469. [CrossRef]

152. Swan, L.E.; Schmidt, M.; Schwarz, T.; Ponimaskin, E.; Prange, U.; Boeckers, T.; Thomas, U.; Sigrist, S.J. Complex interaction of Drosophila GRIP PDZ domains and Echinoid during muscle morphogenesis. *EMBO J.* **2006**, *25*, 3640–3651. [CrossRef] [PubMed]

153. Chanana, B.; Graf, R.; Koledachkina, T.; Pflanz, R.; Vorbrüggen, G. αPS2 integrin-mediated muscle attachment in Drosophila requires the ECM protein Thrombospondin. *Mech. Dev.* **2007**, *124*, 463–475. [CrossRef] [PubMed]

154. Katzemich, A.; Long, J.Y.; Panneton, V.; Fisher, L.A.B.; Hipfner, D.; Schöck, F. Slik phosphorylation of Talin T152 is crucial for proper Talin recruitment and maintenance of muscle attachment in Drosophila. *Development* **2019**, *146*, dev176339. [CrossRef] [PubMed]

155. Pines, M.; Das, R.; Ellis, S.J.; Morin, A.; Czerniecki, S.; Yuan, L.; Klose, M.; Coombs, D.; Tanentzapf, G. Mechanical force regulates integrin turnover in Drosophila in vivo. *Nat. Cell Biol.* **2012**, *14*, 935–943. [CrossRef]

156. Sparrow, J.C.; Schöck, F. The initial steps of myofibril assembly: Integrins pave the way. *Nat. Rev. Mol. Cell Biol.* **2009**, *10*, 293–298. [CrossRef]

157. Gautel, M.; Djinović-Carugo, K. The sarcomeric cytoskeleton: From molecules to motion. *J. Exp. Biol.* **2016**, *219*, 135. [CrossRef]

158. Rhee, D.; Sanger, J.M.; Sanger, J.W. The premyofibril: Evidence for its role in myofibrillogenesis. *Cell Motil. Cytoskeleton* **1994**, *28*, 1–24. [CrossRef]

159. Jirka, C.; Pak, J.H.; Grosgogeat, C.A.; Marchetii, M.M.; Gupta, V.A. Dysregulation of NRAP degradation by KLHL41 contributes to pathophysiology in nemaline myopathy. *Hum. Mol. Genet.* **2019**, *28*, 2549–2560. [CrossRef]

160. Antin, P.B.; Tokunaka, S.; Nachmias, V.T.; Holtzer, H. Role of stress fiber-like structures in assembling nascent myofibrils in myosheets recovering from exposure to ethyl methanesulfonate. *J. Cell Biol.* **1986**, *102*, 1464–1479. [CrossRef]

161. Epstein, H.; Fischman, D. Molecular analysis of protein assembly in muscle development. *Science* **1991**, *251*, 1039–1044. [CrossRef]

162. Rui, Y.; Bai, J.; Perrimon, N. Sarcomere formation occurs by the assembly of multiple latent protein complexes. *PLoS Genet.* **2010**, *6*, e1001208. [CrossRef] [PubMed]

163. Weitkunat, M.; Kaya-Çopur, A.; Grill, S.W.; Schnorrer, F. Tension and Force-Resistant Attachment Are Essential for Myofibrillogenesis in Drosophila Flight Muscle. *Curr. Biol.* **2014**, *24*, 705–716. [CrossRef] [PubMed]

164. Orfanos, Z.; Leonard, K.; Elliott, C.; Katzemich, A.; Bullard, B.; Sparrow, J. Sallimus and the Dynamics of Sarcomere Assembly in Drosophila Flight Muscles. *J. Mol. Biol.* **2015**, *427*, 2151–2158. [CrossRef] [PubMed]

165. Röper, K.; Mao, Y.; Brown, N.H. Contribution of sequence variation in Drosophila actins to their incorporation into actin-based structures in vivo. *J. Cell Sci.* **2005**, *118*, 3937. [CrossRef] [PubMed]

166. Bulgakova, N.A.; Wellmann, J.; Brown, N.H. Diverse integrin adhesion stoichiometries caused by varied actomyosin activity. *Open Biol.* **2017**, *7*, 160250. [CrossRef] [PubMed]

167. Zappia, M.P.; Frolov, M.V. E2F function in muscle growth is necessary and sufficient for viability in Drosophila. *Nat. Commun.* **2016**, *7*, 10509. [CrossRef] [PubMed]

168. Molnár, I.; Migh, E.; Szikora, S.; Kalmár, T.; Végh, A.G.; Deák, F.; Barkó, S.; Bugyi, B.; Orfanos, Z.; Kovács, J.; et al. DAAM is required for thin filament formation and Sarcomerogenesis during muscle development in Drosophila. *PLoS Genet.* **2014**, *10*, e1004166. [CrossRef]

169. Bai, J.; Hartwig, J.H.; Perrimon, N. SALS, a WH2-Domain-Containing Protein, Promotes Sarcomeric Actin Filament Elongation from Pointed Ends during Drosophila Muscle Growth. *Dev. Cell* **2007**, *13*, 828–842. [CrossRef]

170. Mardahl-Dumesnil, M.; Fowler, V.M. Thin filaments elongate from their pointed ends during myofibril assembly in Drosophila indirect flight muscle. *J. Cell Biol.* **2001**, *155*, 1043–1053. [CrossRef]

171. Bloor, J.W.; Kiehart, D.P. zipper Nonmuscle Myosin-II Functions Downstream of PS2 Integrin in Drosophila Myogenesis and Is Necessary for Myofibril Formation. *Dev. Biol.* **2001**, *239*, 215–228. [CrossRef]

172. Volk, T.; Fessler, L.I.; Fessler, J.H. A role for integrin in the formation of sarcomeric cytoarchitecture. *Cell* **1990**, *63*, 525–536. [CrossRef]

173. Kreisköther, N.; Reichert, N.; Buttgereit, D.; Hertenstein, A.; Fischbach, K.-F.; Renkawitz-Pohl, R. Drosophila Rolling pebbles colocalises and putatively interacts with alpha-Actinin and the Sls isoform Zormin in the Z-discs of the sarcomere and with Dumbfounded/Kirre, alpha-Actinin and Zormin in the terminal Z-discs. *J. Muscle Res. Cell Motil.* **2006**, *27*, 93. [CrossRef] [PubMed]

174. Kelemen-Valkony, I.; Kiss, M.; Csiha, J.; Kiss, A.; Bircher, U.; Szidonya, J.; Maróy, P.; Juhász, G.; Komonyi, O.; Csiszár, K.; et al. Drosophila basement membrane collagen col4a1 mutations cause severe myopathy. *Matrix Biol.* **2012**, *31*, 29–37. [CrossRef] [PubMed]

175. Katzemich, A.; Liao, K.A.; Czerniecki, S.; Schöck, F. Alp/Enigma family proteins cooperate in Z-disc formation and myofibril assembly. *PLoS Genet.* **2013**, *9*, e1003342. [CrossRef]

176. Crisp, S.J.; Evers, J.F.; Bate, M. Endogenous patterns of activity are required for the maturation of a motor network. *J. Neurosci. Off. J. Soc. Neurosci.* **2011**, *31*, 10445–10450. [CrossRef]

177. Broadie, K.; Bate, M. Development of the embryonic neuromuscular synapse of Drosophila melanogaster. *J. Neurosci.* **1993**, *13*, 144. [CrossRef]

178. Keshishian, H.; Broadie, K.; Chiba, A.; Bate, M. The Drosophila Neuromuscular Junction: A Model System for Studying Synaptic Development and Function. *Annu. Rev. Neurosci.* **1996**, *19*, 545–575. [CrossRef]

179. Ruiz-Cañada, C.; Budnik, V. Introduction on The Use of The Drosophila Embryonic/Larval Neuromuscular Junction as A Model System to Study Synapse Development and Function, and A Brief Summary of Pathfinding and Target Recognition. In *International Review of Neurobiology*; Academic Press: New York, NY, USA, 2006; pp. 1–31, ISBN 0074-7742.

180. Landgraf, M.; Bossing, T.; Technau, G.M.; Bate, M. The origin, location, and projections of the embryonic abdominal motorneurons of Drosophila. *J. Neurosci. Off. J. Soc. Neurosci.* **1997**, *17*, 9642–9655. [CrossRef]

181. Schmid, A.; Chiba, A.; Doe, C.Q. Clonal analysis of Drosophila embryonic neuroblasts: Neural cell types, axon projections and muscle targets. *Development* **1999**, *126*, 4653.

182. Landgraf, M.; Jeffrey, V.; Fujioka, M.; Jaynes, J.B.; Bate, M. Embryonic Origins of a Motor System: Motor Dendrites Form a Myotopic Map in Drosophila. *PLoS Biol.* **2003**, *1*, e41. [CrossRef]

183. Ritzenthaler, S.; Suzuki, E.; Chiba, A. Postsynaptic filopodia in muscle cells interact with innervating motoneuron axons. *Nat. Neurosci.* **2000**, *3*, 1012–1017. [CrossRef] [PubMed]

184. Nose, A. Generation of neuromuscular specificity in Drosophila: Novel mechanisms revealed by new technologies. *Front. Mol. Neurosci.* **2012**, *5*, 62. [CrossRef] [PubMed]

185. Nose, A.; Umeda, T.; Takeichi, M. Neuromuscular target recognition by a homophilic interaction of connectin cell adhesion molecules in Drosophila. *Development* **1997**, *124*, 1433. [PubMed]

186. Patel, N.H.; Ball, E.E.; Goodman, C.S. Changing role of even-skipped during the evolution of insect pattern formation. *Nature* **1992**, *357*, 339–342. [CrossRef] [PubMed]

187. Labrador, J.P.; O'Keefe, D.; Yoshikawa, S.; McKinnon, R.D.; Thomas, J.B.; Bashaw, G.J. The Homeobox Transcription Factor Even-skipped Regulates Netrin-Receptor Expression to Control Dorsal Motor-Axon Projections in Drosophila. *Curr. Biol.* **2005**, *15*, 1413–1419. [CrossRef] [PubMed]

188. Chen, K.; Featherstone, D.E. Discs-large (DLG) is clustered by presynaptic innervation and regulates postsynaptic glutamate receptor subunit composition in Drosophila. *BMC Biol.* **2005**, *3*, 1–13. [CrossRef] [PubMed]

189. Bachmann, A.; Kobler, O.; Kittel, R.J.; Wichmann, C.; Sierralta, J.; Sigrist, S.J.; Gundelfinger, E.D.; Knust, E.; Thomas, U. A perisynaptic ménage à trois between Dlg, DLin-7, and Metro controls proper organization of Drosophila synaptic junctions. *J. Neurosci. Off. J. Soc. Neurosci.* **2010**, *30*, 5811–5824. [CrossRef]

190. Broadie, K.; Bate, M. Innervation directs receptor synthesis and localization in Drosophila embryo synaptogenesis. *Nature* **1993**, *361*, 350–353. [CrossRef]

191. Kim, M.D.; Wen, Y.; Jan, Y.-N. Patterning and organization of motor neuron dendrites in the Drosophila larva. *Dev. Biol.* **2009**, *336*, 213–221. [CrossRef]

192. Syed, A.; Lukacsovich, T.; Pomeroy, M.; Bardwell, A.J.; Decker, G.T.; Waymire, K.G.; Purcell, J.; Huang, W.; Gui, J.; Padilla, E.M.; et al. Miles to go (mtgo) encodes FNDC3 proteins that interact with the chaperonin subunit CCT3 and are required for NMJ branching and growth in Drosophila. *Dev. Biol.* **2019**, *445*, 37–53. [CrossRef]

193. Beumer, K.J.; Rohrbough, J.; Prokop, A.; Broadie, K. A role for PS integrins in morphological growth and synaptic function at the postembryonic neuromuscular junction of Drosophila. *Development* **1999**, *126*, 5833. [PubMed]

194. Vonhoff, F.; Keshishian, H. In Vivo Calcium Signaling during Synaptic Refinement at the Drosophila Neuromuscular Junction. *J. Neurosci. Off. J. Soc. Neurosci.* **2017**, *37*, 5511–5526. [CrossRef]

195. DePew, A.T.; Aimino, M.A.; Mosca, T.J. The Tenets of Teneurin: Conserved Mechanisms Regulate Diverse Developmental Processes in the Drosophila Nervous System. *Front. Neurosci.* **2019**, *13*, 27. [CrossRef] [PubMed]

196. Bate, M.; Rushton, E.; Currie, D.A. Cells with persistent twist expression are the embryonic precursors of adult muscles in Drosophila. *Development* **1991**, *113*, 79. [PubMed]

197. Figeac, N.; Jagla, T.; Aradhya, R.; Da Ponte, J.P.; Jagla, K. Drosophila adult muscle precursors form a network of interconnected cells and are specified by the rhomboid-triggered EGF pathway. *Development* **2010**, *137*, 1965. [CrossRef] [PubMed]

198. Lavergne, G.; Zmojdzian, M.; Da Ponte, J.P.; Junion, G.; Jagla, K. Drosophila adult muscle precursor cells contribute to motor axon pathfinding and proper innervation of embryonic muscles. *Development* **2020**, *147*, dev183004. [CrossRef]

199. Gunage, R.D.; Dhanyasi, N.; Reichert, H.; VijayRaghavan, K. Drosophila adult muscle development and regeneration. *Skelet. Muscle Dev. 30th Anniv. MyoD* **2017**, *72*, 56–66. [CrossRef]

200. Laurichesse, Q.; Soler, C. Muscle development: A view from adult myogenesis in Drosophila. *Semin. Cell Dev. Biol.* **2020**. [CrossRef]

201. Oas, S.T.; Bryantsev, A.L.; Cripps, R.M. Arrest is a regulator of fiber-specific alternative splicing in the indirect flight muscles of Drosophila. *J. Cell Biol.* **2014**, *206*, 895–908. [CrossRef]

202. DeAguero, A.A.; Castillo, L.; Oas, S.T.; Kiani, K.; Bryantsev, A.L.; Cripps, R.M. Regulation of fiber-specific actin expression by the Drosophila SRF ortholog Blistered. *Dev. Camb. Engl.* **2019**, *146*, dev164129. [CrossRef]

203. Schiaffino, S.; Reggiani, C. Fiber Types in Mammalian Skeletal Muscles. *Physiol. Rev.* **2011**, *91*, 1447–1531. [CrossRef] [PubMed]

204. Hastings, G.A.; Emerson, C.P., Jr. Myosin functional domains encoded by alternative exons are expressed in specific thoracic muscles of Drosophila. *J. Cell Biol.* **1991**, *114*, 263–276. [CrossRef] [PubMed]

205. Figeac, N.; Daczewska, M.; Marcelle, C.; Jagla, K. Muscle stem cells and model systems for their investigation. *Dev. Dyn.* **2007**, *236*, 3332–3342. [CrossRef] [PubMed]

206. Beira, J.V.; Paro, R. The legacy of Drosophila imaginal discs. *Chromosoma* **2016**, *125*, 573–592. [CrossRef] [PubMed]

207. Aradhya, R.; Zmojdzian, M.; Da Ponte, J.P.; Jagla, K. Muscle niche-driven Insulin-Notch-Myc cascade reactivates dormant Adult Muscle Precursors in Drosophila. *eLife* **2015**, *4*, e08497. [CrossRef]

208. Tavi, P.; Korhonen, T.; Hänninen, S.L.; Bruton, J.D.; Lööf, S.; Simon, A.; Westerblad, H. Myogenic skeletal muscle satellite cells communicate by tunnelling nanotubes. *J. Cell. Physiol.* **2010**, *223*, 376–383. [CrossRef]

209. Gunage, R.D.; Reichert, H.; VijayRaghavan, K. Identification of a new stem cell population that generates Drosophila flight muscles. *eLife* **2014**, *3*, e03126. [CrossRef]

210. Vishal, K.; Brooks, D.S.; Bawa, S.; Gameros, S.; Stetsiv, M.; Geisbrecht, E.R. Adult Muscle Formation Requires Drosophila Moleskin for Proliferation of Wing Disc-Associated Muscle Precursors. *Genetics* **2017**, *206*, 199. [CrossRef]

211. Bernard, F.; Dutriaux, A.; Silber, J.; Lalouette, A. Notch pathway repression by vestigial is required to promote indirect flight muscle differentiation in Drosophila melanogaster. *Dev. Biol.* **2006**, *295*, 164–177. [CrossRef]

212. Dutta, D.; Umashankar, M.; Lewis, E.B.; Rodrigues, V.; VijayRaghavan, K. Hox Genes Regulate Muscle Founder Cell Pattern Autonomously and Regulate Morphogenesis Through Motor Neurons. *J. Neurogenet.* **2010**, *24*, 95–108. [CrossRef]

213. Sudarsan, V.; Anant, S.; Guptan, P.; VijayRaghavan, K.; Skaer, H. Myoblast Diversification and Ectodermal Signaling in Drosophila. *Dev. Cell* **2001**, *1*, 829–839. [CrossRef]

214. Maqbool, T.; Soler, C.; Jagla, T.; Daczewska, M.; Lodha, N.; Palliyil, S.; VijayRaghavan, K.; Jagla, K. Shaping leg muscles in Drosophila: Role of ladybird, a conserved regulator of appendicular myogenesis. *PLoS ONE* **2006**, *1*, e122. [CrossRef] [PubMed]

215. Ghazi, A.; Anant, S.; Vijay Raghavan, K. Apterous mediates development of direct flight muscles autonomously and indirect flight muscles through epidermal cues. *Development* **2000**, *127*, 5309. [PubMed]

216. Dutta, D.; Shaw, S.; Maqbool, T.; Pandya, H.; VijayRaghavan, K. Drosophila Heartless Acts with Heartbroken/Dof in Muscle Founder Differentiation. *PLoS Biol.* **2005**, *3*, e337. [CrossRef]

217. Dutta, D.; Anant, S.; Ruiz-Gomez, M.; Bate, M.; VijayRaghavan, K. Founder myoblasts and fibre number during adult myogenesis in Drosophila. *Development* **2004**, *131*, 3761. [CrossRef]

218. Bryantsev, A.L.; Duong, S.; Brunetti, T.M.; Chechenova, M.B.; Lovato, T.L.; Nelson, C.; Shaw, E.; Uhl, J.D.; Gebelein, B.; Cripps, R.M. Extradenticle and homothorax control adult muscle fiber identity in Drosophila. *Dev. Cell* **2012**, *23*, 664–673. [CrossRef] [PubMed]

219. Schönbauer, C.; Distler, J.; Jährling, N.; Radolf, M.; Dodt, H.-U.; Frasch, M.; Schnorrer, F. Spalt mediates an evolutionarily conserved switch to fibrillar muscle fate in insects. *Nature* **2011**, *479*, 406–409. [CrossRef]

220. DeSimone, S.; Coelho, C.; Roy, S.; VijayRaghavan, K.; White, K. ERECT WING, the Drosophila member of a family of DNA binding proteins is required in imaginal myoblasts for flight muscle development. *Development* **1996**, *122*, 31.

221. Fernandes, J.; Bate, M.; Vijayraghavan, K. Development of the indirect flight muscles of Drosophila. *Development* **1991**, *113*, 67.

222. Kuleesha, Y.; Puah, W.C.; Wasser, M. Live imaging of muscle histolysis in Drosophila metamorphosis. *BMC Dev. Biol.* **2016**, *16*, 12. [CrossRef]

223. Fernandes, J.J.; Keshishian, H. Motoneurons regulate myoblast proliferation and patterning in Drosophila. *Dev. Biol.* **2005**, *277*, 493–505. [CrossRef]

224. Currie, D.A.; Bate, M. The development of adult abdominal muscles in Drosophila: Myoblasts express twist and are associated with nerves. *Development* **1991**, *113*, 91. [PubMed]

225. Rivlin, P.K.; Schneiderman, A.M.; Booker, R. Imaginal Pioneers Prefigure the Formation of Adult Thoracic Muscles in Drosophila melanogaster. *Dev. Biol.* **2000**, *222*, 450–459. [CrossRef] [PubMed]

226. Mukherjee, P.; Gildor, B.; Shilo, B.-Z.; VijayRaghavan, K.; Schejter, E.D. The actin nucleator WASp is required for myoblast fusion during adult Drosophila myogenesis. *Dev. Camb. Engl.* **2011**, *138*, 2347–2357. [CrossRef] [PubMed]

227. Ghazi, A.; Paul, L.; VijayRaghavan, K. Prepattern genes and signaling molecules regulate stripe expression to specify Drosophila flight muscle attachment sites. *Mech. Dev.* **2003**, *120*, 519–528. [CrossRef]

228. Laddada, L.; Jagla, K.; Soler, C. Odd-skipped and Stripe act downstream of Notch to promote the morphogenesis of long appendicular tendons in Drosophila. *Biol. Open* **2019**, *8*, bio038760. [CrossRef] [PubMed]

229. Weitkunat, M.; Brasse, M.; Bausch, A.R.; Schnorrer, F. Mechanical tension and spontaneous muscle twitching precede the formation of cross-striated muscle in vivo. *Dev. Camb. Engl.* **2017**, *144*, 1261–1272. [CrossRef] [PubMed]

230. Spletter, M.L.; Schnorrer, F. Transcriptional regulation and alternative splicing cooperate in muscle fiber-type specification in flies and mammals. *Dev. Biol.* **2014**, *321*, 90–98. [CrossRef]

231. Reedy, M.C.; Beall, C. Ultrastructure of Developing Flight Muscle in Drosophila. I. Assembly of Myofibrils. *Dev. Biol.* **1993**, *160*, 443–465. [CrossRef]

232. Spletter, M.L.; Barz, C.; Yeroslaviz, A.; Zhang, X.; Lemke, S.B.; Bonnard, A.; Brunner, E.; Cardone, G.; Basler, K.; Habermann, B.H.; et al. A transcriptomics resource reveals a transcriptional transition during ordered sarcomere morphogenesis in flight muscle. *eLife* **2018**, *7*, e34058. [CrossRef]

233. Shwartz, A.; Dhanyasi, N.; Schejter, E.D.; Shilo, B.-Z. The Drosophila formin Fhos is a primary mediator of sarcomeric thin-filament array assembly. *eLife* **2016**, *5*, e16540. [CrossRef] [PubMed]

234. Fernandes, I.; Schöck, F. The nebulin repeat protein Lasp regulates I-band architecture and filament spacing in myofibrils. *J. Cell Biol.* **2014**, *206*, 559–572. [CrossRef]

235. Qiu, F.; Brendel, S.; Cunha, P.M.F.; Astola, N.; Song, B.; Furlong, E.E.M.; Leonard, K.R.; Bullard, B. Myofilin, a protein in the thick filaments of insect muscle. *J. Cell Sci.* **2005**, *118*, 1527. [CrossRef] [PubMed]

236. Ball, E.; Karlik, C.C.; Beall, C.J.; Saville, D.L.; Sparrow, J.C.; Bullard, B.; Fyrberg, E.A. Arthrin, a myofibrillar protein of insect flight muscle, is an actin-ubiquitin conjugate. *Cell* **1987**, *51*, 221–228. [CrossRef]

237. Becker, K.D.; O'Donnell, P.T.; Heitz, J.M.; Vito, M.; Bernstein, S.I. Analysis of Drosophila paramyosin: Identification of a novel isoform which is restricted to a subset of adult muscles. *J. Cell Biol.* **1992**, *116*, 669–681. [CrossRef] [PubMed]

238. Maroto, M.; Arredondo, J.J.; Román, M.S.; Marco, R.; Cervera, M. Analysis of the Paramyosin/Miniparamyosin Gene: Miniparamyosin is an independently transcribed, distinct paramyosin isoform, widely distributed in invertebrates. *J. Biol. Chem.* **1995**, *270*, 4375–4382. [CrossRef]

239. Vigoreaux, J.O. Alterations in flightin phosphorylation inDrosophila flight muscles are associated with myofibrillar defects engendered by actin and myosin heavy-chain mutant alleles. *Biochem. Genet.* **1994**, *32*, 301–314. [CrossRef]

240. Reedy, M.C.; Bullard, B.; Vigoreaux, J.O. Flightin is essential for thick filament assembly and sarcomere stability in Drosophila flight muscles. *J. Cell Biol.* **2000**, *151*, 1483–1500. [CrossRef]

241. Craig, R.; Woodhead, J.L. Structure and function of myosin filaments. *Curr. Opin. Struct. Biol.* **2006**, *16*, 204–212. [CrossRef]

242. Orfanos, Z.; Sparrow, J.C. Myosin isoform switching during assembly of the Drosophila flight muscle thick filament lattice. *J. Cell Sci.* **2013**, *126*, 139. [CrossRef]

243. Contompasis, J.L.; Nyland, L.R.; Maughan, D.W.; Vigoreaux, J.O. Flightin Is Necessary for Length Determination, Structural Integrity, and Large Bending Stiffness of Insect Flight Muscle Thick Filaments. *J. Mol. Biol.* **2010**, *395*, 340–348. [CrossRef]

244. Sparrow, J.; Reedy, M.; Ball, E.; Kyrtatas, V.; Molloy, J.; Durston, J.; Hennessey, E.; White, D. Functional and ultrastructural effects of a missense mutation in the indirect flight muscle-specific actin gene of Drosophila melanogaster. *J. Mol. Biol.* **1991**, *222*, 963–982. [CrossRef]

245. Burkart, C.; Qiu, F.; Brendel, S.; Benes, V.; Håäg, P.; Labeit, S.; Leonard, K.; Bullard, B. Modular Proteins from the Drosophila sallimus (sls) Gene and their Expression in Muscles with Different Extensibility. *J. Mol. Biol.* **2007**, *367*, 953–969. [CrossRef]

246. González-Morales, N.; Xiao, Y.S.; Schilling, M.A.; Marescal, O.; Liao, K.A.; Schöck, F. Myofibril diameter is set by a finely tuned mechanism of protein oligomerization in Drosophila. *eLife* **2019**, *8*, e50496. [CrossRef]

247. Truman, J.W.; Schuppe, H.; Shepherd, D.; Williams, D.W. Developmental architecture of adult-specific lineages in the ventral CNS of Drosophila. *Development* **2004**, *131*, 5167. [CrossRef]

248. Brierley, D.J.; Blanc, E.; Reddy, O.V.; Vijayraghavan, K.; Williams, D.W. Dendritic targeting in the leg neuropil of Drosophila: The role of midline signalling molecules in generating a myotopic map. *PLoS Biol.* **2009**, *7*, e1000199. [CrossRef]

249. Enriquez, J.; Venkatasubramanian, L.; Baek, M.; Peterson, M.; Aghayeva, U.; Mann, R.S. Specification of Individual Adult Motor Neuron Morphologies by Combinatorial Transcription Factor Codes. *Neuron* **2015**, *86*, 955–970. [CrossRef]

250. Baek, M.; Mann, R.S. Lineage and Birth Date Specify Motor Neuron Targeting and Dendritic Architecture in Adult Drosophila. *J. Neurosci.* **2009**, *29*, 6904. [CrossRef]

251. Fernandes, J.J.; Keshishian, H. Nerve-muscle interactions during flight muscle development in Drosophila. *Development* **1998**, *125*, 1769.

252. Fernandes, J.; VijayRaghavan, K. The development of indirect flight muscle innervation in Drosophila melanogaster. *Development* **1993**, *118*, 215.

253. Rival, T.; Soustelle, L.; Cattaert, D.; Strambi, C.; Iché, M.; Birman, S. Physiological requirement for the glutamate transporter dEAAT1 at the adult Drosophila neuromuscular junction. *J. Neurobiol.* **2006**, *66*, 1061–1074. [CrossRef]

254. Kimura, K.I.; Truman, J.W. Postmetamorphic cell death in the nervous and muscular systems of Drosophila melanogaster. *J. Neurosci. Off. J. Soc. Neurosci.* **1990**, *10*, 403–411. [CrossRef]

255. Soler, C.; Taylor, M.V. The Him gene inhibits the development of Drosophila flight muscles during metamorphosis. *Mech. Dev.* **2009**, *126*, 595–603. [CrossRef] [PubMed]

256. Soler, C.; Han, J.; Taylor, M.V. The conserved transcription factor Mef2 has multiple roles in adult Drosophila musculature formation. *Development* **2012**, *139*, 1270. [CrossRef]

257. Zhang, S.; Bernstein, S.I. Spatially and temporally regulated expression of myosin heavy chain alternative exons during Drosophila embryogenesis. *Mech. Dev.* **2001**, *101*, 35–45. [CrossRef]

258. Swank, D.M.; Bartoo, M.L.; Knowles, A.F.; Iliffe, C.; Bernstein, S.I.; Molloy, J.E.; Sparrow, J.C. Alternative exon-encoded regions of Drosophila myosin heavy chain modulate ATPase rates and actin sliding velocity. *J. Biol. Chem.* **2001**, *276*, 15117–15124. [CrossRef]

259. Karlik, C.C.; Fyrberg, E.A. Two Drosophila melanogaster tropomyosin genes: Structural and functional aspects. *Mol. Cell. Biol.* **1986**, *6*, 1965. [CrossRef]

260. Mateos, J.; Herranz, R.; Domingo, A.; Sparrow, J.; Marco, R. The structural role of high molecular weight tropomyosins in dipteran indirect flight muscle and the effect of phosphorylation. *J. Muscle Res. Cell Motil.* **2006**, *27*, 189–201. [CrossRef]

261. Katzemich, A.; Long, J.Y.; Jani, K.; Lee, B.R.; Schöck, F. Muscle type-specific expression of Zasp52 isoforms in Drosophila. *Gene Expr. Patterns* **2011**, *11*, 484–490. [CrossRef]

262. Katzemich, A.; Kreisköther, N.; Alexandrovich, A.; Elliott, C.; Schöck, F.; Leonard, K.; Sparrow, J.; Bullard, B. The function of the M-line protein obscurin in controlling the symmetry of the sarcomere in the flight muscle of Drosophila. *J. Cell Sci.* **2012**, *125*, 3367. [CrossRef]

263. Marín, M.-C.; Rodríguez, J.-R.; Ferrús, A. Transcription of Drosophila Troponin I Gene Is Regulated by Two Conserved, Functionally Identical, Synergistic Elements. *Mol. Biol. Cell* **2004**, *15*, 1185–1196. [CrossRef] [PubMed]

264. Mas, J.-A.; García-Zaragoza, E.; Cervera, M. Two Functionally Identical Modular Enhancers in Drosophila Troponin T Gene Establish the Correct Protein Levels in Different Muscle Types. *Mol. Biol. Cell* **2004**, *15*, 1931–1945. [CrossRef] [PubMed]

265. Gremke, L.; Lord, P.C.W.; Sabacan, L.; Lin, S.-C.; Wohlwill, A.; Storti, R.V. Coordinate Regulation of Drosophila Tropomyosin Gene Expression Is Controlled by Multiple Muscle-Type-Specific Positive and Negative Enhancer Elements. *Dev. Biol.* **1993**, *159*, 513–527. [CrossRef] [PubMed]

266. Lin, M.H.; Nguyen, H.T.; Dybala, C.; Storti, R.V. Myocyte-specific enhancer factor 2 acts cooperatively with a muscle activator region to regulate Drosophila tropomyosin gene muscle expression. *Proc. Natl. Acad. Sci. USA* **1996**, *93*, 4623. [CrossRef] [PubMed]

267. Reddy, K.L.; Wohlwill, A.; Dzitoeva, S.; Lin, M.-H.; Holbrook, S.; Storti, R.V. The Drosophila PAR Domain Protein 1 (Pdp1) Gene Encodes Multiple Differentially Expressed mRNAs and Proteins through the Use of Multiple Enhancers and Promoters. *Dev. Biol.* **2000**, *224*, 401–414. [CrossRef]

268. Vigoreaux, J.O.; Saide, J.D.; Pardue, M.L. Structurally different Drosophila striated muscles utilize distinct variants of Z-band-associated proteins. *J. Muscle Res. Cell Motil.* **1991**, *12*, 340–354. [CrossRef]

269. Zhao, C.; Swank, D.M. The Drosophila indirect flight muscle myosin heavy chain isoform is insufficient to transform the jump muscle into a highly stretch-activated muscle type. *Am. J. Physiol. Cell Physiol.* **2017**, *312*, C111–C118. [CrossRef]

270. Vigoreaux, J.O.; Perry, L.M. Multiple isoelectric variants of flightin in Drosophila stretch-activated muscles are generated by temporally regulated phosphorylations. *J. Muscle Res. Cell Motil.* **1994**, *15*, 607–616. [CrossRef]

271. Daley, J.; Southgate, R.; Ayme-Southgate, A. Structure of the Drosophila projectin protein: Isoforms and implication for projectin filament assembly11Edited by M. F. Moody. *J. Mol. Biol.* **1998**, *279*, 201–210. [CrossRef]

272. Glasheen, B.M.; Ramanath, S.; Patel, M.; Sheppard, D.; Puthawala, J.T.; Riley, L.A.; Swank, D.M. Five Alternative Myosin Converter Domains Influence Muscle Power, Stretch Activation, and Kinetics. *Biophys. J.* **2018**, *114*, 1142–1152. [CrossRef]

273. Belozerov, V.E.; Ratkovic, S.; McNeill, H.; Hilliker, A.J.; McDermott, J.C. In vivo interaction proteomics reveal a novel p38 mitogen-activated protein kinase/Rack1 pathway regulating proteostasis in Drosophila muscle. *Mol. Cell. Biol.* **2014**, *34*, 474–484. [CrossRef] [PubMed]

274. Haas, K.F.; Woodruff, E., 3rd; Broadie, K. Proteasome function is required to maintain muscle cellular architecture. *Biol. Cell* **2007**, *99*, 615–626. [CrossRef] [PubMed]

275. Nguyen, H.T.; Voza, F.; Ezzeddine, N.; Frasch, M. Drosophila mind bomb2 is required for maintaining muscle integrity and survival. *J. Cell Biol.* **2007**, *179*, 219–227. [CrossRef] [PubMed]

276. Valdez, C.; Scroggs, R.; Chassen, R.; Reiter, L.T. Variation in Dube3a expression affects neurotransmission at the Drosophila neuromuscular junction. *Biol. Open* **2015**, *4*, 776–782. [CrossRef] [PubMed]

277. Marco-Ferreres, R.; Arredondo, J.J.; Fraile, B.; Cervera, M. Overexpression of troponin T in Drosophila muscles causes a decrease in the levels of thin-filament proteins. *Biochem. J.* **2005**, *386*, 145–152. [CrossRef] [PubMed]

278. Firdaus, H.; Mohan, J.; Naz, S.; Arathi, P.; Ramesh, S.R.; Nongthomba, U. A cis-regulatory mutation in troponin-I of Drosophila reveals the importance of proper stoichiometry of structural proteins during muscle assembly. *Genetics* **2015**, *200*, 149–165. [CrossRef] [PubMed]

279. Wójtowicz, I.; Jabłońska, J.; Zmojdzian, M.; Taghli-Lamallem, O.; Renaud, Y.; Junion, G.; Daczewska, M.; Huelsmann, S.; Jagla, K.; Jagla, T. Drosophila small heat shock protein CryAB ensures structural integrity of developing muscles, and proper muscle and heart performance. *Development* **2015**, *142*, 994. [CrossRef]

280. Jabłońska, J.; Dubińska-Magiera, M.; Jagla, T.; Jagla, K.; Daczewska, M. Drosophila Hsp67Bc hot-spot variants alter muscle structure and function. *Cell. Mol. Life Sci. CMLS* **2018**, *75*, 4341–4356. [CrossRef]

281. Wang, S.; Reuveny, A.; Volk, T. Nesprin provides elastic properties to muscle nuclei by cooperating with spectraplakin and EB1. *J. Cell Biol.* **2015**, *209*, 529–538. [CrossRef]

282. Wang, S.; Volk, T. Composite biopolymer scaffolds shape muscle nucleus: Insights and perspectives from Drosophila. *Bioarchitecture* **2015**, *5*, 35–43. [CrossRef]

283. Lorber, D.; Rotkopf, R.; Volk, T. In vivo imaging of myonuclei during spontaneous muscle contraction reveals non-uniform nuclear mechanical dynamics in Nesprin/klar mutants. *bioRxiv* **2019**, 643015. [CrossRef]

284. Elhanany-Tamir, H.; Yu, Y.V.; Shnayder, M.; Jain, A.; Welte, M.; Volk, T. Organelle positioning in muscles requires cooperation between two KASH proteins and microtubules. *J. Cell Biol.* **2012**, *198*, 833–846. [CrossRef] [PubMed]

285. Morel, V.; Lepicard, S.N.; Rey, A.; Parmentier, M.-L.; Schaeffer, L. Drosophila Nesprin-1 controls glutamate receptor density at neuromuscular junctions. *Cell. Mol. Life Sci.* **2014**, *71*, 3363–3379. [CrossRef] [PubMed]

286. Goel, P.; Dufour Bergeron, D.; Böhme, M.A.; Nunnelly, L.; Lehmann, M.; Buser, C.; Walter, A.M.; Sigrist, S.J.; Dickman, D. Homeostatic scaling of active zone scaffolds maintains global synaptic strength. *J. Cell Biol.* **2019**, *218*, 1706–1724. [CrossRef] [PubMed]

287. Goel, P.; Dickman, D. Distinct homeostatic modulations stabilize reduced postsynaptic receptivity in response to presynaptic DLK signaling. *Nat. Commun.* **2018**, *9*, 1856. [CrossRef]

288. Ziegler, A.B.; Augustin, H.; Clark, N.L.; Berthelot-Grosjean, M.; Simonnet, M.M.; Steinert, J.R.; Geillon, F.; Manière, G.; Featherstone, D.E.; Grosjean, Y. The Amino Acid Transporter JhI-21 Coevolves with Glutamate Receptors, Impacts NMJ Physiology, and Influences Locomotor Activity in Drosophila Larvae. *Sci. Rep.* **2016**, *6*, 19692. [CrossRef]

289. Hong, H.; Zhao, K.; Huang, S.; Huang, S.; Yao, A.; Jiang, Y.; Sigrist, S.; Zhao, L.; Zhang, Y.Q. Structural Remodeling of Active Zones Is Associated with Synaptic Homeostasis. *J. Neurosci.* **2020**, *40*, 2817. [CrossRef]

290. James, T.D.; Zwiefelhofer, D.J.; Frank, C.A. Maintenance of homeostatic plasticity at the Drosophila neuromuscular synapse requires continuous IP3-directed signaling. *eLife* **2019**, *8*, e39643. [CrossRef]

291. Mourikis, P.; Gopalakrishnan, S.; Sambasivan, R.; Tajbakhsh, S. Cell-autonomous Notch activity maintains the temporal specification potential of skeletal muscle stem cells. *Dev. Camb. Engl.* **2012**, *139*, 4536–4548. [CrossRef]

292. Boukhatmi, H.; Bray, S. A population of adult satellite-like cells in Drosophila is maintained through a switch in RNA-isoforms. *eLife* **2018**, *7*, e35954. [CrossRef]

293. Siles, L.; Ninfali, C.; Cortés, M.; Darling, D.S.; Postigo, A. ZEB1 protects skeletal muscle from damage and is required for its regeneration. *Nat. Commun.* **2019**, *10*, 1364. [CrossRef] [PubMed]

294. Kuang, S.; Kuroda, K.; Le Grand, F.; Rudnicki, M.A. Asymmetric self-renewal and commitment of satellite stem cells in muscle. *Cell* **2007**, *129*, 999–1010. [CrossRef] [PubMed]

295. de Haro, M.; Al-Ramahi, I.; De Gouyon, B.; Ukani, L.; Rosa, A.; Faustino, N.A.; Ashizawa, T.; Cooper, T.A.; Botas, J. MBNL1 and CUGBP1 modify expanded CUG-induced toxicity in a Drosophila model of myotonic dystrophy type 1. *Hum. Mol. Genet.* **2006**, *15*, 2138–2145. [CrossRef] [PubMed]

296. Picchio, L.; Plantie, E.; Renaud, Y.; Poovthumkadavil, P.; Jagla, K. Novel Drosophila model of myotonic dystrophy type 1: Phenotypic characterization and genome-wide view of altered gene expression. *Hum. Mol. Genet.* **2013**, *22*, 2795–2810. [CrossRef]

297. Yatsenko, A.S.; Shcherbata, H.R. Drosophila miR-9a Targets the ECM Receptor Dystroglycan to Canalize Myotendinous Junction Formation. *Dev. Cell* **2014**, *28*, 335–348. [CrossRef]

298. Kucherenko, M.M.; Marrone, A.K.; Rishko, V.M.; Magliarelli, H.d.F.; Shcherbata, H.R. Stress and muscular dystrophy: A genetic screen for Dystroglycan and Dystrophin interactors in Drosophila identifies cellular stress response components. *Dev. Biol.* **2011**, *352*, 228–242. [CrossRef]

299. Dialynas, G.; Shrestha, O.K.; Ponce, J.M.; Zwerger, M.; Thiemann, D.A.; Young, G.H.; Moore, S.A.; Yu, L.; Lammerding, J.; Wallrath, L.L. Myopathic lamin mutations cause reductive stress and activate the nrf2/keap-1 pathway. *PLoS Genet.* **2015**, *11*, e1005231. [CrossRef]

300. Chandran, S.; Suggs, J.A.; Wang, B.J.; Han, A.; Bhide, S.; Cryderman, D.E.; Moore, S.A.; Bernstein, S.I.; Wallrath, L.L.; Melkani, G.C. Suppression of myopathic lamin mutations by muscle-specific activation of AMPK and modulation of downstream signaling. *Hum. Mol. Genet.* **2019**, *28*, 351–371. [CrossRef]

301. Jungbluth, H.; Gautel, M. Pathogenic mechanisms in centronuclear myopathies. *Front. Aging Neurosci.* **2014**, *6*, 339. [CrossRef]

302. Schulman, V.K.; Folker, E.S.; Rosen, J.N.; Baylies, M.K. Syd/JIP3 and JNK signaling are required for myonuclear positioning and muscle function. *PLoS Genet.* **2014**, *10*, e1004880. [CrossRef]

303. Rosen, J.N.; Azevedo, M.; Soffar, D.B.; Boyko, V.P.; Brendel, M.B.; Schulman, V.K.; Baylies, M.K. The Drosophila Ninein homologue Bsg25D cooperates with Ensconsin in myonuclear positioning. *J. Cell Biol.* **2019**, *218*, 524–540. [CrossRef] [PubMed]

304. Naimi, B.; Harrison, A.; Cummins, M.; Nongthomba, U.; Clark, S.; Canal, I.; Ferrus, A.; Sparrow, J.C. A Tropomyosin-2 Mutation Suppresses a Troponin I Myopathy inDrosophila. *Mol. Biol. Cell* **2001**, *12*, 1529–1539. [CrossRef] [PubMed]

305. Dahl-Halvarsson, M.; Olive, M.; Pokrzywa, M.; Ejeskär, K.; Palmer, R.H.; Uv, A.E.; Tajsharghi, H. Drosophila model of myosin myopathy rescued by overexpression of a TRIM-protein family member. *Proc. Natl. Acad. Sci. USA* **2018**, *115*, E6566–E6575. [CrossRef] [PubMed]

306. Ugur, B.; Chen, K.; Bellen, H.J. Drosophila tools and assays for the study of human diseases. *Dis. Model. Mech.* **2016**, *9*, 235–244. [CrossRef] [PubMed]

307. Day, K.; Shefer, G.; Shearer, A.; Yablonka-Reuveni, Z. The depletion of skeletal muscle satellite cells with age is concomitant with reduced capacity of single progenitors to produce reserve progeny. *Dev. Biol.* **2010**, *340*, 330–343. [CrossRef] [PubMed]

308. Jiang, C.; Wen, Y.; Kuroda, K.; Hannon, K.; Rudnicki, M.A.; Kuang, S. Notch signaling deficiency underlies age-dependent depletion of satellite cells in muscular dystrophy. *Dis. Models Mech.* **2014**, *7*, 997. [CrossRef]

309. Letsou, A.; Bohmann, D. Small flies—Big discoveries: Nearly a century of Drosophila genetics and development. *Dev. Dyn.* **2005**, *232*, 526–528. [CrossRef]
310. Bellen, H.J.; Tong, C.; Tsuda, H. 100 years of Drosophila research and its impact on vertebrate neuroscience: A history lesson for the future. *Nat. Rev. Neurosci.* **2010**, *11*, 514–522. [CrossRef]

7

The Switch from NF-YAl to NF-YAs Isoform Impairs Myotubes Formation

Debora Libetti, Andrea Bernardini, Sarah Sertic, Graziella Messina, Diletta Dolfini and Roberto Mantovani *

Dipartimento di Bioscienze, Università degli Studi di Milano, Via Celoria 26, 20133 Milano, Italy;
debora.libetti@unimi.it (D.L.); andrea.bernardini@unimi.it (A.B.); sarah.sertic@unimi.it (S.S.);
graziella.messina@unimi.it (G.M.); diletta.dolfini@unimi.it (D.D.)
* Correspondence: mantor@unimi.it

Abstract: NF-YA, the regulatory subunit of the trimeric transcription factor (TF) NF-Y, is regulated by alternative splicing (AS) generating two major isoforms, "long" (NF-YAl) and "short" (NF-YAs). Muscle cells express NF-YAl. We ablated exon 3 in mouse C2C12 cells by a four-guide CRISPR/Cas9n strategy, obtaining clones expressing exclusively NF-YAs (C2-YAl-KO). C2-YAl-KO cells grow normally, but are unable to differentiate. Myogenin and—to a lesser extent, MyoD— levels are substantially lower in C2-YAl-KO, before and after differentiation. Expression of the fusogenic Myomaker and Myomixer genes, crucial for the early phases of the process, is not induced. Myomaker and Myomixer promoters are bound by MyoD and Myogenin, and Myogenin overexpression induces their expression in C2-YAl-KO. NF-Y inactivation reduces MyoD and Myogenin, but not directly: the Myogenin promoter is CCAAT-less, and the canonical CCAAT of the MyoD promoter is not bound by NF-Y in vivo. We propose that NF-YAl, but not NF-YAs, maintains muscle commitment by indirectly regulating Myogenin and MyoD expression in C2C12 cells. These experiments are the first genetic evidence that the two NF-YA isoforms have functionally distinct roles.

Keywords: splicing isoforms; CRISPR-Cas9; exon deletion; NF-Y; muscle differentiation; C2C12 cells

1. Introduction

Cell specification and differentiation during development of multicellular organisms is a complex set of events resulting in the formation of organs, whose physiology is maintained by a balance of cell proliferation and differentiation. A paradigmatic example of these phenomena is formation of skeletal muscle. In the case of mammals—mouse in particular—the process begins at early developmental stages, proceeding through embryonic, fetal and adult stages [1,2]. Sequence-specific transcription factors—TFs—play a central role in specifying the identities of myoblasts, their migration to different body locations, organization and the capacity to self-renew and differentiate into myotubes. These properties are key to guarantee maintenance and functionality of the different muscles throughout the lifespan of the organism, including repair after injury in adult life. A set of four key TFs —MyoD, Myf5, Myogenin, MRF4, termed myogenic regulatory factors (MRFs)—have been identified and thoroughly studied by genetic and biochemical means for their capacity to specify myoblasts identity [3,4]. During development, PAX3/7 are located upstream of MRFs [5]; downstream are many TFs, such as the MADS box MEF2A/C/D [6,7], the bHLH ID1/3 [8–10] and SNAI1 [11], the HOX SIX1/4/5 [12–15], STAT3 [16], NFIX [17,18] and the ZNF KLF2/4/5 [19,20]. Unlike MRFs, most of these TFs are not expressed predominantly in muscle cells and are equally important for development and differentiation of other tissues and organs [21–25].

NF-Y is an evolutionarily conserved heterotrimer formed by the sequence-specific NF-YA and the Histone Fold Domain—HFD—NF-YB/NF-YC [26]. The sequence recognized by NF-Y is the CCAAT box, which plays an important role in the activation of 25%–30% of mammalian genes. NF-Y has been classified as "pioneer" TF, in mammals and plants [27–31]. NF-YA is the regulatory subunit; it is alternatively spliced, generating two major isoforms "short" (NF-YAs) and "long" (NF-YAl), differing in 28 amino acids coded by exon 3 [32]. This stretch is located at the N-terminus of the protein, in the Gln-rich transactivation domain (TAD). NF-YAs and NF-YAl have identical subunits-interactions and DNA-binding properties *in vitro*; ChIP-seq from cells harboring predominantly either one of the two isoforms showed recovery of peaks enriched in CCAAT. The isoforms are expressed at various levels in different tissues and cell lines [32,33]. Importantly, no cell line has been so far described lacking NF-YA—nor the HFDs—and NF-YA inactivation was reported to be fatal to cells [28,34]. NF-YAl is the predominant isoform in muscle C2C12 cells: it is abundant in proliferating cells, but it drops to low levels following terminal differentiation to myotubes, unlike the HFD partners [35–37]. Highly reduced NF-YA protein was found in myotubes of adult mice [38]. This suggested that genes up-regulated in the terminal phases of muscle differentiation are either CCAAT-less or not NF-Y-dependent, whereas the trimer activates cell-cycle and growth-promoting genes required during the proliferative state. However, overexpression of NF-YAl led to improved differentiation of C2C12 [39], suggesting that NF-YAl does take part in the differentiation process.

For decades, C2C12 myoblast cells have represented an informative tool to identify genes involved in muscle differentiation [40]. Ablation of the whole NF-YA gene is early embryonic lethal [41], and KO in stable cell lines could not be generated so far. We investigated the role of NF-YAl by genetically ablating exon 3, leading to the production of an intact NF-YAs. We successfully generated homozygous C2C12 lines expressing only NF-YAs and went on to study differentiation properties.

2. Materials and Methods

2.1. Cell Culture and Proliferation Assay

Mouse myoblast cells (C2C12, ATCC) were cultured in Dulbecco's modified Eagle's medium (DMEM) supplemented with 10% Fetal Bovine Serum (FBS, Gibco-Thermo Fisher Scientific), 4 mM L-Glutamine, 100 units/mL penicillin and 100 µg/mL streptomycin (GM, growth medium), in a humidified 5% CO_2 atmosphere at 37 °C. C2C12 cells differentiation was induced plating cells in DMEM with 2% horse serum (Gibco-Thermo Fisher Scientific), 4 mM L-Glutamine, 100 units/mL penicillin and 100 µg/mL streptomycin (DM, differentiation medium). Proliferation assay was performed by plating 1.5×10^5 cells into a 12-well plate and counting every 24 h for 3 days, using the Trypan Blue dye exclusion test. All data were gathered from at least three independent biological replicates. Multiple comparisons were performed using the One-way ANOVA test.

2.2. Derivation of C2-YAl-KO Clones

To delete the exon 3 of NF-YA gene in C2C12 cells, four guide RNAs (gRNAs) were designed to simultaneously target the two flanking introns by using the online tool https://zlab.bio/guide-design-resources. Potential off-target sites were monitored by the online tool https://crispr.cos.uni-heidelberg.de: Table S1 shows the results of such analysis for the four guides. The selected gRNAs had no common off-target sites and were cloned in the two plasmids pX330A_D10A-1x2_ac and pX330A_ D10A-1x2_bd, following the Multiplex CRISPR/Cas9n Assembly System Kit protocol [42]. 1×10^6 C2C12 cells were transfected with 3 µg of the two gRNAs/CRISPR/Cas9n plasmids by electroporation and plated at low density. 72 h after transfection, single clones were picked, expanded and screened.

For DNA extraction, cells from the individual clones were washed with PBS, collected by scraping, lysed in 100 µL ice-cold lysis buffer (40 mM Tris-HCl, 2 mM EDTA, 0.08% SDS, 80 mM NaCl, 0.5 µg/µL Proteinase K) and incubated overnight at 37 °C in agitation. To precipitate DNA, 100 µL of ice-cold 2-propanol and 0.3 M NaAc were added, samples were mixed and centrifuged at 13,000 rpm for 30 min at 4 °C. The pellet was washed with 150 µL of 70% ethanol, centrifuged at 13,000 rpm for 30 min at

4 °C. Supernatant was discarded, the pellet was dried and resuspended in 30 μL H_2O. The resulting DNAs were then screened for positive exon 3 deletion by PCR.

We screened a total of 335 individual clones and obtained 2 independent homozygously edited clones.

2.3. Protein Extraction and Western Blot Analysis

For Whole Cell Extracts preparation, cells were pelleted by centrifugation, resuspended in ice-cold RIPA buffer (10 mM TrisHCl pH 8.0, 1 mM EDTA, 0.5 mM EGTA, 0.1% SDS, 0.1% sodium deoxycholate, 140 mM NaCl, 1% Triton X-100, 1 mM PMSF, Protease inhibitor cocktail) and incubated for 30 min on ice, with occasional shaking. Samples were centrifuged at 13,000 rpm for 10 min at 4°C and the supernatant recovered and quantified using the Bradford protein assay.

20 μg of extracts were loaded on a 4–10% SDS-polyacrylamide gel and analyzed by Western blot using primary antibodies and a peroxidase-conjugate secondary antibody (Sigma-Aldrich). Primary antibodies: anti-NF-YA (G-2, Santa Cruz), anti-NF-YB (GeneSpin), anti-NF-YC (home-made) anti-Vinculin (H-10, Santa Cruz), anti-MyHCs (MF20, DHSB), anti-Myogenin (IF5D, DHSB), anti-MyoD (C-20, Santa Cruz), anti-Myf5 (C-20, Santa Cruz), anti-Pax3 (DHSB), anti-Snail (C15D3, Cell Signaling). Western blot experiments were performed on three independent biological replicates.

2.4. Reverse Transcriptase PCR and Real-Time PCR

RNA was isolated by the Tri Reagent (Sigma-Aldrich) protocol according to the manufacturer's instruction. The cDNA was produced starting from 1 μg of total RNA using the MMLV Reverse Transcription Mix (GeneSpin) and used for real-time PCR (SYBR® Green Master Mix, Bio-rad Laboratories) analysis. Real-time PCRs were performed with oligonucleotides designed to amplify 100–200 bp fragments (Table S2). The housekeeping gene Rsp15a was used to normalize expression data. The relative sample enrichment was calculated with the formula $2^{-(\Delta\Delta Ct)}$, where $\Delta\Delta Ct$ = [(Ct sample – Ct Rps15a)$_x$ – (Ct sample – Ct Rps15a)$_y$], x = sample and y = sample control. RT-qPCR analyses were performed on three independent biological replicates. For ChIP experiments, we figured out the percentage of input immunoprecipitated by NF-YB and nc (negative control) antibodies. Results of three independent experiments were represented as Fold change (Fc) between NF-YB sample and nc sample as: %Input NF-YB/%Input nc.

2.5. Flow Cytometry Analyses

Cells were harvested by trypsinization and washed in PBS, fixed in ice-cold 70% ethanol and stored at 4 °C at least 24 hours. Cells were then washed with 1% BSA in PBS and resuspended in 500 μL of PI-staining solution (20 μg/mL Propidium Iodide, 10 μg/mL RNaseA, 1X PBS) at room temperature for 30 minutes, light protected. FACS analyses were performed using the BD FACSCantoII, analyzed with FACSDiva software and quantified with FlowJo. A total of 10^4 events were acquired for each sample. Three independent FACS experiments were performed.

2.6. Immunofluorescence

For immunofluorescence analyses, cells were washed three times with PBS and fixed 10 min with ice-cold acetone-methanol (1:1) at room temperature. After three washes, cells were permeabilized with 0.25% Triton X-100 in PBS for 5 min and incubated 1 h with the primary antibody anti-sarcomeric MyHCs (MF20, DHSB) at room temperature. Cells were washed three times, permeabilized 5 min with 0.25% Triton X-100 in PBS and incubated with secondary FITC anti-mouse antibody (1:500, Sigma-Aldrich) plus DAPI (2 μg/mL) for 40 min at room temperature, light protected. The acquisition was performed by using the inverted microscope Leica DMI6000 B. Three independent immunofluorescence experiments were performed.

2.7. Overexpression and RNA Interference Experiments

Myogenin overexpression was performed by electroporating 1×10^6 C2C12 cells with 3 μg of plasmid (pEMSV-Empty/pEMSV-Myog) and plating them in DM for 96 h. Cells were then collected and analyzed. Three independent biological replicates were performed.

For small interfering RNA (siRNA)-mediated knockdown of NF-YB [29], 2×10^6 C2C12 cells were transfected by electroporation with 100 nM of NF-YB [29] or scrambled control siRNA (Qiagen, SI01327193) and plated into a 10 cm plate in GM condition. 72 h after transfection, cells were collected by scraping for total protein preparation and RNA extraction. Gene expression was analyzed performing real-time PCR. Two independent biological replicates of siRNA interference were performed.

2.8. Chromatin Immunoprecipitation Assay (ChIP)

ChIPs were performed as described previously [43] with the following modifications. Briefly, 2×10^7 cells were crosslinked using 1% formaldehyde for 7 min, the reaction was quenched with 125 mM glycine and cells were collected by scraping. After lysis, nuclei were resuspended in Sonication buffer (50 mM Tris-HCl pH 8, 10 mM EDTA, 0.1% SDS, 0.5% sodium deoxycholate, protease Inhibitor cocktail) and sonicated (Bioruptor, Diagenode) to obtain fragments of approximately 150–300 bp, verified on agarose gel electrophoresis. Samples were centrifuged at 13,000 rpm for 10 min at 4 °C and supernatants recovered and quantified by Bradford assay. One hundred micrograms of chromatin were immunoprecipitated with 5 μg of anti-NF-YB (GeneSpin) and anti-FLAG (Sigma-Aldrich) antibodies. Protein-G beads (KPL) were used for recovery of antibody-bound proteins. Crosslinking was reversed by incubation at 65 °C overnight. Reactions were digested with RNase A and Proteinase K and DNA purified using the DNA purification kit (PCR clean Up, GeneSpin). The DNA was eluted in TE (10 mM Tris-HCl pH 8, 1 mM EDTA) and used in real-time PCR. Three independent biological replicates of ChIP experiments were performed.

3. Results

3.1. Ablation of NF-YA Exon 3 in C2C12 Cells by a Four Guides CRISPR/Cas9n Strategy

Mouse C2C12 cells mostly express NF-YAl [35–38]. To study the role of this isoform in maintenance and differentiation of C2C12, we set out a strategy to selectively eliminate exon 3, coding for the 28 extra amino acids present in NF-YAl and absent in NF-YAs. We figured that the use of four guides flanking precisely the exon 3 regions and of the single strand-cutting Cas9-nickase (Cas9n) would minimize off-target effects, which potentially affect the outcome of this technology [44]. Figure 1A shows the design of the four guide oligonucleotides, two couples targeting the 5' and 3' intronic DNA flaking exon 3, respectively. The two couples of oligos were first checked for absence of common genomic targets (Table S1) and cloned unpaired in the final pX330A_D10A-1x2_ad and pX330A_D10A-1x2_cb (Figure S1A), also expressing the Cas9n gene. The two plasmids were transfected in growing C2C12 cells by electroporation. Individual clones were isolated, expanded and analyzed by PCR, employing the amplicons shown in Figure 1B. As expected, the strategy was less efficient if compared to the standard use of two guides plus wt Cas9: 335 clones were individually screened and two were positive for correct ablation in homozygosity, as shown in Figure 1C. The results of PCRs of the two positive clones, #83 and #117, show the expected bands for the A, B and C amplicons, absent in the DNA of the parental C2C12 cells. The regions surrounding exon 3 in both clones were then amplified and sequenced: Figure S1B confirms the deletion of coding sequences of exon 3, with somewhat different ends in the two clones. In summary, we successfully ablated NF-YA exon 3, deriving two clones termed C2-YAl-KO. To the best of our knowledge, this is the second system of genome editing describing a clean deletion of an individual exon [45] and the first one employing the Cas9 nickase system coupled with four gRNAs.

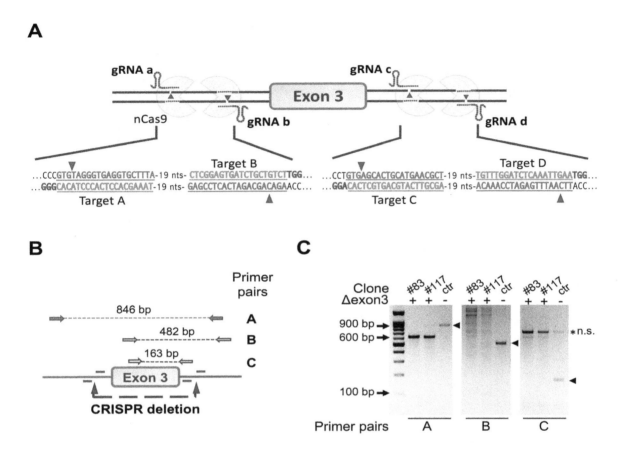

Figure 1. Strategy for ablation of NF-YA exon 3 in C2C12 cells using CRISPR/Cas9n and four gRNAs. (**A**) Gene editing strategy for NF-YA exon 3 deletion using the Cas9-nickase (Cas9n) and four guide RNAs. The targeted sequence by each guide RNA and the deletion sites are shown. Note that Cas9n cuts only the DNA strand that is complementary to and recognized by the gRNA, making necessary the simultaneous presence of two gRNAs/Cas9n complexes to induce a double-strand break (DSB). (**B**) The three primer pairs used to check for positive C2-YAl-KO clones are shown with the specific amplification products highlighted by the dashed lines. (**C**) Example of PCR products run into a 1.2% agarose gel. The expected bands in control cells (ctr) are marked with arrowheads; clones #83 and #117 represent positive C2-YAl-KO clones.

3.2. Characterization of C2-YAl-KO Cells

The two C2-YAl-KO clones were characterized first for expression of NF-YA. We performed qRT-PCR analysis with oligos specific for the individual isoforms [46]; Figure 2A shows that the NF-YAl mRNA is absent in the C2-YAl-KO clones. Extracts were prepared and Western blots performed: as expected, the parental C2C12 cells show expression of NF-YAl (Figure 2B). Instead, the clones express uniquely the NF-YAs isoform. We exposed the blots for long times to verify that no NF-YAl is visible in the two KO clones. Note that the levels of the two isoforms in parental cells—NF-YAl—and edited clones—NF-YAs—are essentially identical, as are the levels of NF-YB and NF-YC: since there is an important level of autoregulation among NF-Y subunits [47], this result indicates that HFD subunits are available for trimer formation and DNA-binding in C2C12 and C2-YAl-KO cells. In summary, genetic ablation of exon 3 in C2C12 was effective, leading to generation of clones that express uniquely the short isoform of NF-YA at physiological levels.

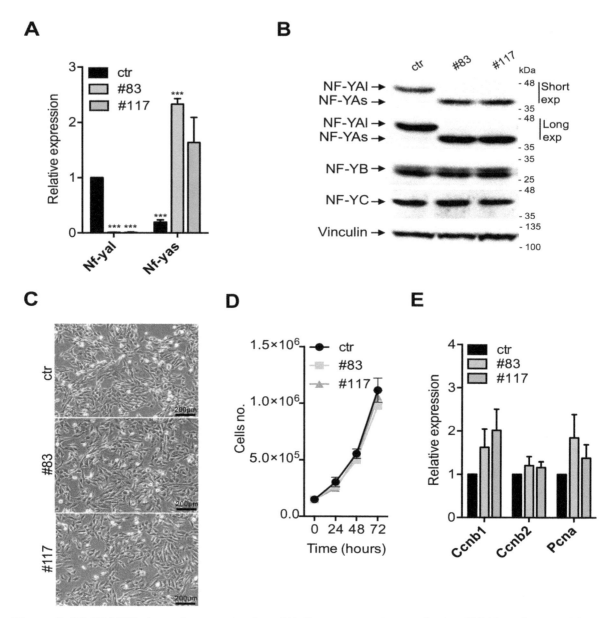

Figure 2. C2-YAl-KO clone characterization. (**A**) Gene expression analysis of NF-YA short and long levels in ctr and C2-YAl-KO clones (#83 and #117) in growth medium (GM) condition. Error bars represent the SD of three independent experiments. P-values were calculated using the one-sample t-test. (**B**) Western blot analysis of NF-Y protein subunits (NF-YA, NF-YB, NF-YC) in ctr cells and C2-YAl-KO clones (#83 and #117) in GM condition. For NF-YA isoforms analysis, short and long exposures are shown. Vinculin was used as loading control. (**C**) Phase contrast analysis of myoblast cells (ctr and C2-YAl-KO clones) morphology in GM condition. Scale bar 200 μm. (**D**) Proliferation assay performed in GM condition counting every 24 h for 3 days using the Trypan Blue dye exclusion test. Error bars represent the SD of three independent experiments. P-values were calculated using the one-way ANOVA test. (**E**) Gene expression analysis of key cell-cycle regulators in ctr and C2-YAl-KO clones (#83 and #117) in GM condition. Error bars represent the SD of three independent experiments. P-values were calculated using the one-sample t-test.

Next, we started to analyze the phenotype of the KO clones: they are stable upon repeated cycles of freezing and thawing and their morphology looks apparently similar to the parental C2C12 cells (Figure 2C). In mouse embryonic stem cells, expression of NF-YAs is associated with growth, and NF-YAl to differentiation [43]: in theory, NF-YAs-expressing C2C12 clones could be enhanced in proliferation. Cells were compared for growth under standard conditions: Figure 2D shows that growth curves are similar, with the two edited clones being marginally slower. In FACS analysis, we did notice some differences: a higher number of S-phase and G2/M cells in the two clones (Figure S2, 21% and 28%, with respect to 18% in C2C12). We checked the mRNA levels of PCNA, Cyclin B1/B2: a slight increase of Cyclin B1 and PCNA in the KO clones is observed (Figure 2E); although not statistically significant, this is consistent with the FACS data. The most noticeable difference, however, was the lower number of sub-G1 cells: 6%–7% in the two clones compared to 12% in the parental C2C12 cells (Figure S2): such non cycling cells are possibly undergoing cell death, suggesting that the switch to NF-YAs is not provoking negative effects on cellular vitality, and, if anything, the opposite. In summary, C2-YAl-KO clones expressing NF-YAs have an apparently normal morphology, grow well, but not faster, with the expected partitioning in cell cycle phases, bar slightly elevated G2/M and decreased sub-G1 populations.

3.3. C2-YAl-KO Cells Fail to Differentiate and Fuse into Myotubes

The levels of NF-YAl drop following terminal differentiation of C2C12 cells and myotubes of mouse muscles show low-to-nil levels of NF-YAl [35–39]. To ascertain whether NF-YAs-expressing cells could form myotubes, we switched the parental C2C12 and the two C2-YAl-KO clones at 70%–80% confluence to a differentiation medium. Before and after 72 h, we monitored cell morphology, performed Immunofluorescence experiments and derived whole cell extracts. Figure 3A shows that parental C2C12 form well organized, multinucleated myotubes, as expected (Upper Panels). The average number of nuclei per fiber is 15, in keeping with an efficient process (Figure 3B). On the other hand, the two edited clones showed a dramatic lack of myotubes formation: cells did not fuse; they were disorganized (Figure 3A, lower panels). We reasoned that the process could be simply slower in these cells and prolonged differentiation up to 5 days: this did not lead to formation of myotubes, nor cell fusion in the C2-YAl-KO clones (not shown). Immunofluorescence and Western blot data are consistent: the MyHCs marker is clearly visible in IFs (Figure 3A, right panels) and WB (Figure 3C) in C2C12 cells after differentiation, but not in the two edited clones. Interestingly, the levels of Myogenin and MyoD were substantially lower both in growing cells and at these late stages of differentiation in C2-YAl-KO clones. As previously reported, NF-YAl, in C2C12, and NF-YAs, in the edited clones, are down-regulated after 72 h of differentiation; NF-YB remained unchanged (Figure 3C). In summary, we conclude that terminal differentiation is completely blocked in C2C12 cells expressing NF-YAs instead of NF-YAl.

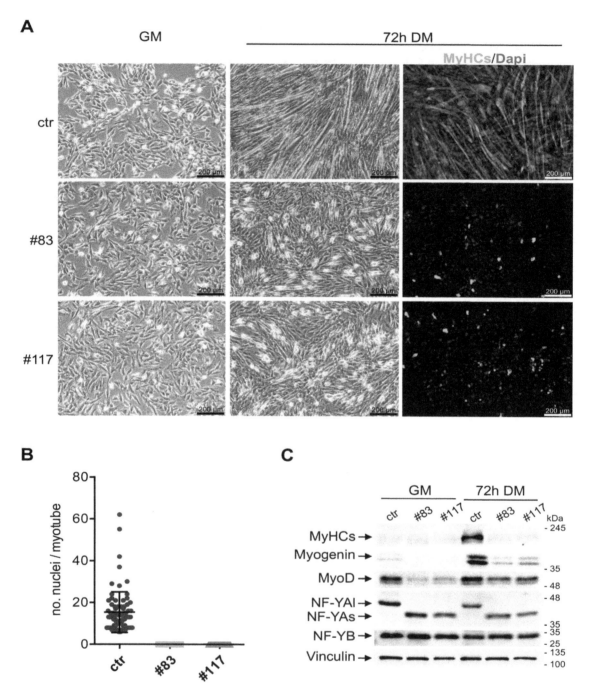

Figure 3. C2-YAl-KO clones fail to differentiate into myotubes. (**A**) Phase contrast analysis of myoblast cells (ctr and C2-YAl-KO clones) before and after 72 h of differentiation (differentiation medium (DM) condition) and immunofluorescence analyses after 72 h of differentiation. Antibody against all sarcomeric MyHCs and DAPI were used. (**B**) Fusion index was calculated as the number of nuclei in each myotube (with three or more nuclei). (**C**) Western blot analysis of key muscle differentiation regulators (MyHCs, MyoD), NF-YA isoforms (NF-YAl, NF-YAs) and NF-YB proteins, before (GM) and after 72 h of differentiation (72 h DM). Vinculin was used as loading control. The experiment was performed three times.

3.4. Expression of TFs in C2-YAl-KO

We analyzed expression of MRFs and TFs with a proven role in differentiation, in the parental and in the C2-YAl-KO cells under growing conditions and 24 h after differentiation. Profiling experiments established this as an early time point to detect significant changes in gene expression [48]. Note that most of the TFs analyzed have CCAAT in promoters and some formally shown to be under NF-Y control. First, we verified expression levels of MRFs in parental C2C12 (Figure S3): Myogenin is robustly induced; MyoD is modestly increased; Myf5 is modestly decreased after differentiation; Mef2C, but not Mef2D, is robustly increased. These changes are in agreement with expectations [49]. At the same time, we analyzed other TFs shown to be important for muscle differentiation: Six1/4/5, Snail, Stat3 and Klf5 are all increased upon C2C12 differentiation, Id1/3 are modestly decreased, Pax3 is unchanged (Figure S3). These results are also in agreement with published data. Having established that our differentiation program runs normally in C2C12 cells, we monitored expression of these genes in the C2-YAl-KO clones. The results are shown in Figure 4A for growing conditions and Figure 4B for differentiation. MRFs show the most conspicuous differences: Myogenin is almost undetectable in growing C2-YAl-KO clones and marginally increased upon differentiation. MyoD basal levels are normal, but induction is reduced upon differentiation, compared to parental C2C12. Myf5 expression is basally similar in the edited clones and higher after differentiation (Figure 4A,B). Mef2C levels are similar in growing conditions, but lower after differentiation: note that the levels are very low basally and differences with parental C2C12 cells are not statistically significant. Mef2D expression is identical in C2C12 and edited clones. As for the other TFs, Six1/4/5, Klf5 and Pax3 show similar expression patterns (Figure 4A,B). Minor changes are observed in growing conditions for Snail, Stat3 and Id1 (one clone only) and for Id1 (same clone) after differentiation. Finally, Id3 shows somewhat higher levels before and after differentiation, but again, these changes are variable in the three experiments and thus not statistically significant.

A

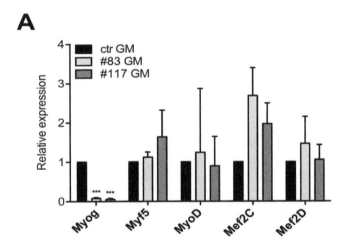
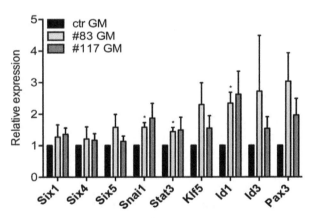

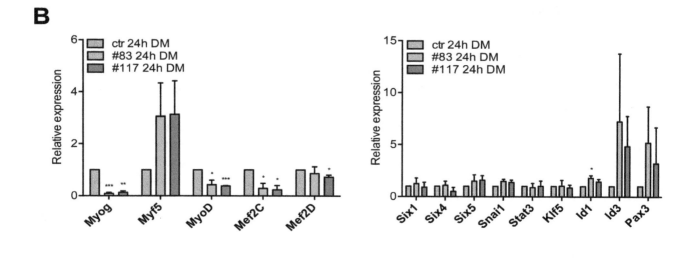

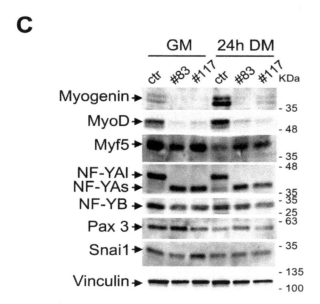

Figure 4. MRFs are downregulated in C2-YAl-KO clones. (**A**) Gene expression analysis of key muscle differentiation regulators (left panel) and other TFs shown to be important for muscle differentiation (right panel) in GM condition. Error bars represent the SD of three independent experiments. P-values were calculated using the one-sample t-test. (**B**) Gene expression analysis of key muscle differentiation regulators (left panel) and other TFs shown to be important for muscle differentiation (right panel) 24 h after differentiation (24 h DM). Error bars represent the SD of three independent experiments. P-values were calculated using the one-sample t-test. (**C**) Western blot analysis of key muscle differentiation regulators (Myogenin, MyoD, Myf5), NF-YA isoforms (NF-YAl, NF-YAs) and NF-YB proteins and other TFs shown to be important for muscle differentiation (Pax3, Snai1), in GM and 24 h DM. Vinculin was used as loading control.

To substantiate these results, protein expression of selected TFs was monitored by Western Blot analysis. Figure 4C shows that Myogenin levels are consistent with the mRNA data, being much lower in C2-YAl-KO clones than in parental cells, both in growing cells and after 24 h of differentiation. MyoD is substantially reduced in growing and differentiating clones, compared to parental C2C12. Note that protein levels were far lower than expected based on the mRNA levels, especially under growing conditions: this calls for post-transcriptional control in edited clones. Myf5 protein is downregulated in C2C12 after differentiation, as expected; in edited clones, it shows lower levels in growing cells, but higher after induction. NF-YA and NF-YB show the expected patterns; Pax3 is very modestly increased in C2-YAl-KO clones and Snail is unchanged. In summary, C2-YAl-KO cells have substantial differences in MRFs levels with respect to C2C12 cells, both before and after differentiation, whereas the other TFs showed rather minor changes.

3.5. Expression of Myomaker and Myomixer Is Activated by Myogenin and It Is Impaired in C2-YAl-KO

We were intrigued by the lack of cell fusion of the C2-YAl-KO clones after induction of differentiation. Myomaker—Mymk—and Myomixer—Mymx—are genes induced transcriptionally during muscle terminal differentiation, including in the C2C12 system [50,51]. Specifically, their expression is essential for the process of myocytes fusion [52]. We checked expression by qRT-PCR in parental C2C12 and in the two edited clones 24 h after differentiation. Figure 5A shows a strong induction—20-fold—of both Myomaker and Myomixer in C2C12 cells. C2-YAl-KO have much lower levels in growing cells (Figure 5B) and even more after differentiation (Figure 5C).

The obvious hypothesis was that these genes are under direct NF-Y control. We surveyed their promoter sequences and verified that no bona fide CCAAT box is present, notably within the evolutionary conserved areas: given the specificity of NF-Y CCAAT recognition, we considered unlikely that it acts directly on their expression. Genetic experiments in zebrafish have recently shown that Myomaker and Myomixer are directly activated by Myogenin [53]. We analyzed ENCODE datasets of C2C12 cells and found that Myogenin and MyoD target both promoters. Myomixer has apparently one promoter, Myomaker has two promoters, some 4 kb distant from each other: Figure 5D shows the overlapping peaks of Myogenin and MyoD. Myogenin binds exclusively after 24 h of differentiation, in accordance with its induced expression. One MyoD peak is visible already under growing conditions on Myomaker, and two additional peaks are found at 24 h. Importantly, the regions bound by MyoD and Myogenin in these two promoters are conserved across vertebrates, as shown by PhastCons data in Figure S4A: this corroborates the functional relevance proven in zebrafish [53]. To verify whether Myogenin activates Myomaker and Myomixer, we overexpressed it in parental C2C12 and in one of the C2-YAl-KO clones (#83) and induced to differentiate: Western blot of Figure 5E shows the increased levels of Myogenin compared to cells transfected with an Empty vector control; q-RT-PCR of Figure 5F shows that Myogenin overexpression has negligible effects on expression of the endogenous Myomaker and Myomixer in parental C2C12, but it increases expression of both genes in the C2-YAl-KO cells. Finally, morphological observation of the edited cells shows —incomplete—improvement in differentiation (Figure S4B).

In essence, we find that the marginal levels of Myogenin in C2-YAl-KO cells could result in lack of induction of the Myomaker and Myomixer targeted genes, entailing lack of cell fusion in NF-YAs-expressing clones.

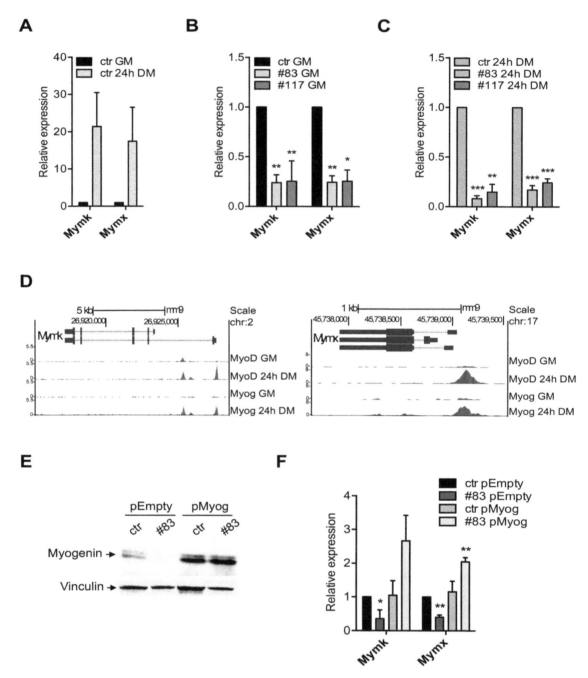

Figure 5. Myogenin directly regulates Myomaker and Myomixer expression. (**A**) Relative expression levels of Myomaker (Mymk) and Myomixer (Mymx) in C2C12 cells before and after 24 h of differentiation (24 h DM). Error bars represent the SD of three independent experiments. P-values were calculated using the one-sample t-test. (**B,C**) Relative expression levels of Myomaker (Mymk) and Myomixer (Mymx) in C2C12 cells before (**B**) and after 24 h of differentiation (**C**) in ctr and the two C2-YAl-KO clones. Error bars represent the SD of three independent experiments. P-values were calculated using the one-sample t-test. (**D**) ChIP-seq peaks of MyoD and Myogenin on Mymk and Mymx promoters in GM and after 24 h of differentiation (24 h DM) (UCSC-genome browser available tracks). Vertical viewing range Mymk: min 0, max 5.5. Vertical viewing range Mymx: min 0, max 8. (**E**) Western blot analysis of Myogenin protein levels in C2C12 cells transfected with a control plasmid (pEmpty) and the Myogenin-overexpressing plasmid (pMyog) 96 h after differentiation induction. Vinculin was used as loading control. (**F**) Relative expression levels of Mymk and Mymx in C2C12 Myog-overexpressing cells after 96 h of differentiation. Error bars represent the SD of three independent experiments. *p*-values were calculated using the one-sample t-test.

3.6. Myogenin and MyoD Are—Indirectly—Regulated by NF-Y

The results shown above beg the question as to whether NF-Y directly regulates MRFs. Myogenin and Myf5 promoters do not contain CCAAT boxes, MyoD does [54]. To verify the NF-Y dependence of these genes, we transitorily inactivated NF-Y activity. In our hands, NF-YA inactivations by shRNA or siRNA were rather inefficient in C2C12 cells (not shown). We thus turned to NF-YB by treating C2C12 cells with an siRNA previously shown to be active and very specific, including in profiling experiments [29]. NF-YB is a necessary component of the DNA-binding trimer: this allows us to inhibit CCAAT-binding activity, upon siRNA treatment. Most importantly, unlike NF-YA, NF-YB inactivation does not trigger apoptosis [29,34], making this a suitable choice for long differentiation processes. Figure 6 shows the results of experiment 1, Figure S5 those of experiment 2: in both, RT-qPCR (Figure 6A and Figure S5A) and Western blots (Figure 6B and Figure S5B) show far lower expression of NF-YB in C2C12 cells treated with NF-YB siRNA, with respect to the control siRNA.

In mRNA analysis, Myogenin, MyoD and Mef2C, but not Myf5 nor Mef2D, are substantially downregulated upon NF-Y inactivation; Myomaker and Myomixer are also reduced. Six1/4/5 a r e reduced: for Six4, this in keeping with an NF-Y dependence predicted from previous data on NF-Y binding to a canonical promoter CCAAT [39]. As for Id1 and Id3, they are somewhat reduced, but the results are borderline significant: Id1 in experiment 2 and Id3 in experiment 1. We conclude that NF-Y removal entails a reduction of MRFs, which, in turn, could explain the observed drop of Myomaker and Myomixer. We also show that members of the Six family are NF-Y targets. Analysis of proteins levels in extracts of siRNA-inactivated cells by Western blots confirmed these results: the levels of NF-YB were lower (although not to the extent of the mRNA) and paralleled by somewhat lower levels of NF-YA. Myogenin is substantially decreased and MyoD is also affected, to a lesser extent (Figure 6B and Figure S5B). We conclude that NF-Y regulates the expression of MyoD and Myogenin in C2C12 cells.

The Myogenin promoter is CCAAT-less and was not bound by NF-Y in C2C12 cells [39] and, despite the presence of a canonical CCAAT, the MyoD promoter was also not bound [39]. To understand whether the positive effect of NF-Y on MyoD is direct, we checked the parental C2C12 cells for the presence of NF-Y in ChIP experiments. Three independent experiments are shown in Figure 6C and Figure S5C. The absence of enrichment of NF-Y on MyoD is indeed confirmed, whereas the Stard4 positive control promoter is clearly bound. Equally positive was the promoter of Id1, but not that of Id3. Note that there is variability in the fold-enrichments in the three experiments: as this is high (from 60 to 800-folds), we consider quantitative changes difficult to interpret, especially when compared to completely negative promoters such as MyoD and Id3. Therefore, we conclude that NF-Y does not regulate MyoD directly—and despite promoter binding—NF-Y has modest effects on Id1 transcription in C2C12 cells.

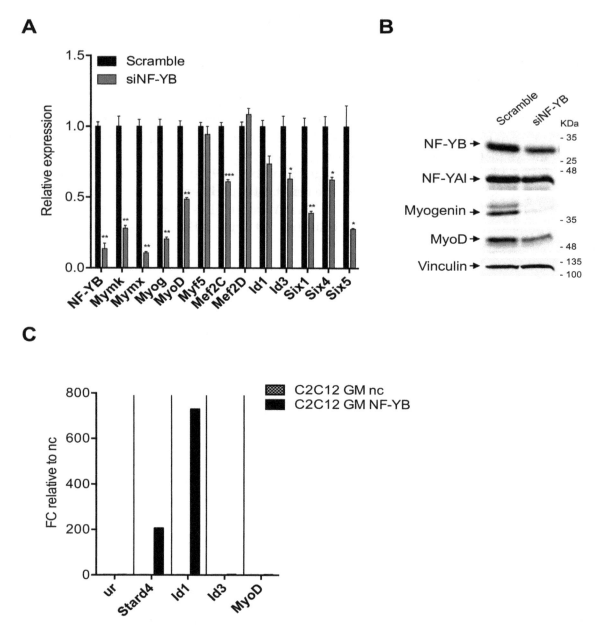

Figure 6. Analysis of NF-Y involvement in muscle specific genes expression. (**A**) Gene expression analysis of NF-YB and key muscle differentiation regulators in C2C12 cells 72 h after NF-YB silencing (siNF-YB) and scrambled siRNA control. Error bars represent the SD of two different RT-qPCR replicates. P-values were calculated using the one-sample t-test. (**B**) Western blot analysis of NF-YB, NF-YA and key muscle differentiation regulators (Myogenin, MyoD) protein levels 72 h after NF-YB silencing (siNF-YB) and the scrambled siRNA control. Vinculin was used as loading control. (**C**) ChIP experiment performed on C2C12 ctr cells in GM condition using NF-YB and negative control (nc) antibodies. The unrelated region (ur) and Stard4 were used as negative and positive control, respectively. Results are represented as the input percentage of each sample normalized to the input percentage of the nc antibody.

4. Discussion

By genome editing, we derived clones of C2C12 cells that express NF-YAs instead of NF-YAl. We verified that NF-YAs—and companion HFDs—are expressed at comparable levels and that it decreases after differentiation. The edited C2C12 clones are stable, grow normally, yet they are completely deficient in differentiation. We report defects of basal and induced expression of Myomaker and Myomixer, early response-genes likely responsible for lack of cell fusion. Their promoters are targeted by MyoD and Myogenin. In turn, we find low—basal and induced—levels of MyoD and Myogenin in the NF-YAs-expressing clones. Finally, expression of both MRFs are indirectly controlled by NF-Y.

4.1. Role of NF-YA Alternative Splicing in Muscle Cells

Specific isoforms of TFs have long been known to impact heavily on transcriptional regulation. Paradigmatic examples are the members of the p53/p63/p73 families, whose isoforms, produced by multiple promoters and alternative splicing, have different targets and often opposing transcriptional effects [55]. The muscle system is no exception [56,57]. Mef2C and Mef2D undergo alternative splicing during muscle differentiation [57,58]: a muscle-specific isoform of Mef2D contains exon α2 rather than α1, both expressed in muscle cells. Growing and early differentiating cells harbors MEF2Dα1; the switch to MEF2Dα2 occurs in terminal stages of C2C12 differentiation, leading to activation of late genes. MEF2Dα1 is phosphorylated at two serines by PKA [59], which mediate association with HDACs, resulting in repression. MEF2Dα2 lacks these residues, functioning as a transcriptional activator. Parallel molecular mechanisms appear to be operating for the related MEF2Cα1/α2 alternative splicing isoforms [58]. The key issue in Mef2 splicing regulation is involvement in late stages of differentiation. Alternative splicing was reported for the master TFs of muscle commitment PAX3 and PAX7, but the functional roles of the single isoforms are less well characterized [60–64].

We show here that a switch from NF-YAl to NF-YAs causes a major difference in the differentiation properties of C2C12 cells. The major NF-YA isoforms, originally reported decades ago [32], are only recently attracting the attention they deserve. In part, this was due to the elusive logic of their expression patterns: in some systems, cells have NF-YAs before—and NF-YAl after—differentiation; in others, such as in muscle cells, NF-YAl is mostly found. In part, it was because of the rather unimpressive nature of the exon 3 amino acids incorporated into NF-YAl: a short stretch rich in glutamines and hydrophobic residues amid the larger transactivation domain. Overexpression experiments suggested differences in gene activation [39,65], but these experiments are to be taken with a grain of salt, because of the large amount of proteins produced, targeting the large number of potential NF-Y sites in the genome. NF-YA AS is likely more complex than what is shown here. First, NF-YAx is another alternatively spliced isoform, recently reported in glioblastomas, devoid of exons 3 and 5: this greatly reduces the activation domain, with important functional consequences [66]. Expression of NF-YAx will have to be monitored in normal cells, to verify whether it is specific for glioblastomas. Second, there are micro differences—6 amino acids—produced in many cell types within the acceptor site of exon 5. Third, some cells show the inclusion of an additional Gln residue at the acceptor splicing site of exon 3, producing a 29 amino acids insertion [32]. Note that a similar situation was reported for PAX3, in which an extra Gln causes differences in DNA-binding affinity [59]. Precise editing techniques, as we have started to use here in C2C12 cells, could sort out the functionality of the various isoforms.

4.2. NF-Y Does Not Target Directly Genes Involved in C2C12 Differentiation

Sequence-specific TFs target specific genomic sites, driven by the discriminatory power of their DNA-binding Domains. However, they are also known to be binding indirectly, being tethered by other TFs or complexes: analysis of genomic locations by ENCODE has shown that this latter mechanism is far from marginal [67]. In addition to ENCODE, several independent ChIP-seq of TFs—and cofactors—identified binding to CCAAT locations [68]. One such example regards the orphan receptor Rev-Erb, important for muscle regeneration, targeting NF-Y sites in C2C12 cells [69]. The reverse, namely NF-Y being tethered to CCAAT-less locations by other TFs, has yet to be described. The issue could theoretically be relevant, since the genes down-regulated after NF-Y removal, or by switching from NF-YAl to NF-YAs, have generally no CCCAT in promoters. The effects appear to be largely indirect, but we do not favor the promoter tethering hypothesis. Rather, we report binding of Myogenin and MyoD to the promoters of Myomaker and Myomixer and show that Myogenin overexpression leads to recovery of their expression in C2-YAl-KO cells. This extends to mouse cells genetic experiments made in zebrafish [53]. It also indicates that NF-Y does not regulate other TFs essential for expression of these two genes. In summary, NF-Y/CCAAT interactions in promoters, which are structurally identical for NF-YAl and NF-YAs, are likely not crucial for genes induced during myotubes formation: rather, the focus is shifted to the control of MRFs, or other TFs.

We have analyzed expression of TFs involved in myoblast/C2C12 differentiation. The majority are not dramatically altered in edited clones. Mef2C induction is impaired, but previous studies indicated that NF-Y is bound to the Mef2D, not to Mef2C promoter [39]. We find that Mef2C, not Mef2D, is regulated by NF-YB RNAi interference. Note that these TFs are also targeted by MyoD and Myogenin, as they play a role in the final stages of differentiation [7,59]. This suggests indirect regulation by NF-Y via MRFs. Id1/Id3 do have bona fide functional CCAAT in promoters [70], bound in cancer cells as per ENCODE data (M. Ronzio, A.B., D.D., R.M., in preparation) and in NTera2 cells [71]: Id1, but not Id3, is bound in vivo by NF-Y in C2C12, parental cells and edited clones. The levels are decreased in C2-YAl-KO upon differentiation, but NF-Y-inactivation brings very marginal decrease in Id1 expression. PAX3, which acts upstream of MyoD, shows variable, somewhat increased mRNA levels in the edited clones, but this is not supported by analysis of protein levels. In summary, there is no clear CCAAT-driven TF that could explain the phenotype: instead, we propose that the decrease of Myogenin and MyoD expression entails a cascade of transcriptional events leading to failure of differentiation (Figure 7).

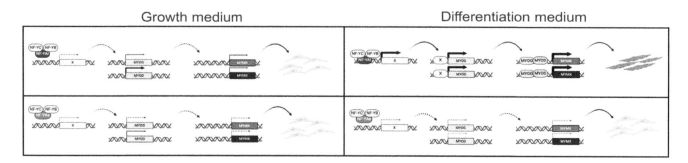

Figure 7. NF-YA isoforms involvement in regulation of expression of muscle genes. Model for NF-YA isoforms mediated regulation of expression of muscle genes in growth condition (left panel) and differentiation condition (right panel).

4.3. NF-Y Regulates MRFs Expression Indirectly

Switching from NF-YAl to NF-YAs—and NF-YB inactivation—negatively affects MRFs expression. Myf5 is moderately down in growing cells, remaining somewhat higher after differentiation. NF-Y-inactivation leads to a severe drop in Myogenin expression and a decrease of MyoD, which indicates an impact of NF-Y on their expression. The regulation appears to be transcriptional for Myogenin, not for MyoD, whose mRNA levels are variable, but overall similar. The Myogenin promoter is CCAAT-less and an indirect effect of NF-Y must be invoked. As for MyoD, the promoter harbors a high affinity NF-Y site, extremely conserved in evolution [54] and at the expected position (at -70 from TSS). Yet, NF-Y is not bound in vivo (Figure 6C). This is the only such example in nearly 200 promoters for which genetic analysis was reported [72]. The combination of an evolutionarily conserved, canonical CCAAT in a standard promoter position might function through NF-Y somewhen during the physiological activation of MyoD in development, while it has become expendable in the C2C12 system. Thus, down-regulation of MyoD in NF-YAs-expressing cells is also an indirect effect. It was proposed that MyoD serves as "pioneer" TF predisposing chromatin configurations for Myogenin to act as powerful activator of terminal differentiation genes and repressor of cell-cycle genes [73]. The latter function might be robustly counteracted by NF-YAs, but we have no evidence of that

(Figure 2). It is now clear that the focus is set on transcriptional regulation of the MyoD and Myogenin units and on which activator TF(s)—or cofactor(s)—is under NF-YAl—but not NF-YAs—direct control. For the time being, the "candidate" TFs approach used here failed to offer a plausible explanation on how NF-YAl regulates MRFs expression, thereby muscle differentiation. We must resolve to more systematic analysis, such as RNA-seq, to identify potential NF-Y-mediated regulators in C2C12. In light of the low intrinsic levels of muscle-commitment by MRFs in C2-YAl-KO clones, such analysis could also shed light on the actual identity of these cells.

Supplementary Materials:
Figure S1: CRISPR/Cas9n system and ablation of NF-YA exon 3 in C2C12 cells. (A) Schematic representation of plasmids construction, following the Multiplex CRISPR/Cas9n Assembly System Kit protocol (Yamamoto lab) [40]. (B) Sequencing of the two C2-YAl-KO clones (#83, #117) compared to the control (ctr). Deleted sequence, targeted sequence and exon 3 sequence are highlighted. Figure S2: Cell-cycle analysis of C2-YAl-KO clones. Flow cytometry analysis of ctr C2C12 cells and the two C2-YAl-KO clones in GM condition. The analysis of three independent experiments and the average of percentage of cells in each cell-cycle phase are shown. Figure S3: Gene expression analysis of TFs in growing and differentiated C2C12 cells. Gene expression analysis by RT-qPCR of key muscle differentiation regulators (left panel) and other TFs shown to be important for muscle differentiation (right panel) in GM condition and 24 h after differentiation in C2C12 ctr cells. Error bars represent the SD of three different experiments. P-values were calculated using the one-sample t-test. Figure S4: Myomaker and Myomixer expression are regulated by MyoD and Myogenin. (A) UCSC view of Mymk and Mymk *loci* showing alignment of ChIP-Seq data and DNA regulatory motifs conserved across Vertebrates by PhastCons. (B) Phase-contrast analysis of C2C12 cells (ctr and #83) morphology transfected with pEmpty or pMyog, 96 h after differentiation. Figure S5: Analysis of NF-Y involvement in muscle specific genes expression. (A) Gene expression analysis by RT-qPCR of NF-YB and key muscle differentiation regulators in C2C12 cells 72 h after NF-YB silencing (siNF-YB) and the scrambled siRNA control (II° experiment). Error bars represent the SD of two different q-PCR replicates. *p*-values were calculated using the one-sample t-test. (B) Western blot analysis of NF-YB, NF-YA and key muscle differentiation regulators (Myogenin, MyoD) protein levels 72 h after NF-YB silencing (siNF-YB) and the scrambled control. Vinculin was used as loading control. (C) Analysis of II° and III° ChIP experiments performed on C2C12 ctr cells in GM condition using NF-YB antibody and the negative control (nc). The unrelated region (ur) and Stard4 were used as negative and positive control, respectively. Results are represented as the input percentage of sample normalized to the nc. Table S1: Off-targets analysis. Analysis of possible off-target sites of each gRNA using the online tool https://crispr.cos.uni-heidelberg.de. For each gRNA the off-target gene name, gene id, position (intronic, intergenic, exonic), mismatches (MM) and the PAM sequence are reported. Table S2: Primers used. The specific sequence of each primer (forward and reverse) used for RT-qPCR and ChIP analysis are reported.

Author Contributions: D.L.: investigation, formal analysis and visualization; A.B.: data curation and methodology; S.S.: investigation; G.M.: resources, writing (review and editing); D.D.: methodology, data curation, writing (review and editing); R.M.: supervision, funding acquisition, writing (Original draft and editing). All authors have read and agreed to the published version of the manuscript.

Acknowledgments: The authors would like to thank prof. Carol Imbriano (Università degli Studi di Modena e Reggio Emilia) for providing antibodies against Myod and Myf5.

References

1. Buckingham, M. Skeletal muscle formation in vertebrates. *Curr. Opin. Genet. Dev.* **2001**, *11*, 440–448. [CrossRef]

2. Buckingham, M.; Rigby, P.W. Gene Regulatory Networks and Transcriptional Mechanisms that Control Myogenesis. *Dev. Cell* **2014**, *28*, 225–238. [CrossRef]

3. Hernández-Hernández, J.M.; García-González, E.G.; Brun, C.E.; Rudnicki, M.A. The myogenic regulatory factors, determinants of muscle development, cell identity and regeneration. *Semin. Cell Dev. Boil.* **2017**, *72*, 10–18. [CrossRef] [PubMed]

4. Zammit, P.S. Function of the myogenic regulatory factors Myf5, MyoD, Myogenin and MRF4 in skeletal muscle, satellite cells and regenerative myogenesis. *Semin. Cell Dev. Boil.* **2017**, *72*, 19–32. [CrossRef] [PubMed]

5. Buckingham, M.; Relaix, F. PAX3 and PAX7 as upstream regulators of myogenesis. *Semin. Cell Dev. Boil.* **2015**, *44*, 115–125. [CrossRef] [PubMed]

6. Black, B.L.; Olson, E.N. Transcriptional Control Of Muscle Development by Myocyte Enhancer Factor-2 (MEF2) Proteins. *Annu. Rev. Cell Dev. Boil.* **1998**, *14*, 167–196. [CrossRef]

7. Taylor, M.V.; Hughes, S.M. Mef2 and the skeletal muscle differentiation program. *Semin. Cell Dev. Boil.* **2017**, *72*, 33–44. [CrossRef]

8. Kumar, D.; Shadrach, J.L.; Wagers, A.J.; Lassar, A.B. Id3 Is a Direct Transcriptional Target of Pax7 in Quiescent Satellite Cells. *Mol. Boil. Cell* **2009**, *20*, 3170–3177. [CrossRef]

9. Wu, J.; Lim, R.W. Regulation of inhibitor of differentiation gene 3 (Id3) expression by Sp2-motif binding factor in myogenic C2C12 cells: Downregulation of DNA binding activity following skeletal muscle differentiation. *Biochim. et Biophys. Acta (BBA) Gene Struct. Expr.* **2005**, *1731*, 13–22. [CrossRef]

10. Atherton, G.T.; Travers, H.; Deed, R.; Norton, J.D. Regulation of cell differentiation in C2C12 myoblasts by the Id3 helix-loop-helix protein. *Cell Growth Differ. Mol. Boil. J. Am. Assoc. Cancer Res.* **1996**, *7*, 1059–1066.

11. Soleimani, V.D.; Yin, H.; Jahani-Asl, A.; Ming, H.; Kockx, C.; Van Ijcken, W.F.J.; Grosveld, F.; Rudnicki, M.A. Snail regulates MyoD binding-site occupancy to direct enhancer switching and differentiation-specific transcription in myogenesis. *Mol. Cell* **2012**, *47*, 457–468. [CrossRef] [PubMed]

12. Grifone, R.; Demignon, J.; Houbron, C.; Souil, E.; Niro, C.; Seller, M.J.; Hamard, G.; Maire, P. Six1 and Six4 homeoproteins are required for Pax3 and Mrf expression during myogenesis in the mouse embryo. *Development* **2005**, *132*, 2235–2249. [CrossRef] [PubMed]

13. Yajima, H.; Motohashi, N.; Ono, Y.; Sato, S.; Ikeda, K.; Masuda, S.; Yada, E.; Kanesaki, H.; Miyagoe-Suzuki, Y.; Takeda, S.; et al. Six family genes control the proliferation and differentiation of muscle satellite cells. *Exp. Cell Res.* **2010**, *316*, 2932–2944. [CrossRef]

14. Santolini, M.; Sakakibara, I.; Gauthier, M.; Aulinas, F.R.; Takahashi, H.; Sawasaki, T.; Mouly, V.; Concordet, J.-P.; Defossez, P.-A.; Hakim, V.; et al. MyoD reprogramming requires Six1 and Six4 homeoproteins: genome-wide cis-regulatory module analysis. *Nucleic Acids Res.* **2016**, *44*, 8621–8640. [CrossRef] [PubMed]

15. Yajima, H.; Kawakami, K. Low Six4 and Six5 gene dosage improves dystrophic phenotype and prolongs life span of mdx mice. *Dev. Growth Differ.* **2016**, *58*, 546–561. [CrossRef]

16. Guadagnin, E.; Mázala, D.; Chen, Y.-W. STAT3 in Skeletal Muscle Function and Disorders. *Int. J. Mol. Sci.* **2018**, *19*, 2265. [CrossRef] [PubMed]

17. Messina, G.; Biressi, S.A.M.; Monteverde, S.; Magli, A.; Cassano, M.; Perani, L.; Roncaglia, E.; Tagliafico, E.; Starnes, L.; Campbell, C.E.; et al. Nfix Regulates Fetal-Specific Transcription in Developing Skeletal Muscle. *Cell* **2010**, *140*, 554–566. [CrossRef]

18. Rossi, G.; Antonini, S.; Bonfanti, C.; Monteverde, S.; Vezzali, C.; Tajbakhsh, S.; Cossu, G.; Messina, G. Nfix Regulates Temporal Progression of Muscle Regeneration through Modulation of Myostatin Expression. *Cell Rep.* **2016**, *14*, 2238–2249. [CrossRef]

19. Hayashi, S.; Manabe, I.; Suzuki, Y.; Relaix, F.; Oishi, Y. Klf5 regulates muscle differentiation by directly targeting muscle-specific genes in cooperation with MyoD in mice. *eLife* **2016**, *5*, 37798. [CrossRef]

20. Sunadome, K.; Yamamoto, T.; Ebisuya, M.; Kondoh, K.; Sehara-Fujisawa, A.; Nishida, E. ERK5 Regulates Muscle Cell Fusion through Klf Transcription Factors. *Dev. Cell* **2011**, *20*, 192–205. [CrossRef]

21. Potthoff, M.J.; Olson, E.N. MEF2: a central regulator of diverse developmental programs. *Dev.* **2007**, *134*, 4131–4140. [CrossRef] [PubMed]

22. Ling, F.; Kang, B.; Sun, X.H. Id proteins: small molecules, mighty regulators. *Curr. Top Dev. Biol.* **2014**, *110*, 189–216. [PubMed]

23. Christensen, K.L.; Patrick, A.N.; McCoy, E.L.; Ford, H.L. Chapter 5 The Six Family of Homeobox Genes in Development and Cancer. *Advances in Cancer Research* **2008**, *101*, 93–126. [PubMed]

24. Bialkowska, A.; Yang, V.W.; Mallipattu, S.K. Krüppel-like factors in mammalian stem cells and development. *Development* **2017**, *144*, 737–754. [CrossRef]

25. Piper, M.; Gronostajski, R.; Messina, G. Nuclear Factor One X in Development and Disease. *Trends Cell Boil.* **2019**, *29*, 20–30. [CrossRef]

26. Dolfini, D.; Gatta, R.; Mantovani, R. NF-Y and the transcriptional activation of CCAAT promoters. *Crit. Rev. Biochem. Mol. Boil.* **2011**, *47*, 29–49. [CrossRef]

27. Fleming, J.D.; Pavesi, G.; Benatti, P.; Imbriano, C.; Mantovani, R.; Struhl, K. NF-Y coassociates with FOS at promoters, enhancers, repetitive elements, and inactive chromatin regions, and is stereo-positioned with growth-controlling transcription factors. *Genome Res.* **2013**, *23*, 1195–1209. [CrossRef]

28. Sherwood, R.I.; Hashimoto, T.; O'Donnell, C.P.; Lewis, S.; A Barkal, A.; Van Hoff, J.P.; Karun, V.; Jaakkola, T.; Gifford, D.K. Discovery of directional and nondirectional pioneer transcription factors by modeling DNase profile magnitude and shape. *Nat. Biotechnol.* **2014**, *32*, 171–178. [CrossRef]

29. Oldfield, A.; Yang, P.; Conway, A.E.; Cinghu, S.; Freudenberg, J.; Yellaboina, S.; Jothi, R. Histone-fold domain protein NF-Y promotes chromatin accessibility for cell type-specific master transcription factors. *Mol. Cell* **2014**, *55*, 708–722. [CrossRef]

30. Oldfield, A.; Henriques, T.; Kumar, D.; Burkholder, A.B.; Cinghu, S.; Paulet, D.; Bennett, B.D.; Yang, P.; Scruggs, B.S.; Lavender, C.A.; et al. NF-Y controls fidelity of transcription initiation at gene promoters through maintenance of the nucleosome-depleted region. *Nat. Commun.* **2019**, *10*, 3072. [CrossRef]

31. Lu, F.; Liu, Y.; Inoue, A.; Suzuki, T.; Zhao, K.; Zhang, Y. Establishing Chromatin Regulatory Landscape during Mouse Preimplantation Development. *Cell* **2016**, *165*, 1375–1388. [CrossRef] [PubMed]

32. Li, X.Y.; Van Huijsduijnen, R.H.; Mantovani, R.; Benoist, C.; Mathis, D. Intron-exon organization of the NF-Y genes. Tissue-specific splicing modifies an activation domain. *J. Boil. Chem.* **1992**, *267*, 8984–8990.

33. Ceribelli, M.; Benatti, P.; Imbriano, C.; Mantovani, R. NF-YC Complexity Is Generated by Dual Promoters and Alternative Splicing. *J. Biol. Chem.* **2009**, *284*, 34189–34200. [CrossRef] [PubMed]

34. Benatti, P.; Dolfini, D.; Vigano, M.A.; Ravo, M.; Weisz, A.; Imbriano, C. Specific inhibition of NF-Y subunits triggers different cell proliferation defects. *Nucleic Acids Res.* **2011**, *39*, 5356–5368. [CrossRef] [PubMed]

35. Farina, A.; Manni, I.; Fontemaggi, G.; Tiainen, M.; Cenciarelli, C.; Bellorini, M.; Mantovani, R.; Sacchi, A.; Piaggio, G. Down-regulation of cyclin B1 gene transcription in terminally differentiated skeletal muscle cells is associated with loss of functional CCAAT-binding NF-Y complex. *Oncogene* **1999**, *18*, 2818–2827. [CrossRef] [PubMed]

36. Gurtner, A.; Manni, I.; Fuschi, P.; Mantovani, R.; Guadagni, F.; Sacchi, A.; Piaggio, G. Requirement for Down-Regulation of the CCAAT-binding Activity of the NF-Y Transcription Factor during Skeletal Muscle Differentiation. *Mol. Boil. Cell* **2003**, *14*, 2706–2715. [CrossRef] [PubMed]

37. Gurtner, A.; Fuschi, P.; Magi, F.; Colussi, C.; Gaetano, C.; Dobbelstein, M.; Sacchi, A.; Piaggio, G. NF-Y Dependent Epigenetic Modifications Discriminate between Proliferating and Postmitotic Tissue. *PLOS ONE* **2008**, *3*, e2047. [CrossRef]

38. Goeman, F.; Manni, I.; Artuso, S.; Ramachandran, B.; Toietta, G.; Bossi, G.; Rando, G.; Cencioni, C.; Germoni, S.; Straino, S.; et al. Molecular imaging of nuclear factor-Y transcriptional activity maps proliferation sites in live animals. *Mol. Boil. Cell* **2012**, *23*, 1467–1474. [CrossRef]

39. Basile, V.; Baruffaldi, F.; Dolfini, D.; Belluti, S.; Benatti, P.; Ricci, L.; Artusi, V.; Tagliafico, E.; Mantovani, R.; Molinari, S.; et al. NF-YA splice variants have different roles on muscle differentiation. *Biochim. et Biophys. Acta (BBA) - Gene Regul. Mech.* **2016**, *1859*, 627–638. [CrossRef]

40. Mauro, A. Satellite cell of skeletal muscle fibers. *J. Cell Boil.* **1961**, *9*, 493–495. [CrossRef]

41. Maity, S.N. NF-Y (CBF) regulation in specific cell types and mouse models. *Biochim. et Biophys. Acta (BBA) Bioenerg.* **2016**, *1860*, 598–603. [CrossRef] [PubMed]

42. Sakuma, T.; Nishikawa, A.; Kume, S.; Chayama, K.; Yamamoto, T. Multiplex genome engineering in human cells using all-in-one CRISPR/Cas9 vector system. *Sci. Rep.* **2014**, *4*, 5400. [CrossRef] [PubMed]

43. Dolfini, D.; Minuzzo, M.; Pavesi, G.; Mantovani, R. The Short Isoform of NF-YA Belongs to the Embryonic Stem Cell Transcription Factor Circuitry. *STEM CELLS* **2012**, *30*, 2450–2459. [CrossRef] [PubMed]

44. Cullot, G.; Boutin, J.; Toutain, J.; Prat, F.; Pennamen, P.; Rooryck, C.; Teichmann, M.; Rousseau, E.; Lamrissi-Garcia, I.; Guyonnet-Duperat, V.; et al. CRISPR-Cas9 genome editing induces megabase-scale chromosomal truncations. *Nat. Commun.* **2019**, *10*, 1136. [CrossRef] [PubMed]

45. Min, Y.-L.; Bassel-Duby, R.; Olson, E.N. CRISPR Correction of Duchenne Muscular Dystrophy. *Annu. Rev. Med.* **2018**, *70*, 239–255. [CrossRef] [PubMed]

46. Bungartz, G.; Land, H.; Scadden, D.T.; Emerson, S.G. NF-Y is necessary for hematopoietic stem cell proliferation and survival. *Blood* **2012**, *119*, 1380–1389. [CrossRef] [PubMed]

47. Belluti, S.; Semeghini, V.; Basile, V.; Rigillo, G.; Salsi, V.; Genovese, F.; Dolfini, D.; Imbriano, C. An autoregulatory loop controls the expression of the transcription factor NF-Y. *Biochim. et Biophys. Acta (BBA) Bioenerg.* **2018**, *1861*, 509–518. [CrossRef]

48. Moran, J.; Li, Y.; Hill, A.A.; Mounts, W.M.; Miller, C.P. Gene expression changes during mouse skeletal myoblast differentiation revealed by transcriptional profiling. *Physiol. Genom.* **2002**, *10*, 103–111. [CrossRef]

49. Clever, J.L.; Sakai, Y.; Wang, R.A.; Schneider, D.B. Inefficient skeletal muscle repair in inhibitor of differentiation knockout mice suggests a crucial role for BMP signaling during adult muscle regeneration. *Am. J. Physiol. Physiol.* **2010**, *298*, C1087–C1099. [CrossRef]

50. Salizzato, V.; Zanin, S.; Borgo, C.; Lidron, E.; Salvi, M.; Rizzuto, R.; Pallafacchina, G.; Donella-Deana, A. Protein kinase CK2 subunits exert specific and coordinated functions in skeletal muscle differentiation and fusogenic activity. *FASEB J.* **2019**, *33*, 10648–10667. [CrossRef]

51. Millay, D.P.; Gamage, D.G.; Quinn, M.E.; Min, Y.-L.; Mitani, Y.; Bassel-Duby, R.; Olson, E.N. Structure–function analysis of myomaker domains required for myoblast fusion. *Proc. Natl. Acad. Sci.* **2016**, *113*, 2116–2121. [CrossRef] [PubMed]

52. Petrany, M.J.; Millay, D.P. Cell Fusion: Merging Membranes and Making Muscle. *Trends Cell Boil.* **2019**, *29*, 964–973. [CrossRef] [PubMed]

53. Ganassi, M.; Badodi, S.; Quiroga, H.P.O.; Zammit, P.S.; Hinits, Y.; Hughes, S.M. Myogenin promotes myocyte fusion to balance fibre number and size. *Nat. Commun.* **2018**, *9*, 4232. [CrossRef] [PubMed]

54. Pedraza-Alva, G.; Zingg, J.M.; Jost, J.P. AP-1 binds to a putative cAMP response element of the MyoD1 promoter and negatively modulates MyoD1 expression in dividing myoblasts. *J. Boil. Chem.* **1994**, *269*, 6978–6985.

55. Murray-Zmijewski, F.; Lane, D.P.; Bourdon, J.C. p53/p63/p73 isoforms: an orchestra of isoforms to harmonise cell differentiation and response to stress. *Cell Death Differ.* **2006**, *13*, 962–972. [CrossRef]

56. Imbriano, C.; Molinari, S. Alternative Splicing of Transcription Factors Genes in Muscle Physiology and Pathology. *Genes* **2018**, *9*, 107. [CrossRef]

57. Nakka, K.; Ghigna, C.; Gabellini, D.; Dilworth, F.J. Diversification of the muscle proteome through alternative splicing. *Skelet. Muscle* **2018**, *8*, 8. [CrossRef]

58. Zhang, M.; Zhu, B.; Davie, J. Alternative Splicing of MEF2C pre-mRNA Controls Its Activity in Normal Myogenesis and Promotes Tumorigenicity in Rhabdomyosarcoma Cells*. *J. Boil. Chem.* **2014**, *290*, 310–324. [CrossRef]

59. Sebastian, S.; Faralli, H.; Yao, Z.; Rakopoulos, P.; Palii, C.; Cao, Y.; Singh, K.; Liu, Q.-C.; Chu, A.; Aziz, A.; et al. Tissue-specific splicing of a ubiquitously expressed transcription factor is essential for muscle differentiation. *Genome Res.* **2013**, *27*, 1247–1259. [CrossRef]

60. Vogan, K.; Underhill, D.A.; Gros, P. An alternative splicing event in the Pax-3 paired domain identifies the linker region as a key determinant of paired domain DNA-binding activity. *Mol. Cell. Boil.* **1996**, *16*, 6677–6686. [CrossRef]

61. Barber, T.D.; Barber, M.C.; Cloutier, T.E.; Friedman, T.B. PAX3 gene structure, alternative splicing and evolution. *Gene* **1999**, *237*, 311–319. [CrossRef]

62. Pritchard, C.; Grosveld, G.; Hollenbach, A.D. Alternative splicing of Pax3 produces a transcriptionally inactive protein. *Gene* **2003**, *305*, 61–69. [CrossRef]

63. Charytonowicz, E.; Matushansky, I.; Castillo-Martin, M.; Hricik, T.; Cordon-Cardo, C.; Ziman, M. Alternate PAX3 and PAX7 C-terminal isoforms in myogenic differentiation and sarcomagenesis. *Clin. Transl. Oncol.* **2011**, *13*, 194–203. [CrossRef] [PubMed]

64. Vorobyov, E.; Horst, J. Expression of two protein isoforms of PAX7 is controlled by competing cleavage-polyadenylation and splicing. *Gene* **2004**, *342*, 107–112. [CrossRef] [PubMed]

65. LiBetti, D.; Bernardini, A.; Chiaramonte, M.L.; Minuzzo, M.; Gnesutta, N.; Messina, G.; Dolfini, D.; Mantovani, R. NF-YA enters cells through cell penetrating peptides. *Biochim. et Biophys. Acta (BBA) Bioenerg.* **2019**, *1866*, 430–440. [CrossRef] [PubMed]

66. Cappabianca, L.; Farina, A.R.; Di Marcotullio, L.; Infante, P.; De Simone, D.; Sebastiano, M.; Mackay, A. Discovery, characterization and potential roles of a novel NF-YAx splice variant in human neuroblastoma. *J. Exp. Clin. Cancer Res.* **2019**, *38*, 1–25. [CrossRef]

67. Wang, J.; Zhuang, J.; Iyer, S.; Lin, X.; Whitfield, T.W.; Greven, M.C.; Pierce, B.G.; Dong, X.; Kundaje, A.; Cheng, Y.; et al. Sequence features and chromatin structure around the genomic regions bound by 119 human transcription factors. *Genome Res.* **2012**, *22*, 1798–1812. [CrossRef]

68. Zambelli, F.; Pavesi, G. Genome wide features, distribution and correlations of NF-Y binding sites. *Biochim. et Biophys. Acta (BBA) Bioenerg.* **2017**, *1860*, 581–589. [CrossRef]

69. Welch, R.D.; Guo, C.; Sengupta, M.; Carpenter, K.J.; Stephens, N.A.; Arnett, S.A.; Meyers, M.J.; Sparks, L.M.; Smith, S.R.; Zhang, J.; et al. Rev-Erb co-regulates muscle regeneration via tethered interaction with the NF-Y cistrome. *Mol. Metab.* **2017**, *6*, 703–714. [CrossRef]

70. Van Wageningen, S.; Ridder, M.C.B.-D.; Nigten, J.; Nikoloski, G.; Erpelinck-Verschueren, C.A.J.; Löwenberg, B.; De Witte, T.; Tenen, D.G.; Van Der Reijden, B.A.; Jansen, J.H. Gene transactivation without direct DNA binding defines a novel gain-of-function for PML-RARα. *Blood* **2008**, *111*, 1634–1643. [CrossRef]

71. Moeinvaziri, F.; Shahhosseini, M. Epigenetic role of CCAAT box-binding transcription factor NF-Y onIDgene family in human embryonic carcinoma cells. *IUBMB Life* **2015**, *67*, 880–887. [CrossRef] [PubMed]

72. Dolfini, D.; Mantovani, R.; Zambelli, F.; Pavesi, G. A perspective of promoter architecture from the CCAAT box. *Cell Cycle* **2009**, *8*, 4127–4137. [CrossRef] [PubMed]

73. Singh, K.; Dilworth, F.J. Differential modulation of cell cycle progression distinguishes members of the myogenic regulatory factor family of transcription factors. *FEBS J.* **2013**, *280*, 3991–4003. [CrossRef]

8

The Survey of Cells Responsible for Heterotopic Ossification Development in Skeletal Muscles— Human and Mouse Models

Łukasz Pulik [1,†], Bartosz Mierzejewski [2,†], Maria A. Ciemerych [2], Edyta Brzóska [2,*] and Paweł Łęgosz [1,*]

[1]   Department of Orthopaedics and Traumatology, Medical University of Warsaw, Lindley 4 St, 02-005 Warsaw, Poland; lukasz.pulik@wum.edu.pl
[2]   Department of Cytology, Faculty of Biology, University of Warsaw, Miecznikowa 1 St, 02-096 Warsaw, Poland; bmierzejewski@biol.uw.edu.pl (B.M.); ciemerych@biol.uw.edu.pl (M.A.C.)
*   Correspondence: edbrzoska@biol.uw.edu.pl (E.B.); pawel.legosz@wum.edu.pl (P.Ł.);

†   These authors contribute equaly to this work.

Abstract: Heterotopic ossification (HO) manifests as bone development in the skeletal muscles and surrounding soft tissues. It can be caused by injury, surgery, or may have a genetic background. In each case, its development might differ, and depending on the age, sex, and patient's conditions, it could lead to a more or a less severe outcome. In the case of the injury or surgery provoked ossification development, it could be, to some extent, prevented by treatments. As far as genetic disorders are concerned, such prevention approaches are highly limited. Many lines of evidence point to the inflammatory process and abnormalities in the bone morphogenetic factor signaling pathway as the molecular and cellular backgrounds for HO development. However, the clear targets allowing the design of treatments preventing or lowering HO have not been identified yet. In this review, we summarize current knowledge on HO types, its symptoms, and possible ways of prevention and treatment. We also describe the molecules and cells in which abnormal function could lead to HO development. We emphasize the studies involving animal models of HO as being of great importance for understanding and future designing of the tools to counteract this pathology.

Keywords: muscles; heterotopic ossification; skeletal muscle stem and progenitor cells; HO precursors

1. Introduction

Heterotopic ossification (HO) is a disregulation of skeletal muscle homeostasis and regeneration, which results in mature bone formation in atypical locations. HO could develop in the skeletal muscles, and also in surrounding tissues such as fascia, tendons, skin, and subcutis [1]. HO can be acquired or have genetic origin. The most prevalent is acquired HO which can occur in response to a direct trauma, burn, or amputations. Similarly, iatrogenic trauma, caused by orthopedic surgery such as hip replacement, often triggers HO development [1,2]. Another acquired form of the disease is neurogenic HO (NHO) which is a frequent complication of central nervous system injury [3]. The knowledge about the molecular mechanisms that leads to HO formation and cell precursors engaged in this process is still limited. HO requires the presence of stem or progenitor cells which are able to follow the osteogenic program, although the identity of these cells remains unclear. Many different populations of progenitor cells could be possible precursors in the HO development. The animal studies suggest that progenitor cells can vary depending on the HO subtype. The studies using mouse HO models show that endothelial cells, mesenchymal cells, pericytes present in the skeletal muscles, tendons and connective tissue cells, or even circulating stem/precursor cells could be a source of HO precursors [1,4,5]. It is also known, that trauma or micro-trauma, which leads to a local inflammatory response, delivers the signals to develop HO. Recent studies showed the role of immune response cells, especially monocytes/macrophages, at the early stages of trauma-induced HO development [6]. They confirm the importance of macrophages in the induction of neurogenic and genetic forms of HO [7]. Activated macrophages express osteoinductive signaling factors in the course of HO pathogenesis. Thus, the presence of the cells reflects increased secretion of HO promoting cytokines/chemokines such as interleukin 6 (IL6), IL10, transforming beta-1 growth factor (TGFβ1), and neurotrophin 3 (NT3). A significant dysregulation of macrophage immune checkpoints was proven in HO animal models [8–10]. Finally, both individual predisposition and risk factors also attribute to HO development [11].

Histologically HO formation is similar to the physiological bone fracture healing. During HO development initially soft tissue is infiltrated with the whole spectrum of inflammatory cells. Such infiltration is followed by enhanced fibroblast proliferation, neovascularization, differentiation of chondrocytes, and results in mature bone formation [12]. HO is formed mainly by endochondral ossification. However, an intramembranous mechanism can also be involved. Typically HO formation is characterized by a zonal bone development model called "eggshell calcification" [13]. HO consists mainly of mechanically weak woven bone with an irregular osteoblasts distribution, but mature lamellar bone with Haversian-like canals can be often found. The bone tissue gradually matures with the outer appearance of the cortical bone [14]. Primarily, HO occurs in soft tissues and has no connection with the skeletal bone, but when it grows in the volume, it can attach to the periosteum.

2. Heterotopic Ossification as a Clinical Issue

HO is a diverse pathologic process and its spectrum can range from mild, clinically irrelevant to severe cases. In most of the patients it is minor and symptomless. Unfortunately, in some patients, extensive HO located around joints can cause restrictions in the range of motion (ROM), resulting even in the total ankylosis of the joint. In this group of patients HO can be associated with a significant limitation of daily activities and disability [1].

2.1. Traumatic HO

HO lesions can occur in response to direct trauma, such as connective tissue injury, bone fractures, burns, amputations, and combat-related blast injuries [2]. Approximately 30% of all fractures and dislocations which were subjected to operative treatment can trigger HO formation. It was a recognized clinical problem, in the acetabular and proximal femur fractures and fractures or dislocations of the elbow [1,15]. HO is also a common complication of traumatic limb amputation, both in civilian (22.8%) and in a military setting (62.9%) [16]. After the isolated burn injury HO incidence is relatively low (1%–4%), but it can be underestimated due to the lack of routine x-ray screening of such patients [17,18]. The typical locations of burn-induced HO are the elbow (50.0%), glenohumeral joint (20.3%), and the hip joint (17.6%) [18].

Recognized risk factors for trauma-induced HO are young age, male sex, severe concomitant injuries, compound fractures, extensive surgical approaches, and postponed surgeries [19,20]. The presence of local wound infection is also a well-established factor associated with HO [21]. In the military setting, the high incidence of HO is associated with concomitant brain injury, multiple wounds, and the severity of the injury [2]. The extent of burns, local wound infection, and the duration of intensive therapy are the risk factors for the formation of burn-induced HO. The role of immobilization and iatrogenic paralysis is also under investigation [18,22].

As far as the symptoms are concerned it can be associated with reduced joint mobility, pain, and decreased limb function. In the upper extremity, HO can limit everyday activities such as eating, dressing, and personal grooming, while in the lower limb it can affect gait and cause limp and difficulties in sitting [15]. Patients with amputation associated HO may experience difficulties with prosthesis fitting. Other local complications can occur, such as ulcers, skin graft necrosis, and neurovascular impairment [16]. The contractures and reduction of joint ROM in burn injuries are often caused by soft tissue scarring. However, HO should always be taken into consideration in differential diagnosis [18].

2.2. Surgery-Induced HO

HO is a well-described complication of orthopedic surgical procedures, typically joint replacements. The main indication for this kind of treatment is symptomatic, end-stage joint osteoarthritis. This type of HO usually involves the tissues where the surgical approach is performed, as unavoidable trauma is done to the muscle and fascia. It is most commonly described after a total hip replacement (THR) and cervical total disc arthroplasty (CTDA). It was also reported after the ankle, knee, and shoulder arthroplasty [23–25]. HO is radiologically present in every second patient after total hip replacement (40%–56%), and cervical total disc arthroplasty (44.6%–58.2%). However, high-grade HO occurs only in 2%–7% of total hip replacement and 11%–16% of cervical total disc arthroplasty patients [24–26].

The risk factors for the development of HO in patients undergoing total hip replacement are young age and male sex. The other predisposing conditions are bone and joint diseases such as ankylosing spondylitis, hypertrophic arthritis, and Paget's disease. The impact of the surgical approach, especially micro-invasive surgery (MIS) techniques, is being intensively discussed, but the results are still inconclusive [24,27,28]. Similarly, in patients after the cervical total disc arthroplasty, the male sex is an independent risk factor for HO development. Another important aspect is an artificial disc device type [29].

In the majority of patients suffering from surgery induced HO, small islands of the bone of no clinical significance are observed. However, extensive lesions can affect the biomechanical function of an endoprosthesis and block the movement in the affected joint. In total hip replacement patients, high-grade HO can significantly impact ROM, especially flexion, abduction, and external rotation, and affect the overall function of the hip [30]. In extreme cases, HO can require surgical intervention and excision (3.3%) [27]. In contrast to total hip replacement, in cervical total disc arthroplasty patients, severe HO does not affect patient-related pain, quality of life, or function [31].

2.3. Neurogenic HO

Neurogenic heterotopic ossification (NHO) can occur after the spinal cord injury (SCI) or traumatic brain injury (TBI). Other clinical conditions, such as cerebral stroke, anoxia, and non-traumatic myelopathies, can also attribute to NHO [32–34]. The incidence of NHO in spinal cord injury (40%–50%) was reported to be higher than in traumatic brain injury patients (8%–23%). However, symptomatic NHO is more frequent in traumatic brain injury than in spinal cord injury patients (11% vs. 4%). The incidence of this type of HO in cerebral stroke patients is relatively low (0.5%–1.2%) [35,36]. In contrast to traumatic lesions, NHO lesions typically occur in locations distant from the site of injury. The NHO lesions are usually located around the hip joints in both spinal cord injury (63%) and traumatic brain injury (40%) [36]. Other possible locations of NHO are the shoulder, knee, and elbow joints [37,38].

The demographic risk factors predisposing to NHO after spinal cord injury are male sex and young age. The complete spinal cord injury, high level of rupture, and spasticity can also be associated with an elevated incidence of NHO. Moreover, urinary tract infections and pneumonia significantly increase the risk of NHO [1,38]. NHO may also be associated with human leukocyte antigen B27 (HLA-B27) presence in spinal cord injury patients [39]. In traumatic brain injury patients, the NHO associated conditions are lower walking abilities, spasticity, pressure ulcers, neurogenic bladder, and systemic infections [40].

NHO usually develops two months after a spinal cord injury or traumatic brain injury [36,41,42]. Initially, it is characterized by inflammation-like prodromal symptoms such as swelling, redness of the joint, and low-grade fever. If there is no sensory impairment, the pain can also be present. Usually, two years after the neurological event, the lesions are fully developed [3,36]. Most of the patients do not suffer from NHO associated symptoms. However, when the lesions are extensive, it can affect joint ROM creating problems with moving from sitting to lying position and nursing. Additionally, the risk of bedsores significantly rises [3,37]. Moreover, patients with severe NHO obtain less satisfactory functional results and require prolonged rehabilitation [43].

2.4. Genetic HO

There are also rare, inherited forms of HO, such as fibrodysplasia ossificans progressiva (FOP) and progressive osseous heteroplasia (POH) [44,45]. FOP is autosomal-dominant disorder caused by up to 14 different mutations localised in the type I bone morphogenic protein (BMP) receptor, i.e., activin type 1 receptor (ACVR1; also called activin-like kinase 2, ALK2) gene [44,46]. However, a single mutation, i.e., arginine to histidine at position 206; R206H, is present in the majority of FOP patients [44,46]. The ossification of skeletal muscles in FOP occurs mostly in early childhood and is characterized by inflammation-like symptoms and episodical flareups [44]. POH is the other autosomal dominant inherited form of HO, which is caused by the mutation in gene encoding guanine nucleotide-binding protein, alpha stimulating (GNAS) [47]. The exact incidence of FOP is estimated to be approximately 1 person per 2 million [47]. The epidemiological data of 299 FOP patients from fifty-four countries participating in the International FOP Association (IFOPA) Global Registry will be published soon [48]. In most cases of FOP, it is caused by de novo mutations, but there is also a risk of parental transmission [49]. The incidence of POH is unknown. Similarly to FOP, in POH family transmissions have been documented, but the majority of the patients have spontaneous mutations [47]. There are no identified predisposing factors for inherited HO, including ethnic, racial, or geographic factors [47,50].

Children suffering from FOP are born with characteristic deformities of the toe and then, usually between 5 and 10 years of age, start to present soft tissue swelling which could be spontaneous or caused by minor injuries. With age, mature bone appears at the site of edema in the muscles and surrounding tissues. HO can appear in any location except for the viscera and thoracic diaphragm. The first affected areas are neck and upper back. Progression of HO over time leads to mobility restriction, respiratory problems, and heart failure associated with intercostal and spinal muscle ossification and chest deformation [50]. Recent studies revealed dysmorphology of the hip, spine, and tibiofibular joint, which can predispose to the high incidence of arthropathy in FOP patients [51]. Other aspects of FOP are malnutrition due to temporomandibular joint ossification and hearing problems due to middle ear HO. Most patients use a wheelchair at the end of their second decade of life [47,49]. In contrast to FOP, the HO lesions in POH usually appear early, i.e., during the first year of life. POH starts from the skin and subcutis and later on affects the deeper-lying striated muscles and fascia. POH is characterized by changeable expressivity and somatic mosaicism, including asymptomatic carriers. In some cases with high expression, it can result in early severe disability with joint ankylosis. The sings of POH can also include growth retardation, osteoporosis, and low body weight. The diagnostic criteria for POH have been proposed [45].

2.5. Diagnostic Imaging

Radiography is a first-line diagnostic tool in routine HO detection. The most commonly used HO classification systems, such as the Brooker classification for the hip and Hastings and Graham classification of the elbow, are based on the X-ray assessment [3]. Computed tomography (CT) can provide a more accurate assessment of the relation of HO lesion to the joint and other vascular and neural structures. CT and X-ray examinations remain the gold standard in the imaging diagnosis due to a low cost, simplicity, and high effectiveness in detecting fully developed HO lesions [52]. Nuclear medicine modalities can also be useful and provide metabolic and functional information on developing HO. The scintigraphy, including planar bone scan and single-photon emission computed tomography (SPECT), is proven to be a highly sensitive method in HO detection [53,54]. Similarly, the positron emission tomography (PET) can be useful in the HO diagnosis and successfully identify early HO and chronic lesions [55]. The other diagnostic imaging techniques include magnetic resonance imaging (MRI) that can identify vascularization and increased density in the early phases of HO as early as two days after the onset of clinical symptoms [38]. Recently, the ultrasonography is gaining popularity in HO detection and monitoring due to its safety profile, low cost, and the possibility of bedside-application [56]. In diagnostic imaging, it is critical to distinguish HO from neoplastic processes such as osteosarcoma, deep venous thrombosis (DVT). HO can also mimic gout, avulsion fracture, or local tissue calcifications like dystrophic and tumoral calcification or calcific tendonitis [11,52].

2.6. Biomarkers

The serum alkaline phosphatase enzyme (ALP) was extensively investigated as a potential biomarker of HO in traumatic HO, NHO after spinal cord injury, and total hip replacement induced HO. The elevated ALP level reflects enhanced bone turnover and increases with osteoclast activity. Detection of ALP could serve as a relatively inexpensive and widely available test for HO. Serum ALP concentration increases about two weeks after the operation reaching the peak concentration at week 10–12 and returns to the base level at week 18. However, ALP levels can be normal in the presence of HO development (55.2%), and the usefulness of ALP in HO screening is being discussed. Similarly, a bone-specific isoform of alkaline phosphatase (BAP) can be elevated in HO patients, but BAP levels are normal in most cases (67.8%). The other tested HO biomarkers are urinary excretion of type I collagen cross-linked C-telopeptide (CTX-1) and prostaglandin E2 (PGE2). The classical inflammation marker C-reactive protein, CRP is elevated in 77.0% of HO patients, but it is not specific [39,57,58]. Additionally, cytokine levels are investigated as biomarkers of HO onset. In the mouse model of FOP, the level of monocyte chemoattractant protein 1 (MCP1) (serum, saliva), IL1β (saliva), and tumor necrosis factor α (TNFα) (serum) were significantly increased compared to control group. In the mouse model of trauma-induced HO, the levels of TNFα, IL1β, IL6, and MCP1 were increased in serum samples [59]. In human studies, HO was associated with the level of serum (IL3, IL12) and wound effluent cytokines (IL3, IL13) in combat-injured patients [60].

Recently proteomic biomarkers were analyzed with mass spectrometry in non-genetic HO patients. Significant differences were found in the levels of certain peptides in patients with HO compared to the non-HO group. The researchers point out the protein fragments of osteocalcin (OC), collagen alpha 1 (COL1), osteomodulin (OMD) as potential clinical biomarkers for HO [61]. Another investigated class of HO biomarkers are small non-coding RNA molecules (miRNA). The disregulation of miRNA homeostasis may play a vital role in HO development. For instance, the decreased expression of miRNA-630, which is responsible for endothelial cells transition towards mesenchymal cells, was observed in HO patients [62]. The decreased level of miRNA-421 in humeral fracture patients is associated with BMP2 overexpression and a higher rate of the HO occurrence [63]. The miRNA-203 downregulation leads to an increase in expression of runt-related transcription factor 2 (Runx2), which is a crucial osteoblast differentiation regulator [64]. The miRNA particles are not only possible HO indicators, but they can also be future therapeutic targets.

2.7. Prophylaxis

The standard HO prophylaxis is pharmacological treatment with nonsteroidal anti-inflammatory drugs (NSAIDs) or local external beam radiotherapy (RT). The NSAIDs or radiotherapy prophylaxis is a well-proven and effective method, but it is not specific. Currently, the more targeted pharmacological strategies are being tested and developed for inhibiting specific pathways and molecules responsible for HO. Once the mature lesion is developed, it is not possible to reverse the changes, and the only remaining treatment option is surgical resection [65]. Despite that NSAIDs are effective prophylaxis of HO, they do not present efficacy when HO is fully developed. There is no difference between non-selective NSAIDs and selective NSAIDs in HO treatment [66]. The selective cyclooxygenase-2 (COX-2) inhibitors can significantly decrease discontinuation of treatment due to gastro-intestinal (GI) side effects [67,68]. However, non-selective NSAIDs are the most commonly used in clinical practice (87%) and remain "golden standard" in HO prevention. Indomethacin non-selective COX inhibitor is the most commonly prescribed NSAID for HO prophylaxis (57%) with a daily dose of 100–150 mg with a mean of 30 days of administration [69,70]. In addition to high efficiency, NSAIDs are approximately 45 times more cost-effective compared to RT [71,72].

RT recommended before the surgery or early, up to 72 h post-surgery, is an equally successful method for prophylaxis of HO development as NSAIDs. The multiple fractions RT is more effective in the reduction of HO. It is dose-dependent, but a modification of a biologically effective radiation dose over the >2500 cGy did not result in better effectiveness [73]. In total hip replacement patients, the combination of NSAIDs and RT may also be beneficial [74]. The RT seems to be a safe method of HO prevention in total hip replacement patients regarding local neoplastic processes and aseptic loosening of the implant [75].

The other prophylaxis modalities were also proposed. Taking into account bacterial contamination of wound in traumatic HO, locally administered vancomycin prophylaxis suppressed HO in trauma-induced rats infected with methicillin—resistant *Staphylococcus aureus* (MRSA) [76]. Bisphosphonates that are mainly used as anti-osteoporosis drugs and act by inhibiting calcification, and bone resorption dependent on osteoclasts, have no significantly higher efficacy than NSAIDs [77]. The aspirin, which has both effects of NSAID and the anti-platelet agents, is often used for venous thromboembolism (VTE) prophylaxis in total hip replacement patients and was also shown to be effective in the HO rate reduction [78].

2.8. Treatment

Surgical removal of lesions is currently the only effective method when HO is already formed and gives clinical symptoms. However, the operation itself may induce the formation of new ossifications. Among the indications of HO are pain and reduction of ROM. In most cases, the treatment also includes NSAIDs or radiotherapy as the prevention of relapse. A common strategy is to change the type of prophylaxis or the application of another type of NSAIDs class if the previously used prophylaxis has failed. The standard procedure is simple excision of HO, but it is unclear whether it should be removed completely or only partially [79]. Some authors recommend HO surgery only when the mature bone tissue is formed. However, early intervention minimizes the development of intra-articular changes and HO recurrence, so ossifications should be removed as soon as the mature bone is formed, without unnecessary delay [80–83]. As a result of surgery, the pain level is reduced and ROM increases, which significantly improves the function and often reduces the level of pain [70,84–88]. The total hip replacement is a promising solution for NHO in the area of the hip joint in patients after traumatic brain injury. The standard procedure is the Girdlestone procedure, but total hip replacement seems to give better results than a simple excision. When using THA, ossification has less tendency to relapse and the patient achieves more satisfactory functional results. [89,90].

3. Heterotopic Ossification Precursor Cells

3.1. Stem and Progenitor Cells in Skeletal Muscles

HO development is a complex process engaging many different cell types. Several lines of evidence suggest that the development of HO in skeletal muscle could be a result of pathological differentiation of stem and progenitor cells present in skeletal muscle. The most important cells responsible for postnatal skeletal muscle growth and regeneration are satellite cells (SCs), i.e., unipotent stem cells located between muscle fibers plasmalemma and basal lamina (Figure 1). These cells are activated in response to skeletal muscle injury which results in the cell cycle re-entry [91]. The signals activating satellite cells are provided by damaged muscle fibers, inflammatory cells, and endothelium [92]. Activated SCs start to proliferate, differentiate into myoblasts, i.e., muscle progenitor cells, and then myocytes. The myocytes fuse with existing myofibers or with each other to form myotubes and then, after innervation, myofibers. Many studies showed that SC presence is essential for skeletal muscle regeneration [93]. This multi-step process is accompanied by changes in expression of pair box transcription factors 7 (Pax7) and myogenic regulatory factors (MRFs), such as MYOD, MRF5, myogenin, MRF4, as well as skeletal muscle structural proteins [94]. Importantly, SCs are able to follow two different fates—they could maintain PAX7 and down-regulate MYOD expression to self-renew their population or down-regulate PAX7 and maintain MYOD expression to upregulate MYOGENIN and initiate differentiation [94]. SCs proliferation is regulated by MYOD and MYF5 which control the activity of the genes involved in DNA replication and cell cycle progression, such as cell division cycle 6 protein (CDC6) and minichromosome maintenance complex component 2 (MCM2). MYOD contribution in the myogenic differentiation also involves the induction of miR206 and miR486 which downregulate PAX7 [95]. Moreover, long non-coding RNA linc-RAM promotes the formation of MYOD complex with chromatin modifier BAF60c which enables MYOD binding to promoters of target genes and marks the chromatin for recruitment of chromatin-remodeling complex, i.e., BRG1-based SWItch/Sucrose NonFermentable (SWI/SNF). This MYOD-BAF60c-BRG1 complex remodels the chromatin and activates transcription of MYOD-target genes [96]. Furthermore, MYOD, as stated above, promotes expression of MYOGENIN and MRF4, i.e., transcription factors responsible for myoblast cell cycle exit and their differentiation into myocytes and myotubes. These differentiation steps are accompanied with expression of myosin heavy chains (MHC), enolase 3 (ENO3), and muscle creatine kinase (MCK) [91].

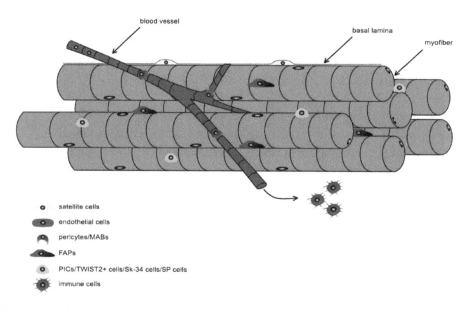

Figure 1. The stem and progenitor cells responsible for skeletal muscle homeostasis. The multinucleated skeletal muscle myofibers are accompanied by several types of stem and progenitor cells, such as satellite cells, endothelial cells, pericytes, mesoangioblasts (MABs), and fibro-adipogenic progenitors (FAPs), which could participate in regeneration. Other populations of muscle interstitial cells, such as, PW1+/PAX7 interstitial cells (PICs), Sk-34 cells, TWIST2+ cells, side population (SP) cells was also shown to be able to follow myogenic program. Moreover, the skeletal muscle reconstruction is accompanied by infiltration by immune cells.

Importantly, the fate of SCs is determined by their interactions with the niche. The quiescent SC niche is formed by myofibers and the extracellular matrix (ECM), i.e., the basal lamina. Such a niche is modified after the skeletal muscle injury and during regeneration. The factors secreted by damaged myofibers, inflammatory cells, endothelial cells, fibroblasts, and fibro-adipogenic progenitors (FAP), present in skeletal muscle, regulate the fate of SCs and myoblasts. Since the inflammation is among the initial responses to muscle injury, resident immune cells, such as mast cells and neutrophils, are activated by factors released by degenerated fibers [97]. The immune cells start to produce pro-inflammatory molecules, such as histamine, TNFα, interferon γ (IFNγ), IL1β, which leads to increased vascular permeability and myeloid cells recruitment. Both neutrophils and macrophages participate in damaged myofibers removal. Simultaneously, factors secreted by neutrophils and macrophages play an important role in the SC activation and myoblast proliferation and differentiation. Thus, the depletion of macrophages reduces the level of hepatocyte growth factor (HGF) and insulin-like growth factor 1 (IGF1), causing impairment of skeletal muscle regeneration [98]. HGF binds with c-met and plays a role in SC activation [99]. IGF-1 promotes myoblasts proliferation and differentiation [100,101]. Macrophages also secrete TNFα and IL6, i.e., factors which promote myoblasts proliferation and differentiation [102]. Other cells that play crucial role in skeletal muscle reconstruction are endothelial cells. They participate in the restoration of vasculature in damaged muscle and secrete pro-angiogenic and pro-myogenic factors, such as apelin, oncostatin, and periostin [103–105]. ECM remodeling that is an important step during muscle regeneration involves fibroblasts and FAPs (also named "mesenchymal progenitors"). These cells also produce pro-myogenic factors, such as: IGF1, IL6, and follistatin [106–108]. FAPs are interstitial non-myogenic progenitors expressing platelet derived growth factor receptor α (PDGFRα) [109–111]. In intact muscle FAPs are quiescent but after an injury they start to proliferate and synthesize ECM proteins, as well as abovementioned factors [112]. In aged muscles and during chronic diseases the FAPs accumulation and differentiation into fibroblasts and adipocytes is observed. Thus, these cells could be engaged in the formation of fibrosis or adipose tissue accumulation [112].

Except for abovementioned cell populations, skeletal muscle interstitium is the source of stem and progenitor cells different form SCs [113]. Their role in skeletal muscle homeostasis is extensively studied using mouse models. However, many studies also focus on human cells [113]. In mouse as well as in human muscles pericytes and mesangioblast are localized peripherally to microvessel endothelium. They are described as PDGFRβ, NG2, CD146 expressing cells [114–119]. Such cells were shown to be able to fuse with myofibers and occupy satellite cell niche in regenerating muscle [114–118]. Moreover, mouse and human pericytes secrete IFG-1 and angiopoetin that are known factors supporting myoblasts differentiation [120]. Other populations detected in mouse muscles are PW1+/PAX7 interstitial cells, i.e., PICs expressing PW1, SCA1, and CD34 [121]. These cells transplanted to injured mouse muscles participated in the regeneration and restoration of SC population [121]. Next, the TWIST2+ progenitor cells expressing transcription factor TWIST2, myoendothelial cells expressing CD34, i.e., Sk34 cells, and side population (SP) cells isolated on the basis of Hoechst day exclusion were identified in mouse muscle interstitium [122–124]. They showed myogenic potential in vitro and formed new myofibers after transplantation into injured muscles [122–124], similarly to CD133+ cells presented in human muscles [125].

3.2. The Osteogenic Potential of Stem and Progenitor Cells Residing in Skeletal Muscle—In Vitro Studies

Few populations of stem and progenitor cells residing in skeletal muscle and described above could follow osteogenic differentiation in vitro. Among them are mouse and human SCs. BMP4 and BMP7 treatment of mouse SCs induced their osteogenic differentiation, which was shown by increased expression of ALP (and also its activity), osteopontin, and osteocalcin, i.e., the markers of osteogenic differentiation. Moreover, SCs were able to undergo spontaneous osteogenic differentiation when cultured in Matrigel [126]. Osteogenic properties were also documented for human SCs after their in vitro culture in osteogenic differentiation medium (OB-1, ZenBio). After 14 days of treatment, cells increased expression of osteogenic differentiation genes, such as, RUNX2 and BGLAP. Moreover, Alizarin Red staining revealed the accumulation of calcium deposits [127]. Further, such staining of mouse skeletal muscle-derived TBX18+ pericytes, cultured in medium supplemented with dexamethasone, L-ascorbic acid-phosphate, β-glycerophosphate, and BMP2, revealed the deposition of mineralized matrix also indicating differentiation in osteogenic lineages [128]. Similarly, human ALP+ pericytes were able to differentiate in osteoblasts after BMP2 treatment in vitro [117]. On the other hand, CD146+/ALP+ progenitors isolated from human skeletal muscles were not able to follow osteogenic program in vivo after transplantation with hydroxyapatite/tricalcium phosphate scaffold [129]. Finally, mouse FAPs characterized by the presence of markers such as TIE2, PDGFRα or SCA1 differentiated into osteoblasts formation after BMP7, BMP2, treatment or when cells were cultured in osteogenic differentiation medium containing dexamethasone, β-glycerophosphate, and ascorbic-acid [109,110,130]. So far, osteogenic differentiation has not been analyzed or documented for other cell populations, such as PIC, TWIST2+ cell, Sk34 cells, as well as human circulating CD133+ cells [121,123,125,131–136].

3.3. The Cells Directly Participating in Heterotropic Ossification Formation In Vivo

Different animal models, which could be divided into two groups, were used to follow the cells responsible for HO development [1,5,21]. The first one consists of genetically modified animals, i.e., mouse engineered to express, in controlled manner, constitutively active ACVR1, which mimic FOP. The second group includes animal models in that trauma was caused by muscle blunt-force or forced ROM damage, muscle dissection, hip surgery or skin burn with Achilles tenotomy. The third group includes animals in which HO develops after BMPs injection or overexpression. The fourth model bases at the spinal cord injury in conjunction with cardiotoxin induced muscle damage. Moreover, a lot of information about the cell types responsible for HO formation was obtained thanks to lineage tracing [1,5,21].

Using the abovementioned models, a few cell populations were designated to be responsible for HO formation. As mentioned, several skeletal muscle cell types, such as human pericytes and mouse SCs, and FAPs present osteogenic potential in vitro. Importantly, in vitro results cannot be directly translated to in vivo situation. Notably, in vivo studies using mouse models proposed that HO precursors could originate from skeletal muscle endothelial, "mesenchymal" or pericyte populations or tendon and connective tissue cells or even circulating stem/precursor cells [1,5,21,137]. Some initial studies suggested that endothelial cells, characterized by the presence of TIE2, which is the tyrosine kinase receptor for angiopoetin, are engaged in HO formation [138,139]. Tracing these cells on the basis of Tie2 expression proved that they participate in HO development after BMP2 intramuscular injection or cardiotoxin induced skeletal muscle injury in transgenic mice that overexpressed BMP4 at neuromuscular junction [138,139]. Importantly, neither SCs (expressing *MyoD*) nor vascular smooth muscle cells (expressing smooth muscle myosin heavy chain) contributed to HO [138]. Moreover, also other lineage tracing and transplantation experiments clearly showed that SCs did not participate in HO development [130,138,140]. The presence of TIE2 expressing cells was observed in human fragments of tissue from FOP patients [139]. However, the studies in which the cells expressing *Cdh5* (VE-cadherin), i.e., endothelial progenitor cells, were traced, showed that in HO lesion such cells were located only peripherally [141]. Thus, the endothelial progenitors did not participate in HO formation [141]. Moreover, it was showed that TIE2 is not unique marker of endothelial cells. It is also expressed by mouse muscle interstitial cells that are able to follow osteogenic program. Next, TIE2+ cells express PDGFRα and SCA1 and do not express CD31 and CD45 [130]. Thus, these cells correspond to the population of FAPs described in human and mouse skeletal muscles [109,142]. The mesodermal origin of HO precursors was also proven by tracing of PRX1+ cells after tenotomy resulting in the formation of HO [143,144]. During embryogenesis *Prx1* gene is expressed in tissues of mesodermal origin and is crucial for cartilage and bone development. *Dermo1* gene expression, on the other hand, is restricted to the perichondrium. Tracing of DERMO+1 cells showed their engagement in HO development [143]. The localization in skeletal muscle interstitium was also demonstrated for MX1 expressing cells that form HO in response to muscle injury in mice expressing constitutively active form of ACVR1 [145]. MX1 is interferon induced GTP binding protein and is expressed in skeletal muscle interstitial cells, bone marrow osteoprogenitors and endothelial cells [145]. Lineage tracing method allowed further characterization of HO precursor cells. Thus, it was shown that GLAST or GLI1 expressing cells form HO [146,147]. GLAST, i.e., glial high affinity glutamate transporter, is expressed in different tissues and among them are interstitial cells of connective tissue and pericytes [147]. GLI1, i.e., glioma-associated oncogene 1, is a transcription factor engaged in HEDGEHOG signaling [146]. In the skeletal muscle interstitium *Glast* or *Gli1* expressing cells were localized close to vasculature, co-expressed fibroblast-specific protein 1 (FSP1), STRO1, and PDGFRα [146,147]. On the other hand, it was also well documented that NG2+ pericytes, similarly to endothelial or hematopoietic cells, did not participate in HO development [145].

The other source of HO precursors is tendon and connective tissue within the skeletal muscle [145,148]. The cells expressing transcription factor scleraxis (*Scx*) were localized in the tendon and ligaments [145]. However, the presence of *Scx* expressing cells was also noticed in the connective tissue within the skeletal muscle [148]. The SCX+ cells also express PDGFRα, SCA1, and S100A4 [148]. *Scx* expressing cells are able to develop HO localized in the tendon and joints spontaneously in mice expressing constitutively active form of ACVR1 and after tendon injury or intramuscular loading of BMP containing-scaffold [145]. In such mice, the HO developed only in injured muscles [148].

Summarizing, the question about the HO precursor cell identity is still open. Evidence presented above allowed us to conclude that potential HO precursors are of mesodermal origin and are located in the skeletal muscle interstitium. In mouse cells able to form HO could be identified on the basis of TIE2, PDGFRα, SCA1, GLAST, FSP1, STRO1, GLI1, and MX1 expression. Moreover, such cells should show many similar features to skeletal muscle FAPs and pericytes. Tendon and connective tissue present within skeletal muscle could be considered as the source of cells responsible for HO formation. In human, however, such cells are not precisely described yet. Moreover, it is also suggested that different types of cells could be responsible for HO development dependently of HO type [1,5,21,137].

4. Possible Signaling Mechanisms of Ectopic Osteogenesis in Skeletal Muscles

The knowledge on molecular mechanisms of HO formation is limited. It is well established that ectopic osteogenesis occurs as a result of traumatic injury, severe burns, and is commonly observed after invasive surgeries, which indicates that it is related to inflammation. However, the precise immune and signaling regulation is poorly understood. One of the best-known regulators of bone development and postnatal bone maintenance are bone morphogenic proteins (BMPs) [149]. BMPs are members of TGFβ superfamily, which also consists of TGFβ, activins or inhibins. Canonical TGFβ/BMP signaling is a linear cascade which involves TGFβ/BMP ligands, two types of receptors (type I and II), and signal transducers—SMADs. Receptor binding to BMP leads to SMADs—SMAD1/5/8, to TGFβ leads to SMAD2/3 phosphorylation. Activated SMADs bind to SMAD4, then the complex is accumulated in nucleus where regulates target gene expression [150]. One of the downstream targets of these pathways is for example gene encoding RUNX2, well-known master regulator of osteogenesis which is also aberrantly expressed in the ossified soft tissues [151–154]. TGFβ dependent activation of SMAD2/3 promotes osteoprogenitors migration and early stages of differentiation, while negatively regulates further steps of osteogenesis. SMAD2/3 phosphorylation inhibits RUNX2 expression and activated SMAD3 recruits class II histone deacetylases (HDACs) 4 and 5 which inhibit RUNX2 function. Although TGFβ-SMAD3 negatively regulates osteoblastogenesis, it also inhibits osteoblast apoptosis and differentiation into osteocytes [155]. On the other hand, there is TGFβ dependent non-SMAD pathway which also contributes to bone formation. TGFβ binding to its receptors can result in activation of MAPK p38 or MAPK ERK1/2 pathways through TAB1-TAK1 complex which leads to positive regulation of RUNX2 activity and favors osteoclast differentiation [156]. It indicates that TGFβ molecule is coupling bone formation, through RUNX2 phosphorylation, osteoprogenitors enrichment or osteoblast proliferation promotion, and inhibition of apoptosis with bone resorption through inhibition of RUNX2 expression and function and osteoclast maturation [157]. BMPs binding to receptor leads to SMAD1/5/8 phosphorylation (except BMP3 which action leads to SMAD2/3 phosphorylation). Activated SMAD1/5/8 bind with SMAD4 and promote expression of many osteogenesis promoting factors like RUNX2, OSX or DLX5. Similarly, to TGFβ, BMPs also can activate SMAD-independent pathway through phosphorylation of TAK1-TAB1 complex and activation of MAPK p38 or MAPK ERK1/2 pathways. In conclusion, most BMP ligands are strong osteogenic agents, acting through both SMAD-dependent and SMAD-independent signaling pathway, which synergize osteogenic transcriptional factors like RUNX2 or OSX [157,158].

In vitro and in vivo exogenous stimulation of TGFβ/BMP signaling (BMP2, BMP4, BMP9 or TGFβ) is commonly used for induction of ossification. Those proteins, especially BMP2 and BMP9, are also highly expressed in human HO [159]. One of the most intensively studied disease which manifests itself in severe HO is FOP. It is still unclear, however, what the cellular and molecular mechanisms are that cause pathological effects. Analyzes of human mesenchymal stromal cells (MSC; expressing CD44, CD73 and CD105), derived from induced pluripotent stem cells (iPSC) obtained from FOP which patients, showed that these cells were characterized by higher activity ofof SMAD1/3/5,

SMAD2/3 and MAPK ERK1/2 when compared to genetically corrected resFOP-iPSCs-MSCs [160]. Most studies suggest that mutation in ACVR1 present in FOP patients cells causes hypersensitivity to BMPs, which results in constitutive phosphorylation of its receptor, and continuous signal transduction via phosphorylation of SMAD1/5/8. As a result downstream targets of BMP signaling, like ID-1, OSX or RUNX2 are expressed [130,161,162]. However, recent report, based on study of murine FAPs, demonstrated that R206H substitution in ACVR1 may be neomorphic and altering signaling specificity to activins. Normally, activins binding to ACVR1 receptor lead to SMAD2/3 phosphorylation. Obtained results suggest that Activin A binding to mutated ACVR1 (R206H) receptor leads to SMAD1/5/8 instead of SMAD2/3 phosphorylation which results in ectopic bone formation [163]. It is well established that TGFβ/BMP signaling crosstalks with other pathways during embryonic and postnatal development, similarly as with MAPK described above. For example, crosstalk between canonical WNT pathway, TLR pathway or mTOR pathway was described [164]. TLR signaling intermediate evolutionary conserved signaling intermediate in toll pathway (ECSIT) is necessary for BMP signaling in formation of mesoderm during mouse embryogenesis [165]. Additionally, β-catenin was shown to be necessary for bone development and osteoblast formation in mouse embryos [151]. Other studies showed that β-catenin complexed with T cell factor 1 (TCF1) directly stimulates Runx2 expression [166]. Another study suggested that β-catenin, together with other proteins like SMAD1, DLX5, Sp7 or SOX6, form an enhanceosome which binds to enhancer of Runx2 gene and promotes its expression [167].

Hypoxia and inflammation are also among the factors implicated in the episodic induction of ectopic bone formation. Notably, mTOR modulates hypoxic and inflammatory signaling during the early stages of HO. At the later stages of HO, however, mTOR signaling is critical for chondrogenesis and osteogenesis [164]. Increase in mTOR signaling was shown using mouse model of FOP, i.e., animals which express constitutively active activin receptor, i.e., ACVR1 [168] and its inhibitor, rapamycin, has been shown to suppress HO formation [168]. Hypoxic environment stabilizes hypoxia-inducible factor 1α (HIF1α) which regulates expression of many proteins, such as VEGF or BMPs, which are involved in HO formation [169]. Analysis of three different mouse FOP/HO models have demonstrated hypoxia and increased HIF1α signaling [144]. Expression of HIF1α was also increased in adipose samples derived from severely burned patients, i.e., those ones being at risk for trauma-induced HO development [144,170]. Interestingly, analysis of human HO tissues, human preosteoblasts (hFOB1.19) and tissues of mice serving as a model of HO, revealed that miRNAs have essential role in osteoblast differentiation and HO development. miRNA-203 have been shown to be negatively correlated with HO and to participate in inhibition of osteoblast differentiation by directly binding to RUNX2 [64]. Nevertheless, the mechanisms underlying the development of HO in patients that not carry any mutations are still obscure. Moreover, even in FOP patients bone formation is not always observed in their soft tissues. Bone formation seems to be rather a result of injuries and inflammation, which strongly suggests a link between immune response and HO. In vivo studies using rabbits showed that bacterial transplantation into tibia bone increased inflammation-driven bone formation. In the same study, lipoteichoic acid (LTA)—the bacterial cell-wall derived toll-like receptor 2 (TLR2) activator—was identified as an osteo-stimulatory factor [171]. Other studies involving FOP patients-derived connective tissue progenitor cells revealed that such cells present much higher expression of TLRs in comparison to cells that are expressing normal ACVR1 receptor. That effect was even more significant after TNFα treatment of examined cells. The same study also revealed that TLR signaling can induce SMAD1/5/8 phosphorylation. Additionally, ECSIT, complex including TAK1 and TRAF6, which plays pivotal role in TLR-mediated NK-kB and SMAD1/5/8 signaling, was identified as a link between TLR-pathway and BMP pathway in human FOP-connective tissue progenitor cells [172,173]. As described above, normal cells, not carrying any mutations in *ACVR1*, can undergo osteogenesis after BMP stimulation. Thus, development of heterotopic bone provides the signaling environment in which BMP level is sufficient enough to stimulate the cells to form the bone [163]. Results of these reports together suggest that main mechanism of HO formation is connected with TGFβ/BMP signaling, especially SMAD1/5/8 action, which leads to expression of osteogenic transcription factors. Factors present in damaged tissue lead also to activation of mTOR, WNT or TLR pathways which may cross-talk with TGFβ/BMP or independently promote osteogenic factors expression and induce HO formation. Even small ossification within tissue provide a BMP rich environment, which further stimulates neighboring cells to follow osteogenic differentiation and support newly creating bone growth. However, it still remains unclear why spontaneous HO is observed or how that process is induced and regulated (Figure 2).

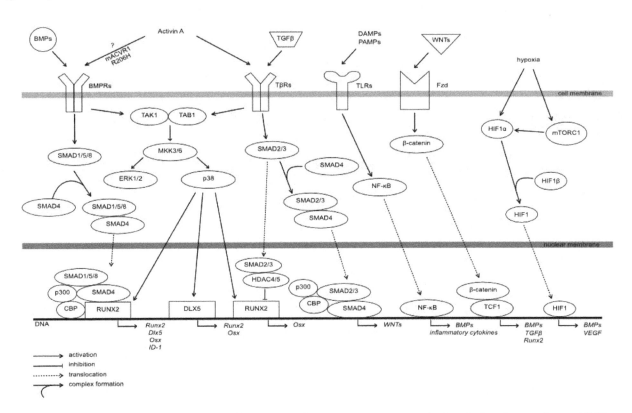

Figure 2. Possible signaling mechanisms of ectopic osteogenesis in skeletal muscles. BMPs bind to homomeric type II receptors which phosphorylate homomeric type I receptor and induce SMAD-dependent and SMAD-independent signaling. In the SMAD-dependent signaling SMADs 1, 5 or 8 complex with SMAD4 and translocate to the nucleus where recruit RUNX2 and other co-factors to regulate osteogenic gene expression. TGFβ binds to complex of two TGFβ types I receptors (TβRI) and two type II receptors (TβRII), which phosphorylate each other and induce SMAD-dependent and SMAD-independent signaling. In the SMAD-dependent signaling activated SMAD2/3 form complex with SMAD4. Complex translocates to the nucleus where recruits co-factors and regulates target gene expression. Activated SMAD3 recruits HDACs which inhbit RUN2 activity. In the SMAD-independent pathway, regardless of the ligand bind to the receptors, TAK1 recruits TAB1 to initiate p38 MAPK or ERK1/2 MAPK signaling cascade. MAPK phosphorylates and activates RUNX2, DLX5, and OSX transcription factors. Activation of TLR singaling pathways by PAMPs and DAMPs lead to activation of nuclear factor-kappaB (NF-κB), which controls the expression of an array of inflammatory cytokine genes and BMPs. WNTs bind to Frizzled (Fzd) receptors and activate the canonical WNT pathway which leads to accumulation of β-catenin in the cytoplasm. β-catenin is translocated to the nucleus where forms complex with TCF1 which acts as transcriptional activator of *Runx2*. Low level of oxygen (hypoxia) induces the mTOR pathway. HIF1α, a downstream intermediate in mTOR signaling, is a key transcriptional regulator of the cellular response to hypoxia. It forms complex with HIF1β and as HIF1 enters to the nuclei where regulates target gene expression.

5. Future Therapeutic Options

Currently, a clinical trial phase 3 of highly specific retinoic acid receptor γ (RARγ) agonist, R667 (palovarotene), carried out by Clementia Pharmaceuticals involves 90 FOP patients (NCT03312634).

RAR is a strong inhibitor of chondrogenesis. Stimulation of its γ subtype reduces in BMP signaling by lowering SMAD1/5/8 phosphorylation and as a result decreases HO formation. The safety profile of this drug is being carefully assessed due to the teratogenic potential of RAR agonists and other side effects, including cheilitis, xerosis, dryness of mucous membranes, inhibition of growth plates in children, hearing and vision impairment [70,174]. Another investigated strategy is blocking mutant ACVR1. The ACRV1 stimulates BMP through SMAD1/5/8 signaling and promote HO. Such approaches involve anti-Activin A antibody (REGN2477) and which is currently at phase 2 of randomized control trial for 44 FOP patients (NCT03188666, Regeneron Pharmaceuticals) [175]. Other ACVR1 direct inhibitors (AZD0530 and PD 161570) are being investigated. The AZD0530 difumarate inhibits both BMP and TGFβ signaling. Phase 2 study involving AZD0530 (Saracatinib) to prevent FOP is currently carried out by VU University Medical Center (NCT04307953) [176]. The other treatment strategies include a local application of apyrase, which influences the BMP-SMAD pathway by the reduction of SMAD1/5/8 phosphorylation [177]. The BMP receptor antagonists, such as noggin, also inhibit HO in animal models [178]. Researchers also suggest that pharmacological inhibition of HIF1α using PX-478, rapamycin, apigenin, or imatinib can reduce pathologic extraskeletal bone formation [144,179]. Recently, gene therapy opportunities raised for HO. Non-virus-mediated transfer of small interfering RNA (siRNA) particles against mRNA encoding *Runx2* and *Smad4* inhibited HO in rats after Achilles tenotomy [180]. The siRNA could also possibly directly block mutant ACVR1 as a therapeutic option in future studies [179]. Additionally, the immune system may be a potential target for HO prevention. Neutralizing antibodies against immune checkpoint proteins (ICs) block limit the extent of HO in animal studies [9].

6. Conclusions

In this review we summarize current knowledge on the development of different forms of HO. Numerous projects involving analysis of patients' tissues and also animal models allowed great advancement in the understanding of this pathology. However, we are still not certain about the precise sources of the osteogenic progenitors involved in this pathology. Additionally, the knowledge on the signaling pathways deregulated despite being enormous is still not sufficient to design the properly targeted treatment. Nevertheless, what we already know allowed us to propose several hope-giving therapeutic approaches which are currently tested. Thus, more work needs to be done, but it seems that we are on the proper path.

Author Contributions: Conceptualization, P.Ł. and E.B.; Writing—Original Draft Preparation, Ł.P., E.B., and B.M.; Writing—Review and Editing, E.B., P.Ł., and M.A.C.; Visualization, B.M.; Supervision, P.Ł. and E.B. All authors have read and agreed to the published version of the manuscript.

Abbreviations

ACVR1/ALK2	Activin A receptor type 1/activin-like kinase 2
ALP	alkaline phosphatase
BAF60c	60 KDa BRG-1/Brm-Associated Factor Subunit C
BAP	bone-specific isoform of alkaline phosphatase
BMP	bone morphogenetic protein
CD	cluster of differentiation
CDC6	cell division cycle 6 protein
COL-1	collagen alpha 1
COX-2	cyclooxygenase-2
CRP	C-reactive protein
CTDA	cervical total disc arthroplasty
CTX-1	type I collagen cross-linked C-telopeptide
Dlx5	Distal-Less Homeobox 5

DVT	deep venous thrombosis
ECM	extracellular matrix
ENO3	enolase 3
ERK	extracellular signal-regulated kinase
FAP	fibro-adipogenic progenitors
FOP	fibrodysplasia ossificans progressive
FSP1	fibroblast-specific protein 1
GLAST	glial high affinity glutamate transporter
GLI1	glioma-associated oncogene 1
GNAS	guanine nucleotide-binding protein, subunit alpha
HDAC	histone deacetylase
HGF	hepatocyte growth factor
HIF1α	hypoxia-inducible factor 1α
HLA	human leukocyte antigen
HO	heterotopic ossification
ID-1	DNA-Binding Protein Inhibitor ID-1
IFN γ	interferon γ
IFOPA	international FOP Association
IGF1	insulin-like growth factor 1
IL	Interleukin
iPSC	induced pluripotent stem cell
LTA	lipoteichoic acid
MAPK	mitogen-activated protein kinases
MCK	muscle creatine kinase
MCM2	minichromosome maintenance complex component 2
MCP-1	monocyte chemoattractant protein-1
MHC	myosin heavy chains
miRNA	microRNA
MIS	micro-invasive surgery
MRF	myogenic regulatory factor
MRI	magnetic resonance imaging
MRSA	methicillin-resistant Staphylococcus aureus
MSC	mesenchymal stromal cell
mTOR	mammalian target of rapamycin
NF-κB	Nuclear factor-κB
NG2	neural-glial antigen 2
NHO	neurogenic heterotopic ossification
NSAID	nonsteroidal anti-inflammatory drug
NT-3	neurotrophin-3
OC/BGLAP	osteocalcin/Bone Gamma-Carboxyglutamate Protein
OMD	Osteomodulin
OSX/Sp7	Osterix
Pax7	paired box transcription factor 7
PDGFRα	platelet derived growth factor receptor α
PGE2	prostaglandin E2
PIC	PW1 interstitial cell
POH	progressive osseous heteroplasia
Prx1	peroxiredoxin Prx1
ROM	range of motion
RT	Radiotherapy
RUNX2	runt-related transcription factor 2
SC	satellite cell
SCA1	stem cell antigen 1
SCI	spinal cord injury

Scx   Scleraxis
Sox6   SRY-Box Transcription Factor 6
SP cell   side population cell
SPECT   single-photon emission computed tomography
SWI/SNF   SWItch/Sucrose NonFermentable
TAB1   TAK1 binding protein
TBI   traumatic brain injury
TBX18   T-box transcription factor 18
TCF1   T cell factor 1
TGFβ   transforming growth factor β
THR   total hip replacement
TIE2   angiopoietin receptor
TLR   toll-like receptor
TNF-α   tumor necrosis factor-α
TRAF6   TNF Receptor Associated Factor 6
TWIST2   Twist Basic Helix-Loop-Helix Transcription Factor 2/DERMO1
VE-cadherin   vascular endothelial cadherin (Cdh15)
VEGF   vascular endothelial growth factor
VTE   venous thromboembolism
WNT   wingless/integrated

References

1. Meyers, C.; Lisiecki, J.; Miller, S.; Levin, A.; Fayad, L.; Ding, C.; Sono, T.; McCarthy, E.; Levi, B.; James, A.W. Heterotopic Ossification: A Comprehensive Review. *JBMR Plus* **2019**, *3*, e10172. [CrossRef] [PubMed]

2. Nauth, A.; Giles, E.; Potter, B.K.; Nesti, L.J.; O'brien, F.P.; Bosse, M.J.; Anglen, J.O.; Mehta, S.; Ahn, J.; Miclau, T.; et al. Heterotopic ossification in orthopaedic trauma. *J. Orthop. Trauma* **2012**, *26*, 684–688. [CrossRef] [PubMed]

3. van Kuijk, A.A.; Geurts, A.C.H.; van Kuppevelt, H.J.M. Neurogenic heterotopic ossification in spinal cord injury. *Spinal Cord.* **2002**, *40*, 313–326. [CrossRef] [PubMed]

4. Łęgosz, P.; Drela, K.; Pulik, Ł.; Sarzyńska, S.; Małdyk, P. Challenges of heterotopic ossification-Molecular background and current treatment strategies. *Clin. Exp. Pharm. Physiol.* **2018**, *45*, 1229–1235. [CrossRef] [PubMed]

5. Lees-Shepard, J.B.; Goldhamer, D.J. Stem cells and heterotopic ossification: Lessons from animal models. *Bone* **2018**, *109*, 178–186. [CrossRef] [PubMed]

6. Convente, M.R.; Wang, H.; Pignolo, R.J.; Kaplan, F.S.; Shore, E.M. The immunological contribution to heterotopic ossification disorders. *Curr. Osteoporos. Rep.* **2015**, *13*, 116–124. [CrossRef]

7. Levesque, J.P.; Sims, N.A.; Pettit, A.R.; Alexander, K.A.; Tseng, H.W.; Torossian, F.; Genet, F.; Lataillade, J.J.; Le Bousse-Kerdiles, M.C. Macrophages Driving Heterotopic Ossification: Convergence of Genetically-Driven and Trauma-Driven Mechanisms. *J. Bone Miner. Res.* **2018**, *33*, 365–366. [CrossRef]

8. Sorkin, M.; Huber, A.K.; Hwang, C.; Carson, W.F.; Menon, R.; Li, J.; Vasquez, K.; Pagani, C.; Patel, N.; Li, S.; et al. Regulation of heterotopic ossification by monocytes in a mouse model of aberrant wound healing. *Nat. Commun.* **2020**, *11*, 722. [CrossRef]

9. Kan, C.; Yang, J.; Na, D.; Xu, Y.; Yang, B.; Zhao, H.; Lu, H.; Li, Y.; Zhang, K.; McGuire, T.L.; et al. Inhibition of immune checkpoints prevents injury-induced heterotopic ossification. *Bone Res.* **2019**, *7*, 33. [CrossRef]

10. Zhang, J.; Wang, L.; Chu, J.; Ao, X.; Jiang, T.; Bin, Y.; Huang, M.; Zhang, Z. Macrophage-derived neurotrophin-3 promotes heterotopic ossification in rats. *Lab. Investig.* **2020**. [CrossRef]

11. Bossche, L.V.; Vanderstraeten, G. Heterotopic ossification: A review. *J. Rehabil. Med.* **2005**, *37*, 129–136. [CrossRef] [PubMed]

12. Foley, K.L.; Hebela, N.; Keenan, M.A.; Pignolo, R.J. Histopathology of periarticular non-hereditary heterotopic ossification. *Bone* **2018**, *109*, 65–70. [CrossRef] [PubMed]

13. Fleckenstein, J.L.; Crues, J.V.; Reimers, C.D. *Muscle Imaging in Health and Disease*; Springer: New York, NY, USA, 1996; ISBN 978-1-4612-2314-6.

14. Ohlmeier, M.; Krenn, V.; Thiesen, D.M.; Sandiford, N.A.; Gehrke, T.; Citak, M. Heterotopic Ossification in Orthopaedic and Trauma surgery: A Histopathological Ossification Score. *Sci. Rep.* **2019**, *9*, 18401. [CrossRef]

15. Barfield, W.R.; Holmes, R.E.; Hartsock, L.A. Heterotopic Ossification in Trauma. *Orthop. Clin. N. Am.* **2017**, *48*, 35–46. [CrossRef] [PubMed]

16. Eisenstein, N.; Stapley, S.; Grover, L. Post-Traumatic Heterotopic Ossification: An Old Problem in Need of New Solutions. *J. Orthop. Res.* **2018**, *36*, 1061–1068. [CrossRef]

17. Chen, H.-C.; Yang, J.-Y.; Chuang, S.-S.; Huang, C.-Y.; Yang, S.-Y. Heterotopic ossification in burns: Our experience and literature reviews. *Burns* **2009**, *35*, 857–862. [CrossRef]

18. Thefenne, L.; de Brier, G.; Leclerc, T.; Jourdan, C.; Nicolas, C.; Truffaut, S.; Lapeyre, E.; Genet, F. Two new risk factors for heterotopic ossification development after severe burns. *PLoS ONE* **2017**, *12*, e0182303. [CrossRef]

19. Hong, C.C.; Nashi, N.; Hey, H.W.; Chee, Y.H.; Murphy, D. Clinically relevant heterotopic ossification after elbow fracture surgery: A risk factors study. *Orthop. Traumatol. Surg. Res.* **2015**, *101*, 209–213. [CrossRef]

20. Firoozabadi, R.; O'Mara, T.J.; Swenson, A.; Agel, J.; Beck, J.D.; Routt, M. Risk Factors for the Development of Heterotopic Ossification After Acetabular Fracture Fixation. *Clin. Orthop. Relat. Res.* **2014**, *472*, 3383–3388. [CrossRef]

21. Dey, D.; Wheatley, B.M.; Cholok, D.; Agarwal, S.; Yu, P.B.; Levi, B.; Davis, T.A. The traumatic bone: Trauma-induced heterotopic ossification. *Transl. Res.* **2017**, *186*, 95–111. [CrossRef]

22. Orchard, G.R.; Paratz, J.D.; Blot, S.; Roberts, J.A. Risk Factors in Hospitalized Patients With Burn Injuries for Developing Heterotopic Ossification—A Retrospective Analysis. *J. Burn Care Res.* **2015**, *36*, 465–470. [CrossRef] [PubMed]

23. Bemenderfer, T.B.; Davis, W.H.; Anderson, R.B.; Wing, K.; Escudero, M.I.; Waly, F.; Penner, M. Heterotopic Ossification in Total Ankle Arthroplasty: Case Series and Systematic Review. *J. Foot Ankle Surg.* **2020**. [CrossRef] [PubMed]

24. Zhu, Y.; Zhang, F.; Chen, W.; Zhang, Q.; Liu, S.; Zhang, Y. Incidence and risk factors for heterotopic ossification after total hip arthroplasty: A meta-analysis. *Arch. Orthop. Trauma Surg.* **2015**, *135*, 1307–1314. [CrossRef] [PubMed]

25. Chen, J.; Wang, X.; Bai, W.; Shen, X.; Yuan, W. Prevalence of heterotopic ossification after cervical total disc arthroplasty: A meta-analysis. *Eur. Spine J.* **2012**, *21*, 674–680. [CrossRef] [PubMed]

26. Lee, K.-B.; Cho, Y.-J.; Park, J.-K.; Song, E.-K.; Yoon, T.-R.; Seon, J.-K. Heterotopic Ossification After Primary Total Ankle Arthroplasty. *JBJS* **2011**, *93*, 751–758. [CrossRef]

27. Łęgosz, P.; Sarzyńska, S.; Pulik, Ł.; Stępiński, P.; Niewczas, P.; Kotela, A.; Małdyk, P. Heterotopic ossification and clinical results after total hip arthroplasty using the anterior minimally invasive and anterolateral approaches. *Arch. Med. Sci.* **2018**. [CrossRef]

28. Anthonissen, J.; Ossendorf, C.; Hock, J.L.; Steffen, C.T.; Goetz, H.; Hofmann, A.; Rommens, P.M. The role of muscular trauma in the development of heterotopic ossification after hip surgery: An animal-model study in rats. *Injury* **2016**, *47*, 613–616. [CrossRef]

29. Yi, S.; Shin, D.A.; Kim, K.N.; Choi, G.; Shin, H.C.; Kim, K.S.; Yoon, D.H. The predisposing factors for the heterotopic ossification after cervical artificial disc replacement. *Spine J.* **2013**, *13*, 1048–1054. [CrossRef]

30. Kocic, M.; Lazovic, M.; Mitkovic, M.; Djokic, B. Clinical significance of the heterotopic ossification after total hip arthroplasty. *Orthopedics* **2010**, *33*, 16. [CrossRef]

31. Sundseth, J.; Jacobsen, E.A.; Kolstad, F.; Sletteberg, R.O.; Nygaard, O.P.; Johnsen, L.G.; Pripp, A.H.; Andresen, H.; Fredriksli, O.A.; Myrseth, E.; et al. Heterotopic ossification and clinical outcome in nonconstrained cervical arthroplasty 2 years after surgery: The Norwegian Cervical Arthroplasty Trial (NORCAT). *Eur. Spine J.* **2016**, *25*, 2271–2278. [CrossRef]

32. McCarthy, E.F.; Sundaram, M. Heterotopic ossification: A review. *Skelet. Radiol.* **2005**, *34*, 609–619. [CrossRef] [PubMed]

33. Nalbantoglu, M.; Tuncer, O.G.; Acik, M.E.; Matur, Z.; Altunrende, B.; Ozgonenel, E.; Ozgonenel, L. Neurogenic heterotopic ossification in Guillain-Barre syndrome: A rare case report. *J. Musculoskelet. Neuronal Interact.* **2020**, *20*, 160–164. [PubMed]

34. Zhang, Y.; Zhan, Y.; Kou, Y.; Yin, X.; Wang, Y.; Zhang, D. Identification of biological pathways and genes associated with neurogenic heterotopic ossification by text mining. *PeerJ* **2020**, *8*, e8276. [CrossRef] [PubMed]

35. Pek, C.H.; Lim, M.C.; Yong, R.; Wong, H.P. Neurogenic heterotopic ossification after a stroke: Diagnostic and radiological challenges. *Singap. Med. J.* **2014**, *55*, e119–e122. [CrossRef]

36. Reznik, J.; Biros, E.; Marshall, R.; Jelbart, M.; Milanese, S.; Gordon, S.; Galea, M. Prevalence and risk-factors of neurogenic heterotopic ossification in traumatic spinal cord and traumatic brain injured patients admitted to specialised units in Australia. *J. Musculoskelet. Neuronal Interact.* **2014**, *14*, 19–28.

37. Citak, M.; Suero, E.M.; Backhaus, M.; Aach, M.; Godry, H.; Meindl, R.; Schildhauer, T.A. Risk Factors for Heterotopic Ossification in Patients With Spinal Cord Injury: A Case-Control Study of 264 Patients. *Spine* **2012**, *37*, 1953–1957. [CrossRef]

38. Sullivan, M.P.; Torres, S.J.; Mehta, S.; Ahn, J. Heterotopic ossification after central nervous system trauma: A current review. *Bone Jt. Res.* **2013**, *2*, 51–57. [CrossRef]

39. Citak, M.; Grasmücke, D.; Suero, E.M.; Cruciger, O.; Meindl, R.; Schildhauer, T.A.; Aach, M. The roles of serum alkaline and bone alkaline phosphatase levels in predicting heterotopic ossification following spinal cord injury. *Spinal Cord.* **2016**, *54*, 368–370. [CrossRef]

40. Dizdar, D.; Tiftik, T.; Kara, M.; Tunç, H.; Ersöz, M.; Akkuş, S. Risk factors for developing heterotopic ossification in patients with traumatic brain injury. *Brain Inj.* **2013**, *27*, 807–811. [CrossRef]

41. Ohlmeier, M.; Suero, E.M.; Aach, M.; Meindl, R.; Schildhauer, T.A.; Citak, M. Muscle localization of heterotopic ossification following spinal cord injury. *Spine J.* **2017**, *17*, 1519–1522. [CrossRef]

42. Suero, E.M.; Meindl, R.; Schildhauer, T.A.; Citak, M. Clinical Prediction Rule for Heterotopic Ossification of the Hip in Patients with Spinal Cord Injury. *Spine* **2018**, *43*, 1572–1578. [CrossRef] [PubMed]

43. Johns, J.S.; Cifu, D.X.; Keyser-Marcus, L.; Jolles, P.R.; Fratkin, M.J. Impact of Clinically Significant Heterotopic Ossification on Functional Outcome after Traumatic Brain Injury. *J. Head Trauma Rehabil.* **1999**, *14*, 269–276. [CrossRef] [PubMed]

44. Shore, E.M.; Xu, M.; Feldman, G.J.; Fenstermacher, D.A.; Cho, T.-J.; Choi, I.H.; Connor, J.M.; Delai, P.; Glaser, D.L.; LeMerrer, M.; et al. A recurrent mutation in the BMP type I receptor ACVR1 causes inherited and sporadic fibrodysplasia ossificans progressiva. *Nat. Genet.* **2006**, *38*, 525–527. [CrossRef] [PubMed]

45. Adegbite, N.S.; Xu, M.; Kaplan, F.S.; Shore, E.M.; Pignolo, R.J. Diagnostic and mutational spectrum of progressive osseous heteroplasia (POH) and other forms of GNAS-based heterotopic ossification. *Am. J. Med. Genet. Part A* **2008**, *146*, 1788–1796. [CrossRef]

46. Valer, J.A.; Sanchez-de-Diego, C.; Pimenta-Lopes, C.; Rosa, J.L.; Ventura, F. ACVR1 Function in Health and Disease. *Cells* **2019**, *8*, 1366. [CrossRef]

47. Pignolo, R.J.; Ramaswamy, G.; Fong, J.T.; Shore, E.M.; Kaplan, F.S. Progressive osseous heteroplasia: Diagnosis, treatment, and prognosis. *Appl. Clin. Genet.* **2015**, *8*, 37–48. [CrossRef]

48. Pignolo, R.J.; Cheung, K.; Kile, S.; Fitzpatrick, M.A.; De Cunto, C.; Al Mukaddam, M.; Hsiao, E.C.; Baujat, G.; Delai, P.; Eekhoff, E.M.W.; et al. Self-reported baseline phenotypes from the International Fibrodysplasia Ossificans Progressiva (FOP) Association Global Registry. *Bone* **2020**. [CrossRef]

49. Pignolo, R.J.; Shore, E.M.; Kaplan, F.S. Fibrodysplasia Ossificans Progressiva: Clinical and Genetic Aspects. *Orphanet J. Rare Dis.* **2011**, *6*, 80. [CrossRef] [PubMed]

50. Kaplan, F.S.; Le Merrer, M.; Glaser, D.L.; Pignolo, R.J.; Goldsby, R.E.; Kitterman, J.A.; Groppe, J.; Shore, E.M. Fibrodysplasia ossificans progressiva. *Best Pr. Res. Clin. Rheumatol.* **2008**, *22*, 191–205. [CrossRef]

51. Towler, O.W.; Shore, E.M.; Kaplan, F.S. Skeletal malformations and developmental arthropathy in individuals who have fibrodysplasia ossificans progressiva. *Bone* **2020**, *130*, 115116. [CrossRef]

52. Mujtaba, B.; Taher, A.; Fiala, M.J.; Nassar, S.; Madewell, J.E.; Hanafy, A.K.; Aslam, R. Heterotopic ossification: Radiological and pathological review. *Radiol. Oncol.* **2019**, *53*, 275–284. [CrossRef] [PubMed]

53. Ghanem, M.A.; Dannoon, S.; Elgazzar, A.H. The added value of SPECT-CT in the detection of heterotopic ossification on bone scintigraphy. *Skelet. Radiol.* **2020**, *49*, 291–298. [CrossRef] [PubMed]

54. Lima, M.C.; Passarelli, M.C.; Dario, V.; Lebani, B.R.; Monteiro, P.H.S.; Ramos, C.D. The use of spect/ct in the evaluation of heterotopic ossification in para/tetraplegics. *Acta Ortopédica Bras.* **2014**, *22*, 12–16. [CrossRef] [PubMed]

55. Botman, E.; Raijmakers, P.G.H.M.; Yaqub, M.; Teunissen, B.; Netelenbos, C.; Lubbers, W.; Schwarte, L.A.; Micha, D.; Bravenboer, N.; Schoenmaker, T.; et al. Evolution of heterotopic bone in fibrodysplasia ossificans progressiva: An [18F]NaF PET/CT study. *Bone* **2019**, *124*, 1–6. [CrossRef]

56. Rosteius, T.; Suero, E.; Grasmücke, D.; Aach, M.; Gisevius, A.; Ohlmeier, M.; Meindl, R.; Schildhauer, T.; Citak, M. The sensitivity of ultrasound screening examination in detecting heterotopic ossification following spinal cord injury. *Spinal Cord.* **2017**, *55*, 71–73. [CrossRef]

57. Shehab, D.; Elgazzar, A.H.; Collier, B.D. Heterotopic ossification. *J. Nucl. Med.* **2002**, *43*, 346–353.

58. Łęgosz, P.; Pulik, Ł.; Stępiński, P.; Janowicz, J.; Wirkowska, A.; Kotela, A.; Sarzyńska, S.; Małdyk, P. The Use of Type I Collagen Cross-Linked C-Telopeptide (CTX-1) as a Biomarker Associated with the Formation of Periprosthetic Ossifications Following Total Hip Joint. Arthroplasty. *Ann. Clin. Lab. Sci.* **2018**, *48*, 183–190.

59. Sung Hsieh, H.H.; Chung, M.T.; Allen, R.M.; Ranganathan, K.; Habbouche, J.; Cholok, D.; Butts, J.; Kaura, A.; Tiruvannamalai-Annamalai, R.; Breuler, C.; et al. Evaluation of Salivary Cytokines for Diagnosis of both Trauma-Induced and Genetic Heterotopic Ossification. *Front. Endocrinol.* **2017**, *8*. [CrossRef]

60. Forsberg, J.A.; Potter, B.K.; Polfer, E.M.; Safford, S.D.; Elster, E.A. Do Inflammatory Markers Portend Heterotopic Ossification and Wound Failure in Combat Wounds? *Clin. Orthop. Relat. Res.* **2014**, *472*, 2845–2854. [CrossRef]

61. Edsberg, L.E.; Crowgey, E.L.; Osborn, P.M.; Wyffels, J.T. A survey of proteomic biomarkers for heterotopic ossification in blood serum. *J. Orthop. Surg. Res.* **2017**, *12*, 69. [CrossRef]

62. Sun, Y.; Cai, J.; Yu, S.; Chen, S.; Li, F.; Fan, C. MiR-630 Inhibits Endothelial-Mesenchymal Transition by Targeting Slug in Traumatic Heterotopic Ossification. *Sci. Rep.* **2016**, *6*, 22729. [CrossRef] [PubMed]

63. Ju, C.; Lv, Z.; Zhang, C.; Jiao, Y. Regulatory effect of miR-421 on humeral fracture and heterotopic ossification in elderly patients. *Exp. Ther. Med.* **2019**, *17*, 1903–1911. [CrossRef] [PubMed]

64. Tu, B.; Liu, S.; Yu, B.; Zhu, J.; Ruan, H.; Tang, T.; Fan, C. miR-203 inhibits the traumatic heterotopic ossification by targeting Runx2. *Cell Death Dis.* **2016**, *7*, e2436. [CrossRef] [PubMed]

65. Li, F.; Mao, D.; Pan, X.; Zhang, X.; Mi, J.; Rui, Y. Celecoxib cannot inhibit the progression of initiated traumatic heterotopic ossification. *J. Shoulder Elb. Surg.* **2019**, *28*, 2379–2385. [CrossRef] [PubMed]

66. Joice, M.; Vasileiadis, G.I.; Amanatullah, D.F. Non-steroidal anti-inflammatory drugs for heterotopic ossification prophylaxis after total hip arthroplasty. *Bone Jt. J.* **2018**, *100*, 915–922. [CrossRef] [PubMed]

67. Xue, D.; Zheng, Q.; Li, H.; Qian, S.; Zhang, B.; Pan, Z. Selective COX-2 inhibitor versus nonselective COX-1 and COX-2 inhibitor in the prevention of heterotopic ossification after total hip arthroplasty: A meta-analysis of randomised trials. *Int. Orthop.* **2011**, *35*, 3–8. [CrossRef]

68. Kan, S.L.; Yang, B.; Ning, G.Z.; Chen, L.X.; Li, Y.L.; Gao, S.J.; Chen, X.Y.; Sun, J.C.; Feng, S.Q. Nonsteroidal Anti-inflammatory Drugs as Prophylaxis for Heterotopic Ossification after Total Hip Arthroplasty: A Systematic Review and Meta-Analysis. *Medicine* **2015**, *94*, e828. [CrossRef]

69. Winkler, S.; Wagner, F.; Weber, M.; Matussek, J.; Craiovan, B.; Heers, G.; Springorum, H.R.; Grifka, J.; Renkawitz, T. Current therapeutic strategies of heterotopic ossification—A survey amongst orthopaedic and trauma departments in Germany. *BMC Musculoskelet. Disord.* **2015**, *16*, 313. [CrossRef]

70. Neal, B.C.; Rodgers, A.; Clark, T.; Gray, H.; Reid, I.R.; Dunn, L.; MacMahon, S.W. A systematic survey of 13 randomized trials of non-steroidal anti-inflammatory drugs for the prevention of heterotopic bone formation after major hip surgery. *Acta Orthop. Scand.* **2000**, *71*, 122–128. [CrossRef]

71. Strauss, J.B.; Chen, S.S.; Shah, A.P.; Coon, A.B.; Dickler, A. Cost of radiotherapy versus NSAID administration for prevention of heterotopic ossification after total hip arthroplasty. *Int. J. Radiat. Oncol. Biol. Phys.* **2008**, *71*, 1460–1464. [CrossRef]

72. Vavken, P.; Dorotka, R. Economic evaluation of NSAID and radiation to prevent heterotopic ossification after hip surgery. *Arch. Orthop. Trauma Surg.* **2011**, *131*, 1309–1315. [CrossRef] [PubMed]

73. Milakovic, M.; Popovic, M.; Raman, S.; Tsao, M.; Lam, H.; Chow, E. Radiotherapy for the prophylaxis of heterotopic ossification: A systematic review and meta-analysis of randomized controlled trials. *Radiother. Oncol.* **2015**, *116*, 4–9. [CrossRef] [PubMed]

74. Wu, F.; Gao, H.; Huang, S.; Wang, G.; Jiang, X.; Li, J.; Shou, Z. NSAIDs combined with radiotherapy to prevent heterotopic ossification after total hip arthroplasty. *Zhongguo Gu Shang China J. Orthop. Traumatol.* **2018**, *31*, 538–542.

75. Pakos, E.E.; Papadopoulos, D.V.; Gelalis, I.D.; Tsantes, A.G.; Gkiatas, I.; Kosmas, D.; Tsekeris, P.G.; Xenakis, T.A. Is prophylaxis for heterotopic ossification with radiation therapy after THR associated with early loosening or carcinogenesis? *Hip. Int.* **2019**, 1120700019842724. [CrossRef] [PubMed]

76. Seavey, J.G.; Wheatley, B.M.; Pavey, G.J.; Tomasino, A.M.; Hanson, M.A.; Sanders, E.M.; Dey, D.; Moss, K.L.; Potter, B.K.; Forsberg, J.A. Early local delivery of vancomycin suppresses ectopic bone formation in a rat model of trauma-induced heterotopic ossification. *J. Orthop. Res.* **2017**, *35*, 2397–2406. [CrossRef]

77. Vasileiadis, G.I.; Sakellariou, V.I.; Kelekis, A.; Galanos, A.; Soucacos, P.N.; Papagelopoulos, P.J.; Babis, G.C. Prevention of heterotopic ossification in cases of hypertrophic osteoarthritis submitted to total hip arthroplasty. Etidronate or Indomethacin? *J. Musculoskelet. Neuronal Interact.* **2010**, *10*, 159–165.

78. Haykal, T.; Kheiri, B.; Zayed, Y.; Barbarawi, M.; Miran, M.S.; Chahine, A.; Katato, K.; Bachuwa, G. Aspirin for venous thromboembolism prophylaxis after hip or knee arthroplasty: An updated meta-analysis of randomized controlled trials. *J. Orthop.* **2019**, *16*, 294–302. [CrossRef]
79. Brouwer, K.M.; Lindenhovius, A.L.; de Witte, P.B.; Jupiter, J.B.; Ring, D. Resection of heterotopic ossification of the elbow: A comparison of ankylosis and partial restriction. *J. Hand Surg.* **2010**, *35*, 1115–1119. [CrossRef]
80. Almangour, W.; Schnitzler, A.; Salga, M.; Debaud, C.; Denormandie, P.; Genet, F. Recurrence of heterotopic ossification after removal in patients with traumatic brain injury: A systematic review. *Ann. Phys. Rehabil. Med.* **2016**, *59*, 263–269. [CrossRef]
81. Genet, F.; Marmorat, J.L.; Lautridou, C.; Schnitzler, A.; Mailhan, L.; Denormandie, P. Impact of late surgical intervention on heterotopic ossification of the hip after traumatic neurological injury. *J. Bone Jt. Surg. Br. Vol.* **2009**, *91*, 1493–1498. [CrossRef]
82. Koh, K.H.; Lim, T.K.; Lee, H.I.; Park, M.J. Surgical treatment of elbow stiffness caused by post-traumatic heterotopic ossification. *J. Shoulder Elb. Surg.* **2013**, *22*, 1128–1134. [CrossRef] [PubMed]
83. Jayasundara, J.A.; Punchihewa, G.L.; de Alwis, D.S.; Renuka, M.D. Short-term outcome after resection of neurogenic heterotopic ossification around the hips and elbow following encephalitis. *Singap. Med. J.* **2012**, *53*, e97–e100.
84. Pontell, M.E.; Sparber, L.S.; Chamberlain, R.S. Corrective and reconstructive surgery in patients with postburn heterotopic ossification and bony ankylosis: An evidence-based approach. *J. Burn Care Res.* **2015**, *36*, 57–69. [CrossRef]
85. Rubayi, S.; Gabbay, J.; Kruger, E.; Ruhge, K. The Modified Girdlestone Procedure With Muscle Flap for Management of Pressure Ulcers and Heterotopic Ossification of the Hip Region in Spinal Injury Patients: A 15-Year Review With Long-term Follow-up. *Ann. Plast. Surg.* **2016**, *77*, 645–652. [CrossRef] [PubMed]
86. Pansard, E.; Schnitzler, A.; Lautridou, C.; Judet, T.; Denormandie, P.; Genet, F. Heterotopic ossification of the shoulder after central nervous system lesion: Indications for surgery and results. *J. Shoulder Elb. Surg.* **2013**, *22*, 767–774. [CrossRef] [PubMed]
87. Mitsionis, G.I.; Lykissas, M.G.; Kalos, N.; Paschos, N.; Beris, A.E.; Georgoulis, A.D.; Xenakis, T.A. Functional outcome after excision of heterotopic ossification about the knee in ICU patients. *Int. Orthop.* **2009**, *33*, 1619–1625. [CrossRef] [PubMed]
88. Akman, S.; Sonmez, M.M.; Erturer, R.E.; Seckin, M.F.; Kara, A.; Ozturk, I. The results of surgical treatment for posttraumatic heterotopic ossification and ankylosis of the elbow. *Acta Orthop. Traumatol. Turc.* **2010**, *44*, 206–211. [CrossRef]
89. Denormandie, P.; de l'Escalopier, N.; Gatin, L.; Grelier, A.; Genêt, F. Resection of neurogenic heterotopic ossification (NHO) of the hip. *Orthop. Traumatol. Surg. Res.* **2018**, *104*, S121–S127. [CrossRef]
90. Łęgosz, P.; Stępiński, P.; Pulik, Ł.; Kotela, A.; Małdyk, P. Total hip replacement vs femoral neck osteotomy in the treatment of heterotopic ossifications, neurogenic in the IV degree by scale Brooker—comparison of treatment results. *Chir. Narz. Ruchu Ortop. Pol.* **2017**, *82*, 28–40.
91. Forcina, L.; Miano, C.; Pelosi, L.; Musaro, A. An Overview about the Biology of Skeletal Muscle Satellite Cells. *Curr. Genom.* **2019**, *20*, 24–37. [CrossRef]
92. Brzoska, E.; Ciemerych, M.A.; Przewozniak, M.; Zimowska, M. Regulation of muscle stem cells activation: The role of growth factors and extracellular matrix. *Vitam. Horm.* **2011**, *87*, 239–276. [CrossRef] [PubMed]
93. Relaix, F.; Zammit, P.S. Satellite cells are essential for skeletal muscle regeneration: The cell on the edge returns centre stage. *Development* **2012**, *139*, 2845–2856. [CrossRef] [PubMed]
94. Zammit, P.S. Function of the myogenic regulatory factors Myf5, MyoD, Myogenin and MRF4 in skeletal muscle, satellite cells and regenerative myogenesis. *Semin. Cell Dev. Biol.* **2017**, *72*, 19–32. [CrossRef] [PubMed]
95. Dey, B.K.; Gagan, J.; Dutta, A. miR-206 and -486 induce myoblast differentiation by downregulating Pax7. *Mol. Cell Biol.* **2011**, *31*, 203–214. [CrossRef] [PubMed]
96. Forcales, S.V.; Albini, S.; Giordani, L.; Malecova, B.; Cignolo, L.; Chernov, A.; Coutinho, P.; Saccone, V.; Consalvi, S.; Williams, R.; et al. Signal-dependent incorporation of MyoD-BAF60c into Brg1-based SWI/SNF chromatin-remodelling complex. *Embo J.* **2012**, *31*, 301–316. [CrossRef]
97. Chazaud, B. Inflammation during skeletal muscle regeneration and tissue remodeling: Application to exercise-induced muscle damage management. *Immunol. Cell Biol.* **2016**, *94*, 140–145. [CrossRef]

98. Liu, X.; Liu, Y.; Zhao, L.; Zeng, Z.; Xiao, W.; Chen, P. Macrophage depletion impairs skeletal muscle regeneration: The roles of regulatory factors for muscle regeneration. *Cell Biol. Int.* **2017**, *41*, 228–238. [CrossRef]

99. Tatsumi, R.; Anderson, J.E.; Nevoret, C.J.; Halevy, O.; Allen, R.E. HGF/SF is present in normal adult skeletal muscle and is capable of activating satellite cells. *Dev. Biol.* **1998**, *194*, 114–128. [CrossRef]

100. Galvin, C.D.; Hardiman, O.; Nolan, C.M. IGF-1 receptor mediates differentiation of primary cultures of mouse skeletal myoblasts. *Mol. Cell Endocrinol.* **2003**, *200*, 19–29. [CrossRef]

101. Tidball, J.G.; Welc, S.S. Macrophage-Derived IGF-1 Is a Potent Coordinator of Myogenesis and Inflammation in Regenerating Muscle. *Mol. Ther. J. Am. Soc. Gene Ther.* **2015**, *23*, 1134–1135. [CrossRef]

102. Chen, S.E.; Jin, B.; Li, Y.P. TNF-alpha regulates myogenesis and muscle regeneration by activating p38 MAPK. *Am. J. Physiol. Cell Physiol.* **2007**, *292*, C1660–C1671. [CrossRef] [PubMed]

103. Latroche, C.; Weiss-Gayet, M.; Chazaud, B. Investigating the Vascular Niche: Three-Dimensional Co-culture of Human Skeletal Muscle Stem Cells and Endothelial Cells. *Methods Mol. Biol.* **2019**, *2002*, 121–128. [CrossRef] [PubMed]

104. Abou-Khalil, R.; Mounier, R.; Chazaud, B. Regulation of myogenic stem cell behavior by vessel cells: The "menage a trois" of satellite cells, periendothelial cells and endothelial cells. *Cell Cycle* **2010**, *9*, 892–896. [CrossRef] [PubMed]

105. Christov, C.; Chretien, F.; Abou-Khalil, R.; Bassez, G.; Vallet, G.; Authier, F.J.; Bassaglia, Y.; Shinin, V.; Tajbakhsh, S.; Chazaud, B.; et al. Muscle satellite cells and endothelial cells: Close neighbors and privileged partners. *Mol. Biol. Cell* **2007**, *18*, 1397–1409. [CrossRef] [PubMed]

106. Fiore, D.; Judson, R.N.; Low, M.; Lee, S.; Zhang, E.; Hopkins, C.; Xu, P.; Lenzi, A.; Rossi, F.M.; Lemos, D.R. Pharmacological blockage of fibro/adipogenic progenitor expansion and suppression of regenerative fibrogenesis is associated with impaired skeletal muscle regeneration. *Stem Cell Res.* **2016**, *17*, 161–169. [CrossRef]

107. Mathew, S.J.; Hansen, J.M.; Merrell, A.J.; Murphy, M.M.; Lawson, J.A.; Hutcheson, D.A.; Hansen, M.S.; Angus-Hill, M.; Kardon, G. Connective tissue fibroblasts and Tcf4 regulate myogenesis. *Development* **2011**, *138*, 371–384. [CrossRef]

108. Murphy, M.M.; Lawson, J.A.; Mathew, S.J.; Hutcheson, D.A.; Kardon, G. Satellite cells, connective tissue fibroblasts and their interactions are crucial for muscle regeneration. *Development* **2011**, *138*, 3625–3637. [CrossRef] [PubMed]

109. Uezumi, A.; Fukada, S.; Yamamoto, N.; Takeda, S.; Tsuchida, K. Mesenchymal progenitors distinct from satellite cells contribute to ectopic fat cell formation in skeletal muscle. *Nat. Cell Biol.* **2010**, *12*, 143–152. [CrossRef] [PubMed]

110. Joe, A.W.; Yi, L.; Natarajan, A.; Le Grand, F.; So, L.; Wang, J.; Rudnicki, M.A.; Rossi, F.M. Muscle injury activates resident fibro/adipogenic progenitors that facilitate myogenesis. *Nat. Cell Biol.* **2010**, *12*, 153–163. [CrossRef] [PubMed]

111. Wosczyna, M.N.; Konishi, C.T.; Perez Carbajal, E.E.; Wang, T.T.; Walsh, R.A.; Gan, Q.; Wagner, M.W.; Rando, T.A. Mesenchymal Stromal Cells Are Required for Regeneration and Homeostatic Maintenance of Skeletal Muscle. *Cell Rep.* **2019**, *27*, 2029–2035.e5. [CrossRef]

112. Forcina, L.; Miano, C.; Scicchitano, B.M.; Musaro, A. Signals from the Niche: Insights into the Role of IGF-1 and IL-6 in Modulating Skeletal Muscle Fibrosis. *Cells* **2019**, *8*, 232. [CrossRef] [PubMed]

113. Mierzejewski, B.; Archacka, K.; Grabowska, I.; Florkowska, A.; Ciemerych, M.A.; Brzoska, E. Human and mouse skeletal muscle stem and progenitor cells in health and disease. *Semin. Cell Dev. Biol.* **2020**. [CrossRef] [PubMed]

114. Birbrair, A.; Delbono, O. Pericytes are Essential for Skeletal Muscle Formation. *Stem Cell Rev. Rep.* **2015**, *11*, 547–548. [CrossRef] [PubMed]

115. Birbrair, A.; Zhang, T.; Wang, Z.M.; Messi, M.L.; Mintz, A.; Delbono, O. Type-1 pericytes participate in fibrous tissue deposition in aged skeletal muscle. *Am. J. Physiol. Cell Physiol.* **2013**, *305*, C1098–C1113. [CrossRef] [PubMed]

116. Dellavalle, A.; Maroli, G.; Covarello, D.; Azzoni, E.; Innocenzi, A.; Perani, L.; Antonini, S.; Sambasivan, R.; Brunelli, S.; Tajbakhsh, S.; et al. Pericytes resident in postnatal skeletal muscle differentiate into muscle fibres and generate satellite cells. *Nat. Commun.* **2011**, *2*, 499. [CrossRef] [PubMed]

117. Dellavalle, A.; Sampaolesi, M.; Tonlorenzi, R.; Tagliafico, E.; Sacchetti, B.; Perani, L.; Innocenzi, A.; Galvez, B.G.; Messina, G.; Morosetti, R.; et al. Pericytes of human skeletal muscle are myogenic precursors distinct from satellite cells. *Nat. Cell Biol.* **2007**, *9*, 255–267. [CrossRef] [PubMed]
118. Gautam, J.; Yao, Y. Pericytes in Skeletal Muscle. *Adv. Exp. Med. Biol.* **2019**, *1122*, 59–72. [CrossRef]
119. Persichini, T.; Funari, A.; Colasanti, M.; Sacchetti, B. Clonogenic, myogenic progenitors expressing MCAM/CD146 are incorporated as adventitial reticular cells in the microvascular compartment of human post-natal skeletal muscle. *PLoS ONE* **2017**, *12*, e0188844. [CrossRef]
120. Kostallari, E.; Baba-Amer, Y.; Alonso-Martin, S.; Ngoh, P.; Relaix, F.; Lafuste, P.; Gherardi, R.K. Pericytes in the myovascular niche promote post-natal myofiber growth and satellite cell quiescence. *Development* **2015**, *142*, 1242–1253. [CrossRef]
121. Mitchell, K.J.; Pannerec, A.; Cadot, B.; Parlakian, A.; Besson, V.; Gomes, E.R.; Marazzi, G.; Sassoon, D.A. Identification and characterization of a non-satellite cell muscle resident progenitor during postnatal development. *Nat. Cell Biol.* **2010**, *12*, 257–266. [CrossRef] [PubMed]
122. Tamaki, T.; Akatsuka, A.; Ando, K.; Nakamura, Y.; Matsuzawa, H.; Hotta, T.; Roy, R.R.; Edgerton, V.R. Identification of myogenic-endothelial progenitor cells in the interstitial spaces of skeletal muscle. *J. Cell Biol.* **2002**, *157*, 571–577. [CrossRef] [PubMed]
123. Liu, N.; Garry, G.A.; Li, S.; Bezprozvannaya, S.; Sanchez-Ortiz, E.; Chen, B.; Shelton, J.M.; Jaichander, P.; Bassel-Duby, R.; Olson, E.N. A Twist2-dependent progenitor cell contributes to adult skeletal muscle. *Nat. Cell Biol.* **2017**, *19*, 202–213. [CrossRef] [PubMed]
124. Gussoni, E.; Soneoka, Y.; Strickland, C.D.; Buzney, E.A.; Khan, M.K.; Flint, A.F.; Kunkel, L.M.; Mulligan, R.C. Dystrophin expression in the mdx mouse restored by stem cell transplantation. *Nature* **1999**, *401*, 390–394. [CrossRef] [PubMed]
125. Torrente, Y.; Belicchi, M.; Sampaolesi, M.; Pisati, F.; Meregalli, M.; D'Antona, G.; Tonlorenzi, R.; Porretti, L.; Gavina, M.; Mamchaoui, K.; et al. Human circulating AC133(+) stem cells restore dystrophin expression and ameliorate function in dystrophic skeletal muscle. *J. Clin. Investig.* **2004**, *114*, 182–195. [CrossRef]
126. Asakura, A.; Komaki, M.; Rudnicki, M. Muscle satellite cells are multipotential stem cells that exhibit myogenic, osteogenic, and adipogenic differentiation. *Differentiation* **2001**, *68*, 245–253. [CrossRef]
127. Castiglioni, A.; Hettmer, S.; Lynes, M.D.; Rao, T.N.; Tchessalova, D.; Sinha, I.; Lee, B.T.; Tseng, Y.H.; Wagers, A.J. Isolation of progenitors that exhibit myogenic/osteogenic bipotency in vitro by fluorescence-activated cell sorting from human fetal muscle. *Stem Cell Rep.* **2014**, *2*, 92–106. [CrossRef]
128. Guimaraes-Camboa, N.; Cattaneo, P.; Sun, Y.; Moore-Morris, T.; Gu, Y.; Dalton, N.D.; Rockenstein, E.; Masliah, E.; Peterson, K.L.; Stallcup, W.B.; et al. Pericytes of Multiple Organs Do Not Behave as Mesenchymal Stem Cells In Vivo. *Cell Stem Cell* **2017**, *20*, 345–359.e5. [CrossRef]
129. Sacchetti, B.; Funari, A.; Remoli, C.; Giannicola, G.; Kogler, G.; Liedtke, S.; Cossu, G.; Serafini, M.; Sampaolesi, M.; Tagliafico, E.; et al. No Identical "Mesenchymal Stem Cells" at Different Times and Sites: Human Committed Progenitors of Distinct Origin and Differentiation Potential Are Incorporated as Adventitial Cells in Microvessels. *Stem Cell Rep.* **2016**, *6*, 897–913. [CrossRef]
130. Wosczyna, M.N.; Biswas, A.A.; Cogswell, C.A.; Goldhamer, D.J. Multipotent progenitors resident in the skeletal muscle interstitium exhibit robust BMP-dependent osteogenic activity and mediate heterotopic ossification. *J. Bone Miner. Res.* **2012**, *27*, 1004–1017. [CrossRef]
131. Pannerec, A.; Formicola, L.; Besson, V.; Marazzi, G.; Sassoon, D.A. Defining skeletal muscle resident progenitors and their cell fate potentials. *Development* **2013**, *140*, 2879–2891. [CrossRef]
132. Tamaki, T.; Akatsuka, A.; Yoshimura, S.; Roy, R.R.; Edgerton, V.R. New fiber formation in the interstitial spaces of rat skeletal muscle during postnatal growth. *J. Histochem. Cytochem.* **2002**, *50*, 1097–1111. [CrossRef] [PubMed]
133. Tamaki, T.; Uchiyama, Y.; Okada, Y.; Ishikawa, T.; Sato, M.; Akatsuka, A.; Asahara, T. Functional recovery of damaged skeletal muscle through synchronized vasculogenesis, myogenesis, and neurogenesis by muscle-derived stem cells. *Circulation* **2005**, *112*, 2857–2866. [CrossRef] [PubMed]
134. Negroni, E.; Riederer, I.; Chaouch, S.; Belicchi, M.; Razini, P.; Di Santo, J.; Torrente, Y.; Butler-Browne, G.S.; Mouly, V. In vivo myogenic potential of human CD133+ muscle-derived stem cells: A quantitative study. *Moleculus* **2009**, *17*, 1771–1778. [CrossRef] [PubMed]

135. Torrente, Y.; Belicchi, M.; Marchesi, C.; D'Antona, G.; Cogiamanian, F.; Pisati, F.; Gavina, M.; Giordano, R.; Tonlorenzi, R.; Fagiolari, G.; et al. Autologous transplantation of muscle-derived CD133+ stem cells in Duchenne muscle patients. *Cell Transpl.* **2007**, *16*, 563–577. [CrossRef] [PubMed]

136. Benchaouir, R.; Meregalli, M.; Farini, A.; D'Antona, G.; Belicchi, M.; Goyenvalle, A.; Battistelli, M.; Bresolin, N.; Bottinelli, R.; Garcia, L.; et al. Restoration of human dystrophin following transplantation of exon-skipping-engineered DMD patient stem cells into dystrophic mice. *Cell Stem Cell* **2007**, *1*, 646–657. [CrossRef]

137. Kaji, D.A.; Tan, Z.; Johnson, G.L.; Huang, W.; Vasquez, K.; Lehoczky, J.A.; Levi, B.; Cheah, K.S.E.; Huang, A.H. Cellular Plasticity in Musculoskeletal Development, Regeneration, and Disease. *J. Orthop. Res.* **2020**, *38*, 708–718. [CrossRef]

138. Lounev, V.Y.; Ramachandran, R.; Wosczyna, M.N.; Yamamoto, M.; Maidment, A.D.; Shore, E.M.; Glaser, D.L.; Goldhamer, D.J.; Kaplan, F.S. Identification of progenitor cells that contribute to heterotopic skeletogenesis. *J. Bone Jt. Surg. Am.* **2009**, *91*, 652–663. [CrossRef]

139. Medici, D.; Shore, E.M.; Lounev, V.Y.; Kaplan, F.S.; Kalluri, R.; Olsen, B.R. Conversion of vascular endothelial cells into multipotent stem-like cells. *Nat. Med.* **2010**, *16*, 1400–1406. [CrossRef]

140. Kan, L.; Liu, Y.; McGuire, T.L.; Berger, D.M.; Awatramani, R.B.; Dymecki, S.M.; Kessler, J.A. Dysregulation of local stem/progenitor cells as a common cellular mechanism for heterotopic ossification. *Stem Cells* **2009**, *27*, 150–156. [CrossRef]

141. Hwang, C.; Marini, S.; Huber, A.K.; Stepien, D.M.; Sorkin, M.; Loder, S.; Pagani, C.A.; Li, J.; Visser, N.D.; Vasquez, K.; et al. Mesenchymal VEGFA induces aberrant differentiation in heterotopic ossification. *Bone Res.* **2019**, *7*, 36. [CrossRef]

142. Uezumi, A.; Fukada, S.; Yamamoto, N.; Ikemoto-Uezumi, M.; Nakatani, M.; Morita, M.; Yamaguchi, A.; Yamada, H.; Nishino, I.; Hamada, Y.; et al. Identification and characterization of PDGFRalpha+ mesenchymal progenitors in human skeletal muscle. *Cell Death Dis.* **2014**, *5*, e1186. [CrossRef] [PubMed]

143. Regard, J.B.; Malhotra, D.; Gvozdenovic-Jeremic, J.; Josey, M.; Chen, M.; Weinstein, L.S.; Lu, J.; Shore, E.M.; Kaplan, F.S.; Yang, Y. Activation of Hedgehog signaling by loss of GNAS causes heterotopic ossification. *Nat. Med.* **2013**, *19*, 1505–1512. [CrossRef] [PubMed]

144. Agarwal, S.; Loder, S.; Brownley, C.; Cholok, D.; Mangiavini, L.; Li, J.; Breuler, C.; Sung, H.H.; Li, S.; Ranganathan, K.; et al. Inhibition of Hif1alpha prevents both trauma-induced and genetic heterotopic ossification. *Proc. Natl. Acad. Sci. USA* **2016**, *113*, E338–E347. [CrossRef] [PubMed]

145. Dey, D.; Bagarova, J.; Hatsell, S.J.; Armstrong, K.A.; Huang, L.; Ermann, J.; Vonner, A.J.; Shen, Y.; Mohedas, A.H.; Lee, A.; et al. Two tissue-resident progenitor lineages drive distinct phenotypes of heterotopic ossification. *Sci. Transl. Med.* **2016**, *8*, 366ra163. [CrossRef]

146. Kan, C.; Chen, L.; Hu, Y.; Ding, N.; Li, Y.; McGuire, T.L.; Lu, H.; Kessler, J.A.; Kan, L. Gli1-labeled adult mesenchymal stem/progenitor cells and hedgehog signaling contribute to endochondral heterotopic ossification. *Bone* **2018**, *109*, 71–79. [CrossRef]

147. Kan, L.; Peng, C.Y.; McGuire, T.L.; Kessler, J.A. Glast-expressing progenitor cells contribute to heterotopic ossification. *Bone* **2013**, *53*, 194–203. [CrossRef]

148. Agarwal, S.; Loder, S.J.; Cholok, D.; Peterson, J.; Li, J.; Breuler, C.; Cameron Brownley, R.; Hsin Sung, H.; Chung, M.T.; Kamiya, N.; et al. Scleraxis-Lineage Cells Contribute to Ectopic Bone Formation in Muscle and Tendon. *Stem Cells* **2017**, *35*, 705–710. [CrossRef]

149. Chen, D.; Zhao, M.; Mundy, G.R. Bone morphogenetic proteins. *Growth Factors* **2004**, *22*, 233–241. [CrossRef]

150. Guo, X.; Wang, X.F. Signaling cross-talk between TGF-beta/BMP and other pathways. *Cell Res.* **2009**, *19*, 71–88. [CrossRef]

151. Komori, T. Runx2, an inducer of osteoblast and chondrocyte differentiation. *Histochem. Cell Biol.* **2018**, *149*, 313–323. [CrossRef]

152. Montecino, M.; Stein, G.; Stein, J.; Zaidi, K.; Aguilar, R. Multiple levels of epigenetic control for bone biology and pathology. *Bone* **2015**, *81*, 733–738. [CrossRef]

153. Uchida, K.; Yayama, T.; Cai, H.X.; Nakajima, H.; Sugita, D.; Guerrero, A.R.; Kobayashi, S.; Yoshida, A.; Chen, K.B.; Baba, H. Ossification process involving the human thoracic ligamentum flavum: Role of transcription factors. *Arthritis Res. Ther.* **2011**, *13*, R144. [CrossRef] [PubMed]

154. Lin, L.; Shen, Q.; Xue, T.; Yu, C. Heterotopic ossification induced by Achilles tenotomy via endochondral bone formation: Expression of bone and cartilage related genes. *Bone* **2010**, *46*, 425–431. [CrossRef] [PubMed]

155. Kang, J.S.; Alliston, T.; Delston, R.; Derynck, R. Repression of Runx2 function by TGF-beta through recruitment of class II histone deacetylases by Smad3. *Embo J.* **2005**, *24*, 2543–2555. [CrossRef] [PubMed]

156. Lee, K.S.; Hong, S.H.; Bae, S.C. Both the Smad and p38 MAPK pathways play a crucial role in Runx2 expression following induction by transforming growth factor-beta and bone morphogenetic protein. *Oncogene* **2002**, *21*, 7156–7163. [CrossRef]

157. Wu, M.; Chen, G.; Li, Y.P. TGF-beta and BMP signaling in osteoblast, skeletal development, and bone formation, homeostasis and disease. *Bone Res.* **2016**, *4*, 16009. [CrossRef]

158. Rahman, M.S.; Akhtar, N.; Jamil, H.M.; Banik, R.S.; Asaduzzaman, S.M. TGF-beta/BMP signaling and other molecular events: Regulation of osteoblastogenesis and bone formation. *Bone Res.* **2015**, *3*, 15005. [CrossRef]

159. Grenier, G.; Leblanc, E.; Faucheux, N.; Lauzier, D.; Kloen, P.; Hamdy, R.C. BMP-9 expression in human traumatic heterotopic ossification: A case report. *Skelet. Muscle* **2013**, *3*, 29. [CrossRef]

160. Matsumoto, Y.; Ikeya, M.; Hino, K.; Horigome, K.; Fukuta, M.; Watanabe, M.; Nagata, S.; Yamamoto, T.; Otsuka, T.; Toguchida, J. New Protocol to Optimize iPS Cells for Genome Analysis of Fibrodysplasia Ossificans Progressiva. *Stem Cells* **2015**, *33*, 1730–1742. [CrossRef]

161. Medici, D.; Olsen, B.R. The role of endothelial-mesenchymal transition in heterotopic ossification. *J. Bone Miner. Res.* **2012**, *27*, 1619–1622. [CrossRef]

162. Agarwal, S.; Loder, S.; Li, J.; Brownley, C.; Peterson, J.R.; Oluwatobi, E.; Drake, J.; Cholok, D.; Ranganathan, K.; Sung, H.H.; et al. Diminished Chondrogenesis and Enhanced Osteoclastogenesis in Leptin-Deficient Diabetic Mice (ob/ob) Impair Pathologic, Trauma-Induced Heterotopic Ossification. *Stem Cells Dev.* **2015**, *24*, 2864–2872. [CrossRef] [PubMed]

163. Lees-Shepard, J.B.; Yamamoto, M.; Biswas, A.A.; Stoessel, S.J.; Nicholas, S.E.; Cogswell, C.A.; Devarakonda, P.M.; Schneider, M.J., Jr.; Cummins, S.M.; Legendre, N.P.; et al. Activin-dependent signaling in fibro/adipogenic progenitors causes fibrodysplasia ossificans progressiva. *Nat. Commun.* **2018**, *9*, 471. [CrossRef] [PubMed]

164. Wu, J.; Ren, B.; Shi, F.; Hua, P.; Lin, H. BMP and mTOR signaling in heterotopic ossification: Does their crosstalk provide therapeutic opportunities? *J. Cell Biochem.* **2019**, *120*, 12108–12122. [CrossRef] [PubMed]

165. Moustakas, A.; Heldin, C.H. Ecsit-ement on the crossroads of Toll and BMP signal transduction. *Genes Dev.* **2003**, *17*, 2855–2859. [CrossRef]

166. Gaur, T.; Lengner, C.J.; Hovhannisyan, H.; Bhat, R.A.; Bodine, P.V.; Komm, B.S.; Javed, A.; van Wijnen, A.J.; Stein, J.L.; Stein, G.S.; et al. Canonical WNT signaling promotes osteogenesis by directly stimulating Runx2 gene expression. *J. Biol. Chem* **2005**, *280*, 33132–33140. [CrossRef] [PubMed]

167. Kawane, T.; Komori, H.; Liu, W.; Moriishi, T.; Miyazaki, T.; Mori, M.; Matsuo, Y.; Takada, Y.; Izumi, S.; Jiang, Q.; et al. Dlx5 and mef2 regulate a novel runx2 enhancer for osteoblast-specific expression. *J. Bone Miner. Res.* **2014**, *29*, 1960–1969. [CrossRef]

168. Hino, K.; Horigome, K.; Nishio, M.; Komura, S.; Nagata, S.; Zhao, C.; Jin, Y.; Kawakami, K.; Yamada, Y.; Ohta, A.; et al. Activin-A enhances mTOR signaling to promote aberrant chondrogenesis in fibrodysplasia ossificans progressiva. *J. Clin. Investig.* **2017**, *127*, 3339–3352. [CrossRef]

169. Huang, Y.; Wang, X.; Lin, H. The hypoxic microenvironment: A driving force for heterotopic ossification progression. *Cell Commun. Signal.* **2020**, *18*, 20. [CrossRef]

170. Peterson, J.R.; De La Rosa, S.; Sun, H.; Eboda, O.; Cilwa, K.E.; Donneys, A.; Morris, M.; Buchman, S.R.; Cederna, P.S.; Krebsbach, P.H.; et al. Burn injury enhances bone formation in heterotopic ossification model. *Ann. Surg.* **2014**, *259*, 993–998. [CrossRef]

171. Croes, M.; Kruyt, M.C.; Boot, W.; Pouran, B.; Braham, M.V.; Pakpahan, S.A.; Weinans, H.; Vogely, H.C.; Fluit, A.C.; Dhert, W.J.; et al. The role of bacterial stimuli in inflammation-driven bone formation. *Eur. Cells Mater.* **2019**, *37*, 402–419. [CrossRef]

172. Wang, H.; Behrens, E.M.; Pignolo, R.J.; Kaplan, F.S. ECSIT links TLR and BMP signaling in FOP connective tissue progenitor cells. *Bone* **2018**, *109*, 201–209. [CrossRef] [PubMed]

173. Wi, S.M.; Moon, G.; Kim, J.; Kim, S.T.; Shim, J.H.; Chun, E.; Lee, K.Y. TAK1-ECSIT-TRAF6 complex plays a key role in the TLR4 signal to activate NF-kappaB. *J. Biol. Chem* **2014**, *289*, 35205–35214. [CrossRef] [PubMed]

174. Shimono, K.; Tung, W.E.; Macolino, C.; Chi, A.H.; Didizian, J.H.; Mundy, C.; Chandraratna, R.A.; Mishina, Y.; Enomoto-Iwamoto, M.; Pacifici, M.; et al. Potent inhibition of heterotopic ossification by nuclear retinoic acid receptor-gamma agonists. *Nat. Med.* **2011**, *17*, 454–460. [CrossRef] [PubMed]

175. Chakkalakal, S.A.; Uchibe, K.; Convente, M.R.; Zhang, D.; Economides, A.N.; Kaplan, F.S.; Pacifici, M.; Iwamoto, M.; Shore, E.M. Palovarotene Inhibits Heterotopic Ossification and Maintains Limb Mobility and Growth in Mice With the Human ACVR1(R206H) Fibrodysplasia Ossificans Progressiva (FOP) Mutation. *J. Bone Miner. Res.* **2016**, *31*, 1666–1675. [CrossRef]

176. Hino, K.; Zhao, C.; Horigome, K.; Nishio, M.; Okanishi, Y.; Nagata, S.; Komura, S.; Yamada, Y.; Toguchida, J.; Ohta, A. An mTOR signaling modulator suppressed heterotopic ossification of Fibrodysplasia Ossificans Progressiva. *Stem Cell Rep.* **2018**, *11*, 1106–1119. [CrossRef] [PubMed]

177. Peterson, J.R.; De La Rosa, S.; Eboda, O.; Cilwa, K.E.; Agarwal, S.; Buchman, S.R.; Cederna, P.S.; Xi, C.; Morris, M.D.; Herndon, D.N.; et al. Treatment of heterotopic ossification through remote ATP hydrolysis. *Sci. Transl. Med.* **2014**, *6*, 255ra132. [CrossRef]

178. Hannallah, D.; Peng, H.; Young, B.; Usas, A.; Gearhart, B.; Huard, J. Retroviral delivery of Noggin inhibits the formation of heterotopic ossification induced by BMP-4, demineralized bone matrix, and trauma in an animal model. *J. Bone Jt. Surg. Am. Vol.* **2004**, *86*, 80–91. [CrossRef]

179. Kaplan, F.S.; Pignolo, R.J.; Al Mukaddam, M.M.; Shore, E.M. Hard targets for a second skeleton: Therapeutic horizons for fibrodysplasia ossificans progressiva (FOP). *Expert Opin. Orphan Drugs* **2017**, *5*, 291–294. [CrossRef]

180. Xue, T.; Mao, Z.; Lin, L.; Hou, Y.; Wei, X.; Fu, X.; Zhang, J.; Yu, C. Non-virus-mediated transfer of siRNAs against Runx2 and Smad4 inhibit heterotopic ossification in rats. *Gene Ther.* **2010**, *17*, 370–379. [CrossRef]

9

Genetic Associations with Aging Muscle

Jedd Pratt [1,2,*], Colin Boreham [1], Sean Ennis [2,3], Anthony W. Ryan [2] and Giuseppe De Vito [1,4]

[1]   Institute for Sport and Health, University College Dublin, Dublin, Ireland;
      colin.boreham@ucd.ie (C.B.); giuseppe.devito@ucd.ie (G.D.V.)
[2]   Genomics Medicine Ireland, Dublin, Ireland; sean.ennis@ucd.ie (S.E.);
      anthony.ryan@genomicsmed.ie (A.W.R.)
[3]   UCD ACoRD, Academic Centre on Rare Diseases, University College Dublin, Dublin, Ireland
[4]   Department of Biomedical Sciences, University of Padova, Via F. Marzolo 3, 35131 Padova, Italy
*   Correspondence: jedd.pratt@ucdconnect.ie

Abstract: The age-related decline in skeletal muscle mass, strength and function known as 'sarcopenia' is associated with multiple adverse health outcomes, including cardiovascular disease, stroke, functional disability and mortality. While skeletal muscle properties are known to be highly heritable, evidence regarding the specific genes underpinning this heritability is currently inconclusive. This review aimed to identify genetic variants known to be associated with muscle phenotypes relevant to sarcopenia. PubMed, Embase and Web of Science were systematically searched (from January 2004 to March 2019) using pre-defined search terms such as "aging", "sarcopenia", "skeletal muscle", "muscle strength" and "genetic association". Candidate gene association studies and genome wide association studies that examined the genetic association with muscle phenotypes in non-institutionalised adults aged ≥50 years were included. Fifty-four studies were included in the final analysis. Twenty-six genes and 88 DNA polymorphisms were analysed across the 54 studies. The *ACTN3*, *ACE* and *VDR* genes were the most frequently studied, although the *IGF1/IGFBP3*, *TNFα*, *APOE*, *CNTF/R* and *UCP2/3* genes were also shown to be significantly associated with muscle phenotypes in two or more studies. Ten DNA polymorphisms (rs154410, rs2228570, rs1800169, rs3093059, rs1800629, rs1815739, rs1799752, rs7412, rs429358 and 192 bp allele) were significantly associated with muscle phenotypes in two or more studies. Through the identification of key gene variants, this review furthers the elucidation of genetic associations with muscle phenotypes associated with sarcopenia.

Keywords: genotype; genetic variation; muscle phenotypes; sarcopenia; aging

1. Introduction

Sarcopenia refers to the progressive deterioration in skeletal muscle mass, strength and physical function with advancing age [1]. The simultaneous presence of low muscle strength, muscle mass and/or physical function forms the diagnostic basis of the recommendations from the European Working Group on Sarcopenia in Older People [2]. These criteria are strong predictors of a multitude of adverse health outcomes, such as cardiovascular disease [3], functional disability [4], fall incidence [5], hospitalisation [6], stroke [7] and mortality [8]. Up to 10% of individuals aged 60–69 years are affected by sarcopenia, with this proportion rising considerably to 40% for adults over 80 years of age [9,10]. The fundamental loss of independence and susceptibility to additional diseases caused by sarcopenia also places a significant burden on public health systems worldwide. This burden is anticipated to grow considerably in coming decades, in line with increases in longevity and the consequent rise in the proportion of elderly [11]. Thus, the consequences of age-related muscle deterioration will become increasingly relevant globally.

While sarcopenia is generally more prevalent among individuals over the age of 60, strong evidence suggests that pronounced changes in muscle tissue begin from around 50 years of age [12]. From this age, muscle mass and strength begin to deteriorate at an annual rate of 1–2% and 1.5–5% respectively [12–14]. Developing an understanding of why and how skeletal muscle deteriorates from this age will be critical to reducing the burden of sarcopenia for patients as well as public health systems.

Currently, it is known that inter-individual variation in muscle phenotypes may be attributed to genetic factors, environmental factors and/or, gene-environment interactions [15,16]. While environmental factors such as physical activity, protein intake [17], sleep quality [18], smoking status [15] and alcohol consumption [19] have been shown to affect muscle phenotypes, heritability studies have highlighted the importance of genetic factors in determining inter-individual variability in skeletal muscle traits [20,21]. These studies have found that genetic factors account for 46–76% and 32–67% of fat-free mass (FFM) and muscle strength variability, respectively [20,21]. Additional longitudinal studies have observed heritability estimates of 64% for change in muscle strength with advancing age [22]. However, while the overall heritability of skeletal muscle phenotypes is well established, the genetic mechanisms underpinning this heritability remain unclear.

Thus, developing a deeper understanding of genetic associations underpinning skeletal muscle phenotypes is of paramount importance in the development of effective treatment interventions to manage age-related changes in muscle structure and function. Furthermore, understanding the genetic mechanisms regulating muscle accrual and loss will help facilitate early screening for susceptibility to sarcopenia, which could allow for preventative measures to be implemented prior to predicted muscle degradation.

Therefore, the purpose of this systematic review was to identify and synthesize the genetic variants associated with muscle phenotypes relevant to sarcopenia in humans.

2. Materials and Methods

Reporting followed the Preferred Reporting Items for Systematic Reviews and Meta-Analyses (PRISMA) statement [23].

2.1. Literature Search and Eligibility Criteria

2.1.1. Inclusion and Exclusion Criteria

To be included in this review, studies had to meet the following criteria:

1. Published between January 2004 and March 2019.
2. Full English text available.
3. Participants must be non-institutionalised human adults, aged 50 years or above.
4. Subjects must have been free from any significant cardiovascular, metabolic or musculoskeletal disorders at the time of the study.
5. Candidate gene association study or genome wide association study (GWAS).

2.1.2. Search Strategy

A systematic literature search of three online databases, PubMed, EMBASE and Web of Science, was conducted on 18 March 2019, for the period between January 2004 and March 2019. This time limit ensured the inclusion of the most pertinent literature. Search terms were selected based off the PEO framework and combined using Boolean operators ("AND", "OR"). Filters were used to limit results to those using human subjects, written in the English language and published within the desired time-frame. The search strategy used was as follows: ("ageing" OR "aged" OR "elderly" OR "older persons" OR "community dwelling") AND ("sarcopenia" OR "skeletal muscle" OR "muscle phenotype" OR "muscle mass" OR "muscle atrophy" OR "muscle strength" OR "grip strength" OR "physical performance" OR "muscle quality" OR "lean mass") AND ("single nucleotide polymorphism" OR "genetic polymorphism" OR "allele" OR "genetic variation" OR "gene variant" OR "mutation" OR "genes" OR "chromosome" OR "genetic predisposition" OR "genetic susceptibility") AND ("genetic association studies" OR "genome-wide association study" OR "GWAS" OR "candidate gene study" OR "genotype" OR "haplotype" OR "heritability"). The scope of the online search was further expanded by assessing bibliographic references of the eligible full text articles for relevant studies.

2.2. Study Selection and Data Extraction

Following the removal of duplicates, titles and abstracts were screened for relevance to the scope of this review. To determine inclusion in this review, the full text of every potentially relevant article was scrutinised for overall content and compliance with the eligibility criteria outlined above. The following data were extracted from each eligible article: authors, year of publication, study design, studied population (number, ethnicity, nationality, sex), gene name, polymorphism, muscle phenotype, main findings of the study.

2.3. Phenotypes

Phenotypic outcomes included in this systematic review were skeletal muscle mass, muscle strength, physical function and sarcopenia prevalence.

2.4. Quality Assessment

The quality and risk of bias of the included studies were assessed using the Quality of Genetic Association Studies (Q-Genie) tool [24]. The Q-Genie tool consists of 11 items that cover the following areas: "rationale for study", "selection and definition of outcome of interest", "selection and comparability of comparison groups", "technical classification of the exposure", "non-technical classification of the exposure", "other source of bias", "sample size and power", "a priori planning of analysis", "statistical methods and control for confounding", "testing of assumptions and inferences for genetic analysis" and "appropriateness of inferences drawn from results". Each area was rated using a 7-point Likert scale ("1 = poor"; "2", "3 = good"; "4", "5 = very good"; "6", "7 = excellent"). The overall quality of the included articles was classified by collating the scores for each theme. Studies with control groups were classified as "poor quality" if the score was ≤ 35, "moderate quality" if the score was > 35 and ≤ 45, and "good quality" if the score was > 45. For studies without control groups, scoring ≤ 32, > 32 and ≤ 40, and > 40 reflected classifications of "poor quality", "moderate quality" and "good quality", respectively.

3. Results

3.1. Search Strategy

The systematic search of the online databases identified 771 papers. Following the addition of filters, removal of duplicates and screening for eligibility, 48 studies remained. Six additional articles were retrieved through the manual search of reference lists, leaving a total of 54 articles to be included in this systematic review. Figure 1 highlights the identification and selection process in accordance with the PRISMA statement.

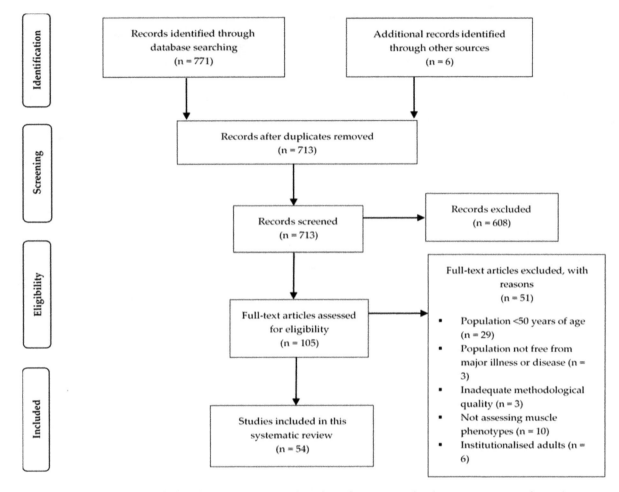

Figure 1. PRISMA flow chart presenting the identification and selection process of articles.

3.2. Quality Assessment

A detailed quality classification for each article is displayed in Table 1. Studies scored between 33 and 50 in the Q-Genie checklist. For studies with control groups ($n = 12$), five were classified as "moderate quality" and seven as "good quality". For non-control group studies ($n = 42$), 17 were classified as "moderate quality" and 25 as "good quality".

Table 1. Q-Genie quality assessment scores for the included studies.

Studies	Items											Total
	1	2	3	4	5	6	7	8	9	10	11	
Arkin, et al., 2006. [25]	4	4	N/A	4	4	3	3	5	4	5	4	40
Bahat, et al., 2010. [26]	4	4	3	4	3	3	3	4	5	4	4	41
Barr, et al., 2010. [27]	5	3	N/A	4	5	2	4	5	5	4	5	42
Bjork, et al., 2019. [28]	4	4	N/A	5	4	3	5	5	5	4	4	43
Buford, et al., 2014. [29]	5	4	3	4	5	3	3	4	6	4	6	47
Bustamante-Ara, et al., 2010. [30]	6	5	N/A	6	5	4	2	4	5	3	5	45
Charbonneau, et al., 2008. [31]	5	5	N/A	6	5	4	2	5	5	3	4	44
Cho, et al., 2017. [32]	4	4	N/A	5	4	3	3	3	4	3	4	37
Crocco, et al., 2011. [33]	5	5	N/A	5	4	3	5	5	5	4	3	44
Da Silva, et al., 2018. [34]	5	4	3	5	4	3	2	4	4	3	5	42
Dato, et al., 2012. [35]	6	5	N/A	5	4	3	4	5	4	4	5	45
De Mars, et al., 2007. [36]	6	5	N/A	5	4	3	3	5	5	4	5	45
Delmonico, et al., 2007. [37]	4	4	N/A	2	3	3	2	4	4	3	4	33
Delmonico, et al., 2008. [38]	5	3	N/A	3	4	3	5	4	5	3	4	39
Garatachea, et al., 2012. [39]	6	5	N/A	7	6	4	2	3	5	3	5	46
Giaccaglia, et al., 2008. [40]	5	5	5	5	4	5	3	4	5	5	4	50

Table 1. *Cont.*

Studies	1	2	3	4	5	6	7	8	9	10	11	Total
Gonzalez-Freire, et al., 2010. [41]	5	5	N/A	5	4	3	2	3	4	4	5	40
Gussago, et al., 2016. [42]	5	6	4	5	4	3	3	5	4	4	5	48
Hand, et al., 2007. [43]	5	4	N/A	6	5	3	3	4	6	3	5	44
Heckerman, et al., 2017. [44]	5	4	N/A	5	5	4	2	4	5	5	4	43
Hopkinson, et al., 2008. [45]	4	5	3	4	4	3	3	3	4	4	4	41
Judson, et al., 2010. [46]	5	4	N/A	5	5	2	4	3	4	4	4	40
Keogh, et al., 2015. [47]	5	4	N/A	5	4	3	2	4	3	4	5	39
Klimentidis, et al., 2016. [48]	4	4	N/A	2	4	4	5	5	5	4	4	41
Kikuchi, et al., 2015. [49]	5	4	3	4	4	4	5	5	5	4	5	48
Kostek, et al., 2005. [50]	5	5	N/A	5	5	3	3	4	5	4	5	44
Kostek, et al., 2010. [51]	5	3	3	5	4	2	3	5	5	4	5	44
Kritchevsky, et al., 2005. [52]	5	3	N/A	5	4	4	5	4	5	4	5	44
Li, et al., 2016. [53]	5	6	N/A	4	4	3	5	4	5	3	4	43
Lima, et al., 2011. [54]	5	3	4	5	3	4	3	4	5	4	5	45
Lin, et al., 2014. [55]	5	4	3	5	3	4	4	5	5	4	5	47
Lin, et al., 2014. [56]	5	5	4	5	4	3	3	5	5	5	4	48
Lunardi, et al., 2013. [57]	4	6	N/A	4	3	3	4	5	4	3	5	41
Ma, et al., 2018. [58]	6	5	N/A	5	5	4	5	4	5	3	4	46
McCauley, et al., 2010. [59]	5	5	N/A	5	3	4	3	4	3	3	5	40
Melzer, et al., 2005. [60]	5	5	N/A	4	2	3	4	4	4	4	5	40
Mora, et al., 2011. [61]	4	3	N/A	4	4	4	3	4	5	4	5	40
Onder, et al., 2008. [62]	5	4	N/A	4	4	3	2	5	3	4	4	38
Pereira, et al., 2013. [63]	5	3	N/A	4	4	4	4	3	4	3	5	39
Pereira, et al., 2013. [64]	6	4	N/A	6	4	4	4	5	5	4	5	47
Pereira, et al., 2013. [65]	6	5	N/A	6	5	3	3	5	5	4	5	47
Prakash, et al., 2019. [66]	4	4	3	5	5	3	4	5	4	5	4	46
Roth, et al., 2004. [67]	5	5	N/A	4	3	3	5	4	5	4	5	43
Skoog, et al., 2016. [68]	6	5	N/A	4	3	3	4	4	3	3	5	40
Tiainen, et al., 2012. [69]	6	5	N/A	4	3	4	2	3	3	3	4	37
Urano, et al., 2014. [70]	5	4	N/A	5	3	4	4	4	5	4	5	43
Verghese, et al., 2013. [71]	5	4	N/A	4	3	3	5	4	4	4	5	41
Walsh, et al., 2005. [72]	5	5	N/A	5	4	4	2	4	5	4	4	42
Wu, et al., 2014. [73]	5	5	N/A	4	4	3	4	4	5	3	4	41
Xia, et al., 2019. [74]	5	5	N/A	4	3	4	4	4	5	3	6	43
Yang, et al., 2015. [75]	5	4	N/A	4	3	4	3	4	5	4	5	41
Yoshihara, et al., 2009. [76]	3	4	N/A	3	3	3	4	3	4	3	3	33
Zempo, et al., 2010. [77]	4	4	N/A	3	3	4	3	4	5	4	4	38
Zempo, et al., 2011. [78]	5	4	N/A	3	3	3	4	4	5	4	4	39

Items: 1: Rationale for study, 2: Selection and definition of outcome of interest, 3: Selection and comparability of comparison groups, 4: Technical classification of the exposure, 5: Non-technical classification of the exposure, 6: Other sources of bias, 7: Sample size and power, 8: A priori planning of analysis, 9: Statistical methods and control for confounding, 10: Testing of assumptions and inferences for genetic analyses, 11: Appropriateness of inferences drawn from results. Scoring: 1 to 7, 1 being poor and 7 being excellent. N/A: not applicable.

3.3. Study and Subject Characteristics

Of the 54 studies included in this systematic review, 35 were cross sectional studies while the remaining 19 were longitudinal. A comprehensive description of the characteristics of the cross-sectional studies are presented in Table 2. Of the longitudinal studies, 11 were intervention studies while 8 were observational follow-up studies. The average intervention length was 21.3 weeks (range 10–72 weeks) while the average follow-up was 4.2 years (range 1–10 years). Table 3 presents a detailed description of the characteristics of the longitudinal studies. Out of the 54 studies, 53 were candidate gene association studies and the remaining article was a genome-wide association study.

Table 2. Cross-sectional studies on genetic associations with muscle phenotypes.

Gene	Polymorphism	Population Data	N	Muscle Phenotype	Results	Reference
				Hormone Genes		
VDR	rs2228570 (Fok1) rs1544410 (Bsm1)	Caucasians 46 males and 58 females Mean age 61.8 ± 8.5 years	104	Muscle strength (KE strength)	Individuals homozygous for the F allele of the rs2228570 polymorphism displayed significantly lower KE strength than carriers of ≥ 1 f allele ($p = 0.007$). KE strength did not differ significantly across rs1544410 genotypes.	Hopkinson, et al., 2008. [45]
VDR	rs2228570 rs1544410	Caucasians (Italians) 87 males and 172 females Aged ≥ 80 years Mean age 85.0 ± 4.5 years	259	Physical function (fall incidence)	Participants homozygous for the b allele of the rs1544410 polymorphism were significantly less likely to fall than carriers of ≥ 1 B allele ($p = 0.02$). Fall incidence did not differ significantly across rs2228570 genotypes.	Onder, et al., 2008. [62]
VDR	rs2228570 rs1544410	Caucasian females (OPUS cohort) Mean age 66.9 ± 7.0 years	2363	Muscle strength (lower limb power) Physical function (fall incidence, rise from chair)	Individuals with a bb genotype of the rs1544410 polymorphism were significantly less likely to fall than carriers of ≥ 1 B allele ($p = 0.025$). These individuals also performed significantly better in rise from chair and lower limb power tests ($p = 0.03, 0.044$ respectively). Fall incidence, muscle power did not differ significantly across rs2228570 genotypes.	Barr, et al., 2010. [27]
VDR	rs2228570 rs1544410 rs731236 (Taq1)	Males living in Turkey Aged 65-93 years Mean age 69 ± 6.9 years	120	Muscle strength (KE and KF peak torque)	KE strength was significantly higher in BB homozygotes compared to carriers of ≥ 1 b allele of the rs1544410 polymorphism ($p = 0.038$). No significant associations were found for rs2228570 and rs731236 genotypes.	Bahat, et al., 2010. [26]
				Hormone Genes		
VDR	rs2228570 (Fok1) rs1544410 (Bsm1) rs731236 (Taq1) rs7975232 (Apa1) rs7136534 rs9729	Caucasian male centenarians (Italian) Mean age 102.3 ± 0.3 years	120	Muscle strength (HG strength)	FF homozygotes displayed significantly greater HG than individuals with ≥ 1 f allele of the rs2228570 polymorphism ($p = 0.021$). HG did not differ significantly between rs1544410, rs7975232 and rs731236 genotypes.	Gussago, et al., 2016. [42]
VDR	rs17882106 rs10735810 rs4516035 rs11568820 rs11574024	Males living in Sweden Aged 69-81 years Mean age 75.4 ± 3.2 years	2844	Muscle strength (HG strength) Physical function (fall incidence, 6 m walk test, 20 cm narrow walk test, timed-stand test)	AA homozygotes were significantly less likely to fall compared to carriers of ≥ 1 G allele of rs716534 ($p = 0.002$). No other significant associations were found between polymorphism and muscle strength or function tasks.	Bjork, et al., 2019. [28]
VDR	rs2228570 rs1544410	Caucasian males Aged 58-93 years	302	Body composition (FFM, AFFM, SMI) Muscle Strength (KE torque) Sarcopenia (SMI < 7.26 kg/m^2)	Men homozygous for the F allele of the rs2228570 polymorphism had significantly less FFM, AFFM and SMI compared to Ff/ff genotypes ($p = 0.002, 0.009, 0.001$ respectively). FF homozygotes also had 2.17-fold higher risk of sarcopenia than carriers of ≥ 1 f allele ($p = 0.03$). No similar associations were found between rs1544410 genotypes.	Roth, et al., 2004. [67]

Table 2. *Cont.*

Gene	Polymorphism	Population Data	N	Muscle Phenotype	Results	Reference
Hormone Genes						
VDR	rs7975232 (Apa1) rs1544410 (Bsm1) rs2239185 rs3782905	Taiwanese 215 males and 154 females Mean age 74.4 ± 6.3 years (males) and 71.7 ± 4.7 years (females)	369	Muscle strength (HG strength)	Females carrying the AC genotype of rs7975232 polymorphism had significantly lower HG than CC homozygotes ($p < 0.05$). In both men and women, physical inactivity and the minor allele of each polymorphism were jointly associated with increased risk of low HG.	Wu, et al., 2014. [73]
VDR	rs2228570 (Fok1)	Chinese 275 males and 510 females Aged 63.2–72.5 years (males) and 63.1–71.9 years (females)	785	Muscle strength (HG strength) Physical function (4 m gait speed) Body composition (FFM, AFFM, SMI) Sarcopenia (SMI < 7.0 kg/m² for men and < 5.4 kg/m² for women and either low HG < 26 kg for men and < 18 kg for women or low gait speed < 0.8 m/s for both sexes)	Males who were homozygous for the f allele of the rs2228570 polymorphism had significantly greater HG and SMI when compared to carriers of ≥1 F allele ($p =$ 0.03, 0.04 respectively). These individuals also had a significantly lower risk of sarcopenia ($p = 0.03$). No similar association was found in the female population.	Xia, et al., 2019. [74]
AR	rs3032358 (CAG repeat)	Caucasian males (STORM cohort) Aged 55-93 years Subjects grouped by repeat number (120 males had < 22 and 174 had ≥ 22)	294	Body composition (total FFM and SMI) Muscle strength (KE isometric strength and HG strength)	Men who had ≥22 repeats exhibited significantly greater total FFM and SMI than men with < 22 repeats ($p < 0.027$, < 0.019 respectively). A similar association was not found in females. No significant association was observed between repeat number and muscle strength phenotypes.	Walsh, et al., 2005. [72]
TRHR	rs1689496 rs7832552	Brazilian females Aged between 60-82 years Mean age 66.6 ± 5.5 years	241	Body composition (FFM, AFFM and SMI) Muscle strength (KE peak torque) Sarcopenia (SMI < 5.45 kg/m²)	Subjects who carried the CC variant of rs1689496 had significantly less AFFM and SMI than AA/AC carriers ($p <0.05$). No significant differences were observed for rs7832552 variants.	Lunardi, et al., 2013. [57]
Growth Factor and Cytokine Genes						
IGF1	rs35767	Health ABC study cohort Blacks (533 males and 705 females) Whites (925 males and 836 females) Aged 70-79 years	2999	Body composition (FFM) Muscle volume (quadriceps CSA) Muscle strength (KE and HG strength, elbow flexor MVC and 1RM) Physical function (gait speed and single leg chair stands)	Black females with a CC genotype had significantly less FFM and quadriceps CSA compared to TT counterparts (both $p < 0.05$). White males with a CC genotype performed significantly worse in the single leg chair stands compared to CT counterparts ($p < 0.05$).	Kostek, et al., 2010. [51]
IGF1	192 bp allele	Caucasians (Spanish) 144 males and 148 females Mean age 76.7 ± 5.4 years (males) and 77.3 ± 6.4 years (females)	292	Muscle strength (KE isometric strength and HG strength)	No significant associations were observed in either males or females with relation to homozygosity, heterozygosity or non-carrier condition of the 192 bp allele ($p = 0.24$).	Mora, et al., 2011. [61]
IGF1 IGFBP3 IGFBP5	rs6214 rs35767 rs3110697 rs2854744 rs11977526 rs1978346 rs12474719	Taiwanese 251 males and 221 females Aged ≥ 65 years Mean age 74.7 ± 6.4 years (males) and 72.8 ± 5.5 years (females)	472	Body composition (SMI)	Individuals carrying the CC genotype of rs2854744 had a 4.3-fold risk of having low SMI compared with those with the AA genotype ($p < 0.05$). No other significant associations were observed for the other polymorphisms.	Yang, et al., 2015. [75]

Table 2. *Cont.*

Gene	Polymorphism	Population Data	N	Muscle Phenotype	Results	Reference
				Growth Factor and Cytokine Genes		
CNTF	rs948562 rs1800169 rs550942 rs4319530 rs1944055 rs2510559 rs2275993 rs1938596	Caucasian females (North American) Aged 70–79 years	363	Muscle strength (KE, HE and HG strength)	5 polymorphisms (rs948562, rs1800169, rs550942, rs4319530, rs1938596) were associated with HG (p <0.05). Haplotype analysis revealed rs1800169 null allele to fully explain relationship with the haplotype and HG under a recessive model, with homozygotes for the null allele exhibiting 3.80kg lower HG (p<0.01).	Arking, et al., 2006. [25]
CNTF CNTFR	rs1800169 rs3808871 rs2070802 C-174T	Caucasians 99 males and 102 females Aged 60–78 years (males) and 60–80 years (females)	201	Body composition (FFM) Muscle strength (isometric and concentric KE and KF at 60°, 120°, 150°, 180°, 240°)	Females who were G/A heterozygotes for the rs1800169 polymorphism produced significantly lower KE at 150° than both G/G and A/A homozygotes (p = 0.029). Males who carried the T allele of the rs3808871 polymorphism produced significantly higher KE and KF isometric torque at 120° when compared to CC homozygotes (p < 0.05). Females who carried the T allele of the rs2070802 polymorphism performed better on KF concentric torques at 60°, 180° and 240° than the A/A homozygotes (p = 0.03, 0.04, 0.04 respectively). No significant associations were observed between polymorphisms and FFM.	De Mars, et al. 2007. [36]
				Growth Factor and Cytokine Genes		
CRP IL6 TNFα ICAM1	rs1800947 rs2069829 rs361525 rs5498 rs2794520 rs1205 rs1130864	Danish twins 200 males and 400 females Aged 73–95 years	600	Physical function (self-reported during a 2-hour interview using a 11-item checklist)	Males who carried ≥1 A allele of the TNFα rs361525 polymorphism had a significantly better physical performance level compared to GG homozygotes (p < 0.001). No other associations were observed between polymorphisms and physical performance.	Tiainen, et al., 2012. [69]
CRP TNFα LTA	rs1800947 rs3093059 rs1799964 rs1800629 rs3093662 rs2239704 rs909253 rs1041981	Taiwanese 251 males and 221 females Aged ≥ 65 years Mean age 74.7 ± 6.4 years (males) and 72.8 ± 5.5 years (females)	472	Muscle strength (HG strength)	In females, the main effect of polymorphisms (rs1800947, rs3093059, rs1799964, rs1800629, rs909253, rs1041981) reflected lower HG. In the male population, polymorphisms (rs1130864, rs2239704) produced the same effect.	Li, et al., 2016. [53]
CRP	rs2794520 rs1205 rs1130864 rs1800947 rs3093059	Taiwanese 251 males and 221 females Aged ≥ 65 years Mean age 74.7 ± 6.4 years (males) and 72.8 ± 5.5 years (females)	472	Muscle strength (HG strength)	HG of subjects carrying the CC variant of polymorphisms rs2794520 and rs1205 was lower by 1.24 kg and 1.28 kg, respectively, compared with TT homozygotes. HG was 1.01 kg lower for every additional C allele of rs3093059 polymorphism. Haplotype C-C-C-C was significantly associated with lower HG than any other haplotypic formation (p = 0.015).	Lin, et al., 2014. [55]

Table 2. *Cont.*

Gene	Polymorphism	Population Data	N	Muscle Phenotype	Results	Reference
				Growth Factor and Cytokine Genes		
CAV1	rs1997623 rs3807987 rs12672038 rs3757733 rs7804372 rs3807992	Taiwanese 265 males and 237 females Aged ≥ 65 years 327 controls, 56 pre-sarcopenic, 63 sarcopenic, 56 severely sarcopenic	502	Body composition (FFM, AFFM, SMI) Muscle strength (HG strength) Muscle function (15 ft walk test) Sarcopenia (SMI < 6.87 kg/m² and 5.46 kg/m² for males and females, respectively and lowest quintile for muscle strength and function tests)	Subjects carrying ≥ 1 A allele of rs3807987 were at a significantly higher risk of sarcopenia than GG homozygotes ($p = 0.0235$). No other significant associations were observed between the remaining polymorphisms.	Lin, et al., 2014. [56]
MSTN	rs1805065 rs35781413 rs1805086 rs368949692 rs143242500	Caucasian nonagenarians 8 males and 33 females Aged 90-97 years	41	Muscle strength (1RM leg press) Physical function (Tinetti scale measured gait and balance, Barthel index) Body Composition (FFM estimated)	Carriers of the rs1805086 KR genotype were associated with lower FFM compared to KK carriers. The RR homozygote was below the 25th sex specific percentile for FFM and functional capacity.	Gonzalez-Freire, et al., 2010. [41]
ACVR2B	rs2276541	Hispanic (354) and Non-Hispanic (2406) females Mean age 64.1 ± 7.4 years	2760	Body composition (FFM, AFFM)	Subjects carrying the A allele of rs2276541 had significantly more FFM than G allele carriers ($p = 0.006$).	Klimentidis, et al., 2016. [49]
				Structural and Metabolic Genes		
ACTN3 ACE	rs1815739 (R577X) rs1799752 (I/D)	Caucasians (Spanish) 8 males and 33 females Aged 90-97 years Mean age 92 ± 2 years	41	Muscle strength (HG strength and 6-7 RM leg press) Physical function (8 m walk test and 4 step stairs test)	Study phenotypes did not differ significantly between ACE or ACTN3 genotypes (all $p > 0.05$).	Bustamante, et al., 2010. [30]
				Structural and Metabolic Genes		
ACTN3	rs1815739 (R577X)	Japanese 183 males and 238 females Aged ≥ 55 years	421	Muscle strength (HG strength) Physical function (chair stand test, 8 ft walking test)	XX homozygotes performed significantly worse in the chair stand test than RR/RX carriers ($p = 0.024, 0.005$ respectively). No significant association was found between ACTN3 genotype and 8 ft walk test or HG.	Kikuchi, et al., 2014. [48]
ACTN3	rs1815739	Koreans 62 males and 270 females Aged ≥ 65 years Mean age 74.4 ± 4.6 years (males) and 74.4 ± 6.6 years (females)	332	Body composition (FFM, AFFM, SMI) Sarcopenia (SMI <7.0 kg/m² and < 5.4 kg/m² for men and women respectively)	Sarcopenia prevalence was significantly associated with RX/XX genotypes ($p = 0.037, 0.038$ respectively). This association remained significant under both a dominant and recessive model ($p = 0.043, 0.029$ respectively).	Cho, et al., 2017. [32]
ACE	rs1799752 (I/D)	Brazilians 38 males and 53 females Aged 60-95 years Mean age 70.6 ± 7.2 years	91	Body composition (FFM, AFFM, SMI) Muscle strength (HG strength) Physical function (TUG test) Sarcopenia (based off FFM, muscle strength and physical function)	Sarcopenia prevalence was significantly higher in II genotype carriers compared to individuals with ≥ 1 D allele ($p = 0.015$).	Da Silva, et al., 2018. [34]
ACTN3 ACE	rs1815739 rs1799752	Caucasians (Spanish) 22 males and 59 females Aged 71-93 years Mean age 82.8 ± 4.8 years	81	Muscle strength (HG strength) Physical function (30s chair stand test, Barthel index) Muscle volume (thigh muscle CSA and muscle quality)	No significant associations were noted between any ACE rs1799752 or ACTN3 rs1815739 genotypes and the tested phenotypes in either males or females ($p > 0.05$).	Garatachea, et al., 2012. [39]

Table 2. *Cont.*

Gene	Polymorphism	Population Data	N	Muscle Phenotype	Results	Reference
Structural and Metabolic Genes						
ACTN3	rs1815739 (R577X)	Chinese 686 males and 777 females Aged 70-87 years 2 age groups (70-79 years and 80-87 years)	1463	Muscle strength (HG strength) Physical function (TUG, 5m walk test) Frailty measure (frailty index containing 23 variables)	In the 70-79 age group, male XX homozygotes performed significantly worse than RR carriers in HG, 5 m walk test and TUG (p = 0.012, 0.011 and 0.039 respectively). Females in this age group who carried the XX genotype had a significantly higher frailty index than RR carriers (p = 0.004).	Ma, et al., 2018. [58]
ACTN3 ACE	rs1815739 rs1799752 (I/D)	Caucasian males (British) Aged 60-70 years Mean age 65 ± 3 years	100	Body composition (FFM and thigh FFM) Muscle strength (isometric and isokinetic KE strength) Contractile properties (time to peak tension, half-relaxation time, peak rate of force development)	There were no significant associations between either ACE or ACTN3 genotypes and the studied phenotypes.	McCauley, et al., 2010. [59]
ACE	rs1799752	Japanese 228 males and 203 females Aged 76 years	431	Muscle strength (HG strength, isokinetic KE) Physical function (10 s maximal stepping rate, single leg standing time with eyes open, maximum walking speed over 10 m)	Individuals homozygous for the I allele had significantly lower HG than carriers of the D allele (p = 0.004). Although not significant, the ACE rs1799752 polymorphism was also positively associated with 10 m maximum walking speed.	Yoshihara, et al., 2009. [76]
ACTN3	rs1815739	Japanese females Aged 50-78 years Mean age 64.1 ± 6 years	109	Body composition (mid-thigh CSA) Physical function (physical activity was measured using an uniaxial accelerometer)	Thigh muscle CSA was significantly lower in XX homozygotes compared to RX/RR carriers (p = 0.04). Physical activity did not significantly differ between genotypes.	Zempo, et al., 2010. [77]
Structural and Metabolic Genes						
ACTN3	rs1815739 (R577X)	Japanese females Middle aged group (n = 82) mean age 50.6 ± 0.9 years Older group (n = 80) mean age 66.8 ± 0.5 years	162	Body composition (mid-thigh CSA) Physical activity (physical activity was measured using an uniaxial accelerometer)	In the middle-aged group, no association was observed between ACTN3 genotypes and thigh muscle CSA or physical activity. In the older group, XX homozygotes had significantly lower thigh muscle CSA than RX/RR carriers (p < 0.05).	Zempo, et al., 2010. [78]
UCP3	rs1800849 rs15763	Caucasians (Italians) 221 males and 211 females Aged 65-105 years Mean age 73.37 ± 7.46 years (males) and 73.37 ± 7.69 years (females)	432	Muscle strength (HG strength)	Carriers of the CC genotype of rs1800849 exhibited significantly lower HG than CT/TT genotypes (p = 0.010). No significant association was observed between rs15763 genotypes and HG.	Crocco, et al., 2011. [33]
UCP3	rs11235972 rs1685354 rs3781907 rs647126	Caucasians (Danish 1905 cohort) 265 males and 643 females Aged 93 years	908	Muscle strength (HG strength)	Individuals carrying the AA genotype of rs11235972 showed significantly lower HG than GG homozygotes (p < 0.001). Subjects carrying a GA genotype of rs1685354 displayed significantly greater HG than AA homozygotes (p = 0.016).	Dato, et al., 2012. [35]
PRDM16	rs12409277	Japanese females Mean age 65.1 ± 9.4 years	1081	Body composition (total FFM%)	Individuals who carried CT/CC variants of rs12409277 had a significantly greater FFM% compared to TT homozygotes (p = 0.003).	Urano, et al., 2014. [70]

KE: knee extensor, HE: hip extensor, KF: knee flexor, HG: handgrip, FFM: fat-free mass, AFFM: appendicular fat-free mass, SMI: skeletal muscle index, CSA: cross sectional area, MVC: maximal voluntary contraction, TUG: timed up and go.

Table 3. Longitudinal studies on genetic association with muscle phenotypes.

Gene	Polymorphism	Study Design	Population Data	N	Muscle Phenotype	Results	Reference
Hormone Genes							
RAMP3	rs3757575 rs2074654 rs1294935 rs11982639 rs12702121	5- and 10-year follow-up	Swedish females (OPRA cohort) Aged 75 years Mean age 75.2 ± 0.1 years	1044	Body composition (total, legs and trunk FFM)	At baseline, C allele carriers of rs2074654 had significantly greater amounts of total and leg FFM ($p = 0.041$, 0.038 respectively) when compared to TT homozygotes. There were no significant associations at follow up.	Prakash, et al., 2019. [66]
Growth Factor and Cytokine Genes							
IGF1	192 bp allele	10-week intervention of single leg KE RT	Caucasians 32 males and 35 females Mean age 70 ± 6 years (males) and 67 ± 8 years (females)	67	Muscle strength (KE 1RM) Muscle volume (using CT) Muscle quality (1RM/muscle volume)	Carriers of the 192 allele achieved significantly greater KE 1RM improvements than non-carriers ($p = 0.02$). Although not significant, a trend towards greater muscle volume was noted between 192 carriers and non-carriers ($p = 0.08$).	Kostek, et al., 2005. [50]
IGF1	192 bp allele	10-week intervention of single leg KE RT	Blacks (12 males and 21 females) Whites (46 males and 49 females) Aged 50–85 years	128	Muscle strength (KE 1RM) Muscle volume (using CT) Muscle quality (1RM/muscle volume)	Significantly greater KE 1RM improvements were observed in individuals with ≥ 1 192 allele compared to non-carriers ($p < 0.01$). No significant differences in muscle volume or quality were noted.	Hand, et al., 2007. [43]
Growth Factor and Cytokine Genes							
TNFα IL6 IL10	rs1800629 rs1800795 rs1800896	10-week intervention of either RT or AE	Brazilian females Aged ≥ 65 years 229 RT group and 222 AE group	451	Physical function (TUG and 10 m walking speed test)	Individuals homozygous for the G allele of polymorphism rs1800629 of TNFα achieved significantly greater TUG improvements with exercise compared to AA/AG genotypes ($p < 0.001$). A significant interaction was displayed between the 3 polymorphisms and TUG performance post exercise ($p < 0.001$). No significant interaction was observed between polymorphisms and 10 m walking speed test.	Pereira, et al., 2013. [65]
Structural and Metabolic Genes							
ACE	rs1799752 (I/D)	10-week intervention of unilateral KE RT	North Americans Whites (65%) and Blacks (35%) 86 males and 139 females Aged 50–85 years (mean age 62 years)	225	Body composition (FFM) Muscle volume (quadriceps) Muscle strength (KE 1RM)	At baseline, carriers of the DD genotype had significantly greater FFM than II homozygotes ($p < 0.05$). DD homozygotes also had greater baseline muscle volume in both the trained and untrained leg than II carriers ($p = 0.02$, 0.01 respectively). No significant associations were observed between genotypes and either 1RM or muscle volume adaptations to RT in either males or females.	Charbonneau, et al., 2008. [31]
ACE	rs1799752	12-month intervention of either PA or health education	Caucasians 97 males and 186 females Aged 70–89 years Mean age 77.2 ± 4.3 years	283	Physical function (400 m gait speed test and SPPB)	A significant difference was observed in gait speed and SPPB post PA in carriers of ≥ 1 D allele ($p = 0.018$, 0.015 respectively), but not in II homozygotes ($p = 0.930$, 0.275 respectively).	Buford, et al., 2014. [29]

Table 3. *Cont.*

Gene	Polymorphism	Study Design	Population Data	N	Muscle Phenotype	Results	Reference
Structural and Metabolic Genes							
ACTN3	rs1815739 (R577X)	10-week intervention of unilateral KE RT	Caucasians 71 males and 86 females Aged 50–85 years Mean age 65 ± 8 years (males) and 64 ± 9 years (females)	157	Body composition (FFM) Muscle volume (quadriceps) Muscle strength (KE 1RM, peak power and velocity)	At baseline, female XX homozygotes had significantly higher absolute and relative KE peak power and peak velocity than carriers of ≥ 1 R allele ($p < 0.05$). In males, change in absolute KE peak power post RT approached significance in RR homozygotes compared to XX carriers ($p = 0.07$). In females, change in relative KE peak power post RT was significantly higher in RR homozygotes compared to XX carriers ($p = 0.02$). At follow-up, male XX homozygotes had a significantly greater increase in 400 m walk time when compared to RX/RR carriers ($p = 0.03$).	Delmonico, et al., 2007. [37]
ACTN3	rs1815739	5-year follow-up	White North Americans 726 males and 641 females (Health ABC cohort) Aged 70–79 years Loss to follow-up (372)	1367	Muscle volume (thigh muscle CSA) Muscle strength (KE isokinetic torque) Physical function (400 m walk test, SPPB, self-reported functional limitation)	Female XX carriers had a 35% greater risk of functional limitation compared to RR homozygotes. No significant associations were noted between genotype and phenotypes at baseline in either males or females ($p > 0.05$).	Delmonico, et al., 2008. [38]
Structural and Metabolic Genes							
ACE	rs1799752 (I/D)	18-month intervention of exercise training (AE and RT)	Caucasians (75%), African-American (22%), Native American, Asian/Pacific Islander, Hispanic (3%)63 males and 150 femalesAged ≥ 65 yearsLoss to follow-up (37)	213	Muscle strength (concentric KE isokinetic strength) Physical function (6 min walk test, self-reported FAST)	Carriers of the DD genotype showed significantly greater improvements in concentric KE strength in response to exercise training than II homozygotes ($p < 0.05$). At baseline, no significant associations were noted between genotypes and measures of muscle strength and physical performance.	Giaccaglia, et al., 2008. [40]
ACTN3	rs1815739 (R577X)	Follow-up (NOSOS 1 year follow up, APOSS 2 year follow up)	Caucasian females (Scottish) NOSOS cohort ($n = 1245$) APOSS cohort ($n = 2918$) Mean age (NOSOS 69.6 ± 5.5 years and APOSS 54.8 ± 2.2 years)	4163	Fall incidences (self-reported for previous year)	In both NOSO and APOSS cohorts, baseline falls were significantly associated with carrying RX/XX genotypes ($p = 0.049$, 0.02 respectively). In a pooled analysis, follow-up fall incidences in the previous year were associated with X allele carriers ($p = 0.01$).	Judson, et al., 2011. [46]

Table 3. *Cont.*

Gene	Polymorphism	Study Design	Population Data	N	Muscle Phenotype	Results	Reference
Structural and Metabolic Genes							
ACE	rs1799752 (I/D)	Follow-up (4.1 year average)	Whites and Blacks 1439 males and 1527 females Aged 70–79 years	2966	Muscle volume (thigh muscle CSA) Muscle strength (maximal and mean isokinetic KE strength) Physical function (physical activity questionnaire, self-reported mobility limitations)	Among individuals with high levels of physical activity II homozygotes developed limitation at a 45% faster rate when compared to ID/DD carriers ($p = 0.01$). ACE genotype did not affect mobility limitation in inactive individuals, nor did it affect any other phenotype in either active or inactive individuals.	Kritchevsky, et al., 2005. [52]
ACTN3 ACE	rs1815739 (R577X) rs1799752	24-week intervention of RT	Brazilian females Mean age 66.7 ± 5.5 years	246	Body composition (FFM, relative total FFM, AFFM and SMI) Muscle strength (KE isokinetic peak torque at 60°s)	At baseline, ACE DD homozygotes had significantly greater SMI than I/ID carriers ($p = 0.044$). ACTN3 X allele carriers had significantly more relative total FFM at baseline than RR homozygotes ($p = 0.04$). In response to RT, only ACE II homozygotes significantly increased AFFM ($p < 0.001$).	Lima, et al., 2011. [54]
Structural and Metabolic Genes							
ACTN3 ACE	rs1815739 (R577X) rs1799752 (I/D)	12-week intervention of high-speed power training	Caucasian females Mean age 65.5 ± 8.2 years	139	Muscle strength (1RM bench press and leg extension and vertical jump) Physical function (sit-to-stand test)	Post intervention, ACE DD homozygotes showed significantly greater improvements in 1RM bench press and sit-to-stand tests ($p = 0.019, 0.013$ respectively) than II carriers. The same interaction approached significance for vertical jump ($p = 0.052$). ACTN3 RR homozygotes displayed significantly greater improvements across all measures than XX carriers ($p < 0.05$). At baseline, there were no significant differences between ACE or ACTN3 genotype for any phenotype.	Pereira, et al., 2013. [63]
ACTN3 ACE	rs1815739 rs1799752	12-week intervention of high-speed power training	Caucasian females Mean age 65.5 ± 8.2 years	139	Muscle function (10 m maximal effort sprints, TUG test)	ACE DD homozygotes displayed significantly greater improvements in 10 m sprint time ($p = 0.012$) than II carriers, but not in GUG performance ($p = 0.331$). Similarly, ACTN3 RR homozygotes improved significantly more than XX carriers in 10m sprint time ($p = 0.044$) but not in TUG performance ($p = 0.477$). At baseline, there were no significant differences between ACE or ACTN3 genotype for any phenotype.	Pereira, et al., 2013 [64]

Table 3. *Cont.*

Gene	Polymorphism	Study Design	Population Data	N	Muscle Phenotype	Results	Reference
			Structural and Metabolic Genes				
ACE/UCP2	rs1799752 (I/D) rs659366	12-week intervention of RT, balance and cardiovascular exercises	Caucasians 18 males and 40 females Aged > 60 years Mean age 70.0 ± 5.9 years (males) and 69.7 ± 5.3 years (females)	58	Muscle strength (HG strength) Physical function (30 s sit to stand, 30 s bicep curls, 8 ft TUG, 6 min walk, Purdue pegboard test)	At baseline, ACE II homozygotes performed significantly worse than ID/DD carriers in the 6 min walk and 8 ft TUG tests ($p = 0.008$, $p < 0.001$ respectively). GG carriers of rs659366 performed significantly worse in the 8 ft TUG test compared with AA/GA genotypes ($p = 0.045$). Post intervention, GG carriers of rs659366 had the greatest improvements in 8 ft TUG performance compared to AA/GA carriers ($p = 0.023$), while a trend for greater improvements in bicep strength was noted for ID/DD carriers compared to II carriers ($p = 0.099$).	Keogh, et al., 2015. [47]
APOE	rs7412 rs429358 (ε4 status)	6-year follow-up	Caucasians (Dutch) 553 males and 709 females Aged > 65 years Mean age 74.9 ± 5.8 years Loss to follow-up (449)	1262	Physical function (5 chair stand test, 3 m gait speed, self-reported mobility)	At baseline, ε4 carriers displayed significantly worse gait speed and chair stand performance ($p = 0.006$, 0.015 respectively) than the e3 group. At follow-up, ε4 status was associated with significantly worse chair stand performance ($p = 0.034$) compared to e3 carriers.	Melzer, et al., 2005. [60]
			Structural and Metabolic Genes				
APOE	rs7412 rs429358 (ε4 status)	4-year follow-up	Swedish 245 males and 364 females Aged 75 years Loss to follow-up (28)	609	Muscle strength (HG strength) Physical function (20 m maximum gait speed, 5 chair stand test, 30 s single leg stand)	Subjects who carried the APOE ε4 allele had a significantly larger decline in HG between age 75 and 79 compared to non-carriers ($p = 0.015$). Carriers of the APOE ε4 allele had significantly lower HG at age 79 compared to non-carriers ($p = 0.006$). The effect of ε4 allele on HG was significantly larger at age 79 than age 75 ($p = 0.033$).	Skoog, et al., 2016. [68]
APOE	rs7412 rs429358 (ε4 status)	Follow-up (3-year average)	North Americans (67.8% White and Blacks 27.1%) 235 males and 392 females Mean age 79.4 ± 5.2 years	627	Physical function (15 ft and 20 ft gait speed, disability scale examining ability to perform ADL's)	Males carrying the ε4 allele showed a significantly more rapid decline in gait speed than male non-carriers ($p = 0.04$). This was most significant in white males only ($p = 0.007$). Similarly, males who carried the ε4 allele had a significantly greater risk of disability than non-carriers ($p = 0.007$).	Verghese, et al., 2013. [71]

Table 3. *Cont.*

Gene	Polymorphism	Study Design	Population Data	N	Muscle Phenotype	Results	Reference
			Structural and Metabolic Genes				
ZNF295 C2CD2	rs928874 rs1788355	GWAS 2-year follow-up	Italians ilSIRENTE cohort (*n* = 286) 116 males and 170 females Mean age 86.1 ± 4.9 years Replication cohort inCHIANTI (*n* = 1055) 440 males and 615 females Mean age 67.8 ± 15.7 years	1341	Body composition (calf circumference, mid-arm muscle circumference) Muscle strength (HG strength) Physical function (4 m walk test, SPPB, ADL)	In the ilSIRENTE cohort, rs928874 and rs1788355 were significantly associated with 4 m gait speed ($p = 5.61 \times 10^{-8}$, 5.73×10^{-8} respectively). This association was not replicated in the inCHIANTI cohort.	Heckerman, et al., 2017. [44]

KE: knee extensor, HG: handgrip, FFM: fat-free mass, AFFM: appendicular fat-free mass, SMI: skeletal muscle index, RT: resistance training, AE: aerobic exercise, CT: computed tomography, CSA: cross sectional area, 1RM: 1 repetition maximum, PA: physical activity, TUG: timed up and go, ADL: activity of daily living, SPPB: short physical performance battery.

A total of 38,112 subjects participated across the 54 studies. Of these, 24,890 (65.3%) were female and 13,222 (34.7%) were male. Thirty-two studies included Caucasians, 13 assessed Asian subjects and the remaining nine studies included Hispanic and African-American participants. As described in the inclusion criteria, all subjects were older than 50 years of age. Thirteen studies included subjects over 50 years of age, 22 studies recruited subjects over 60 years of age and 19 studies included individuals aged 70 years or older.

3.4. Phenotypes and Genotypes

Of the included studies, 26 reported skeletal muscle mass outcomes, 39 studies included muscle strength testing, 27 articles analysed physical function and six examined sarcopenia prevalence. A full description of the phenotypic outcomes in each study are presented in Tables 2 and 3.

In total, 88 DNA polymorphisms in or near to 26 different genes were analysed across the 54 studies included in this review. The Alpha-actinin 3 (*ACTN3*), Angiotensin Converting Enzyme (*ACE*), and Vitamin D Receptor (*VDR*) genes were the most frequently researched, present in 14, 13 and nine articles, respectively. For clarity and ease of interpretation in the present review, genes are categorised into three main groups: hormone genes, growth factor and cytokine genes and structural and metabolic genes.

3.5. Synthesis of Results

3.5.1. Hormone Genes

VDR

Nine studies analysed the association between *VDR* polymorphisms and muscle phenotypes. The first, conducted in 2004 by Roth et al. [67], highlighted a significant association between the rs2228570 (*Fok1*) polymorphism and FFM. Male FF homozygotes had significantly less FFM, appendicular fat-free mass (AFFM) and skeletal muscle index (SMI) compared to f allele carriers ($p = 0.002$, $p = 0.009$, $p = 0.001$ respectively). Furthermore, when classified as sarcopenic, FF carriers were at a two-fold higher risk of being sarcopenic when compared to carriers of the f allele ($p = 0.03$). Hopkinson et al. [45] also found significant interactions between the rs2228570 polymorphism and muscle phenotypes with male FF homozygotes displaying significantly lower knee extensor (KE) strength than f allele carriers ($p = 0.007$). Similarly, Xia et al. [74] found subjects carrying one or more F alleles to have significantly lower handgrip (HG) strength, and FFM ($p = 0.03$, $p = 0.04$ respectively). Furthermore, these individuals had a significantly higher risk of sarcopenia than ff homozygotes ($p = 0.03$). In contrast, a study conducted by Gussago et al. [42] found FF homozygotes to have significantly greater HG strength than f allele carriers ($p = 0.021$).

Significant associations were also identified between the rs1544410 (*Bsm1*) polymorphism and muscle performance phenotypes although, in keeping with the above findings, results were conflicting. In a study conducted by Onder et al. [62], bb homozygotes were significantly less likely to fall than carriers of the B allele ($p = 0.02$). Similarly, in 2010, Barr et al. [27] found females who were homozygous for the b allele to have a significantly lower risk of falling than Bb/BB carriers. These individuals also performed significantly better in the rise from chair and power tests when compared to carriers of B allele ($p = 0.03$, $p = 0.044$ respectively). Contrarily to the above studies, Bahat et al. [26] found KE strength to be significantly higher in BB homozygotes compared to carriers of one or more b alleles ($p = 0.038$).

Additional *VDR* polymorphisms rs7136534 and rs7975232 (*Apa1*) were significantly associated with fall incidence and HG strength respectively ($p = 0.002$, $p < 0.05$) [28,73]. No significant associations were found for the rs731236 (*Taq1*) polymorphism.

Other Genes

Genes encoding the androgen receptor (*AR*), thyrotropin-releasing hormone receptor (*TRHR*) and receptor activity-modifying protein 3 (*RAMP3*) were also shown to associate significantly with skeletal muscle traits (Tables 2 and 3) [57,66,72].

3.5.2. Growth Factor and Cytokine Genes

IGF1 and *IGFBP3*

The interaction between the Insulin-like Growth Factor 1 (*IGF1*) gene and muscle phenotypes was particularly evident in the intervention studies (Table 3). Both Kostek et al. [50] and Hand et al. [43] demonstrated that carriers of one or more 192 alleles achieved significantly greater KE strength improvements in response to resistance training (RT), compared to non-carriers ($p = 0.02$, $p < 0.01$). However, in a cross-sectional study conducted by Mora et al. [61], no significant differences were observed in muscle strength between carriers and non-carriers of the 192 allele ($p = 0.024$).

Significant associations were also noted for polymorphisms rs35767 of the *IGF1* gene and rs2854744 of the Insulin-like Growth Factor Binding Protein 3 (*IGFBP3*) gene. Kostek et al. [51] observed black females carrying the CC genotype of the rs35767 polymorphism to have significantly less total FFM and muscle cross sectional area (CSA) than TT carriers (both $p < 0.05$). Furthermore, male CC homozygotes performed significantly worse in the single leg chair stand test than carriers of the T allele ($p < 0.05$). In a study conducted by Yang et al. [75], CC carriers of the rs2854744 polymorphism had a 4.3 times higher risk of having low SMI compared to AA carriers ($p < 0.05$).

CNTF and *CNTFR*

Two studies examined the Ciliary Neurotrophic Factor (*CNTF*) and Ciliary Neurotrophic Factor Receptor (*CNTFR*) genes (Table 2). In 2006, Arking et al. [25] observed five DNA polymorphisms (rs948562, rs1800169, rs550942, rs4319530, rs1938596) of the *CNTF* gene to be significantly associated with HG strength ($p < 0.05$). Further haplotype analysis revealed the null allele (A) of rs1800169 to fully explain this relationship under a recessive model. Individuals homozygous for the A allele had 3.8 kg lower HG strength than G allele carriers ($p < 0.01$). Interestingly, De Mars et al. [36] found only G/A carriers of the rs1800169 polymorphism to have significantly lower KE strength than G/G or A/A carriers ($p = 0.0229$). Additionally, male T allele carriers of the rs3808871 polymorphism produced significantly higher KE and knee flexor (KF) isometric torque at 120° when compared to CC homozygotes ($p < 0.05$). Furthermore, females who carried the T allele of the rs2070802 polymorphism produced greater KF concentric torques than the A/A homozygotes ($p = 0.04$).

TNFα

Three studies were included in this review which investigated the Tumour Necrosis Factor Alpha (*TNFα*) gene, each with significant findings. In 2013, Pereira et al. [65] observed that G allele homozygotes of the rs1800629 polymorphism achieved significantly faster timed up and go (TUG) test results in response to 10 weeks of RT compared to A allele carriers ($p < 0.001$). Additionally, Tiainen et al. [69] found the A allele of the rs361525 polymorphism to be associated with a significantly better physical performance level compared to GG homozygotes ($p < 0.001$). Finally, Li et al. [53] highlighted the interaction between the A allele of the rs1799964 polymorphism with either the G allele of the Tumour Necrosis Factor Beta (*TNF-β*) rs909253 polymorphism or the A allele of the *TNF-β* rs1041981 polymorphism to result in significantly lower handgrip strength among females ($p = 0.005$, $p = 0.006$ respectively).

Other Genes

Polymorphisms rs2276541 of the activin A type IIB receptor (*ACVR2B*) gene, rs3807987 of Caveolin 1 (*CAV1*) gene and rs1805086 of the Myostatin (*MSTN*) gene were all significantly associated with FFM (Table 2) [41,49,56].

3.5.3. Structural and Metabolic Genes

ACTN3 (The Sprint Gene)

In this review, fourteen studies were included which examined the association between the *ACTN3* rs1815739 (*R577X*) polymorphism and skeletal muscle phenotypes. Carrying the X allele was often associated with lower baseline muscle strength and function (Table 2). For example, in a study conducted by Kikuchi et al. [48], homozygosity for the X allele was associated with significantly poorer performance in the chair stand test compared to RR carriers ($p = 0.024$). Ma et al. [58] also found XX homozygotes to perform significantly worse in HG strength ($p = 0.012$), 5 m walk ($p = 0.011$) and TUG ($p = 0.039$) tests and to also have a significantly higher frailty index ($p = 0.004$). Similar results were observed by Judson et al. [46] in a group of 4163 females where RX and XX genotypes were significantly associated with fall incidence ($p = 0.049$, $p = 0.02$ respectively). In contrast, Delmonico et al. [37] found female XX homozygotes to have significantly higher absolute and relative KE peak power and peak velocity than carriers of the R allele ($p < 0.05$).

Individuals carrying the XX genotype were also shown to have significantly lower improvements in one repetition maximum (1RM) bench press and leg extension, vertical jump and sit-to-stand performance in response to speed and power training when compared to RR carriers (all $p < 0.05$) [63]. Pereira et al. [64] also demonstrated XX carriers to have significantly poorer improvements in 10 m sprint times in response to high speed and power training compared to RR homozygotes ($p = 0.044$). Similarly, female XX carriers were observed to have significantly lower improvements in relative KE peak power following RT compared to RR homozygotes ($p = 0.02$) [37]. In the male population, change in absolute KE peak power post RT approached significance when comparing RR and XX genotypes ($p = 0.07$) [37]. In contrast to the above studies, Delmonico et al. [38] found male XX homozygotes had a significantly greater increase in 400 m walk time when compared to RX/RR carriers ($p = 0.03$).

In a study conducted by Zempo et al. [77] XX homozygotes were observed to have significantly lower thigh muscle CSA compared to RR carriers ($p = 0.04$). Interestingly, in a secondary analysis comparing a middle age group with an old age group, XX homozygosity was only associated with low thigh muscle CSA in the old age group ($p < 0.05$), suggesting that the influence of ACTN3 deficiency is heightened with age [78]. Similar results were noted in 2017 by Cho et al. [32], where sarcopenia prevalence was significantly associated with the XX genotype ($p = 0.038$). In contrast, Lima et al. [54] found X allele carriers to have significantly more relative total FFM than RR homozygotes ($p = 0.04$).

Three studies found no significant differences in muscle phenotypes between *ACTN3* rs1815739 genotypes [30,39,59].

ACE

The relationship between the *ACE* rs1799752 (insertion/deletion) polymorphism and skeletal muscle traits has been extensively investigated since the original study of Montgomery et al. in 1998 [79]. Thirteen articles are included in this review. Firstly, Charbonneau et al. [31] found that carriers of the DD genotype had significantly greater total FFM ($p < 0.05$) and lower limb muscle volume ($p = 0.01$) than II homozygotes. Similarly, in a study of 246 Brazilian females, Lima et al. [54] noted DD homozygotes to have a significantly greater SMI than I allele carriers ($p = 0.044$). These findings were further strengthened by Da Silva et al. [34], who demonstrated sarcopenia prevalence to be significantly higher in II genotype carriers compared to D allele carriers ($p = 0.015$) (Table 2). Interestingly, Lima et al. [54] showed that in response to RT, only *ACE* II homozygotes significantly increased AFFM ($p < 0.001$).

The II genotype was also associated with lower muscle strength and functional performance. For example, within a group of 431 Japanese individuals, Yoshihara et al. [76] found II homozygosity to be associated with significantly lower HG strength compared to D allele carriers ($p = 0.004$). Homozygosity for the I allele was also shown to associate with significantly poorer performance in the 6-min walking test and 8 ft TUG test ($p = 0.008$, $p < 0.001$ respectively) when compared to ID/DD genotypes. Furthermore, in response to RT, DD carriers achieved significantly greater improvements in 1RM bench press and sit-to-stand performance ($p = 0.019$, $p = 0.013$ respectively) [63]. Giaccaglia et al. [40] also found that DD genotype carriers achieved significantly greater improvements in concentric KE strength in response to RT compared to II homozygotes ($p < 0.05$). Similarly, Pereira et al. [64] observed that DD homozygotes became significantly quicker performing 10 m sprints ($p = 0.012$) compared to II carriers. Buford et al. [29] also reported that a 12-month exercise intervention evoked significant improvements in 400 m walking speed ($p = 0.018$) and short physical performance battery test (SPPB) scores ($p = 0.015$), but only in D allele carriers. Interestingly, II homozygosity was also significantly associated with developing mobility limitation at a 45% faster rate when compared to ID/DD carriers ($p = 0.01$) [52].

As with the *ACTN3* rs1815739 genotypes, three studies found rs1799752 genotypes to have no significant influence on skeletal muscle traits [30,39,59].

APOE

Three studies demonstrated significant associations between the Apolipoprotein E (*APOE*) gene and muscle phenotypes (Table 3). A 6-year follow-up study conducted by Melzer et al. [60] found that e4 carriers displayed significantly slower gait speed and chair stand performance ($p = 0.006$, $p = 0.015$ respectively) at baseline and significantly slower chair stand performance ($p = 0.034$) at the end of the 6-year follow-up, compared to e3 carriers. The *APOE* e4 allele was also shown to be associated with a significantly larger decline in HG strength between the ages of 75 and 79 over a 4-year period, compared to non-carriers ($p = 0.015$) [68]. Furthermore, carriers of the e4 allele had significantly lower HG strength at age 79 compared to non-carriers ($p = 0.006$). Interestingly, the effect of the e4 allele on HG strength was significantly larger at age 79 than age 75 ($p = 0.033$), suggesting that the e4 allele becomes increasingly influential with age. In a 3-year follow-up study conducted by Verghese et al. [71], males carrying the e4 allele showed a significantly more rapid decline in gait speed and greater risk of disability than male non-carriers ($p = 0.04$, $p = 0.007$ respectively).

UCP2 and *UCP3*

Three studies reported significant interactions between Uncoupling Proteins 2/3 (*UCP2/3*) polymorphisms and skeletal muscle traits. Firstly, in a group of 432 Caucasians, Crocco et al. [33] found carriers of the CC genotype of the *UCP3* rs1800849 polymorphism to exhibit significantly lower HG strength than carriers of the T allele ($p = 0.010$). Dato et al. [35], then showed that individuals carrying the AA genotype of *UCP3* rs11235972 polymorphism have significantly lower HG strength than GG homozygotes ($p < 0.001$). In 2015, Keogh et al. [47] demonstrated that GG carriers of *UCP2* rs659366 polymorphism perform significantly worse in the 8 ft TUG test compared with AA/GA genotypes ($p = 0.045$). However, post RT intervention, GG homozygotes of *UCP2* rs659366 had the greatest improvements in 8 ft TUG performance ($p = 0.023$).

Genome-wide Studies

Other genes that demonstrated significant associations with muscle phenotypes included the PR domain containing 16 (*PRDM16*) gene, Zinc finger protein 295 (*ZNF295*) gene and C2 calcium dependent domain containing 2 (*C2CD2*) gene (Tables 2 and 3) [44,70].

Moreover, a recent GWAS by Hernandez-Cordero et al. [80] evaluated genetic contribution to ALM in the UK Biobank dataset, comparing middle-aged (38–49 years) and elderly (60–74 years) individuals. A total of 182 genome-wide significant regions, many with multiple variants within them, were associated with ALM in middle-aged individuals. Of these, 78% were also associated with ALM in elderly individuals. Variants at three genes, *VCAM*, *ADAMTSL3* and *FTO*, had previously been associated with lean body mass in the UK Biobank [81]. Hernandez Cortez et al. also confirmed, in vitro, a functional role for *CPNE1* and *STC2* in myogenesis. In addition, the study highlighted five genomic regions, containing multiple genes, that are associated with muscle mass in both mice and humans.

4. Discussion

To the best of the authors' knowledge, this is the first systematic review to collate literature on genetic associations with muscle phenotypes relevant to sarcopenia. To date, most research targeting genetic associations with muscle phenotypes has not focused on elderly subjects, and thus, the genetic mechanisms underpinning the age-related changes in skeletal muscle traits are largely uncharted.

Given that the deterioration of skeletal muscle with advancing age can have profound consequences for patients and public health systems, improving our understanding of how genes influence this process is of paramount importance. This review has enhanced our knowledge surrounding the key genes and gene variants that may prove crucial in further developing our understanding of the pathogenesis of sarcopenia and improving prognosis and treatment interventions alike.

4.1. Summary of Findings

The systematic literature search identified 24 genes and 46 DNA polymorphisms whose expression was significantly associated with muscle phenotypes in older adults. Ten of these DNA polymorphisms (rs154410, rs2228570, rs1800169, rs3093059, rs1800629, rs1815739, rs1799752, rs7412, rs429358 and 192 bp allele) were significantly associated with muscle phenotypes in two or more studies. The complex and multifactorial mechanisms underpinning muscle regulation suggest that the accrual and loss of muscle mass and muscle strength is not reducible to one single gene or gene variant. The dynamic interactions between inhibitory and promotory pathways within the human body further highlight the importance of a holistic approach when considering genetic associations with skeletal muscle traits.

Nevertheless, the findings of this systematic review demonstrate that the most compelling current evidence in the field exists for the *ACTN3*, *ACE* and *VDR* genotypes.

4.1.1. ACTN3 (The Sprint Gene)

The *ACTN3* gene is among the most extensively researched genes in relation to muscle phenotypes, and appeared most frequently within this review. The ACTN3 protein encoded by the *ACTN3* gene forms an integral part of the sarcomere Z-line in fast twitch muscle fibres and further aids in coordinating myofiber contractions [82,83]. Up to 20% of humans are deficient in this protein, due to homozygosity for the premature stop codon at the rs1815739 polymorphism [84]. This significant proportion of ACTN3 deficiency among the population suggests that X allele status is a key factor in variability in muscle phenotypes. In this regard, much of the research surrounding the *ACTN3* genotype has focused on athletic performance [85]. Association studies have repeatedly found reduced X allele frequency among elite sprint/power athletes [85–87]. This suggests that the presence of ACTN3 is crucial for the optimal generation of force. Considering that fast twitch muscle fibres are particularly susceptible to age-related atrophy [88], it is plausible that regulation of this protein may also be an important factor in understanding age-related changes in muscle phenotypes. To date, however, limited research has been conducted within elderly populations, with the result that the true impact of the *ACTN3* gene on age-related changes in muscle phenotypes remains inconclusive. Despite this, fourteen of the studies included in this review examining the *ACTN3* genotype reported promising findings. Carriers of the X allele were often found to display lower skeletal muscle mass, strength and functional abilities. This was particularly evident among the Asian population. All five cross-sectional studies that examined Asian participants found significant associations between X allele status and muscle phenotypes [32,48,58,77]. No such association was found in the other three cross-sectional studies that targeted Caucasian individuals [30,39,59], therefore suggesting ethnicity may determine the degree to which *ACTN3* genotypes effect aging muscle. This coincides with existing research whereby X allele frequency and fast twitch fibre composition have been shown to vary across different ethnic groups [89–92]. The Asian population have the highest frequency of the X allele [89], while having the lowest percentage of fast twitch muscle fibres [90–92], two likely contributing factors in the ethnic group having the highest sarcopenia prevalence globally [93]. Unlike above, X allele status was significantly associated with training adaptation within Caucasian, North-American and South-American individuals. Thus, the inconsistencies within this review highlight the need for future research to provide clarification on how ethnicity, *ACTN3* genotypes and muscle phenotypes are associated within the elderly.

4.1.2. ACE

Like the *ACTN3* gene, the *ACE* gene has been widely researched within athletic populations, and knowledge within older populations is limited. There are, however, compelling molecular pathways controlled by the *ACE* gene that suggest its importance in age-related changes in muscle phenotypes. The ACE is expressed by skeletal muscle endothelial cells, and catalyses the production of angiotensin II, known to enhance skeletal muscle hypertrophy [94,95]. To date, research in relation to muscle phenotypes has centred around the *ACE* rs1799752 polymorphism. The D and I alleles have been associated with higher and lower ACE activity respectively [96–98]. The D allele is suggested, therefore, to associate with greater muscle performance. To support this hypothesis, recent studies have focused on the rs1799752 polymorphism in elite athletes, with interesting findings. The I allele has been repeatedly associated with endurance performance, while the D allele associates with strength/power capabilities [99,100]. Findings from this systematic review further strengthen these observations. The D allele was consistently associated with higher baseline muscle strength and functional performance, as well as greater improvements in muscle strength and function in response to RT. Evidence of the association between the *ACE* rs1799752 polymorphism and muscle mass is less definitive. While the D allele was often associated with greater amounts of FFM, contradictory findings were also in evidence, and thus, further research is needed in this area to reach a consensus. Like with *ACTN3* genotypes, frequency of the I and D allele of the *ACE* gene are highly determined by ethnic background. Asians have been shown to have the highest frequency for the undesirable I allele [101], while African-American have the lowest [101], aligning with global sarcopenia prevalence estimates where Asians and African-Americans have the highest and lowest risk respectively [93]. While evidence in this review is insufficient in highlighting a true ethnic impact on the association between *ACE* genotypes and aging muscle phenotypes, the disparity in allele frequency among different ethnicities is promising.

4.1.3. VDR

The true significance of the association between the *VDR* gene and muscle phenotypes is currently unknown. While the *VDR* gene has been extensively researched, findings are often contradictory. Furthermore, due to its crucial role in regulating calcium absorption, much of the existing research has focused on the association between *VDR* genotypes and bone health [102]. However, the *VDR* gene is also known to stimulate changes in muscle protein synthesis through its key regulatory role in the transcription of messenger RNA [103], and thus, the potential of the *VDR* gene as a candidate gene for muscle phenotype associations has been suggested. More specifically, the rs2228570 polymorphism is the only known VDR polymorphism where variation results in structural changes within the VDR protein due to differences in translational initiation sites [104]. The *VDR* f allele results in a full length VDR protein of 427 amino acids [105], while a *VDR* F allele results in a truncated VDR protein with three amino acids less [106]. Interestingly, three of four studies that examined the rs2228570 polymorphism in this review found F allele carriers to perform significantly worse across a range of muscle phenotypes [45,67,74], suggesting the potential importance of the rs2228570 polymorphism.

While compelling evidence exists supporting the importance of the *VDR* gene for muscle phenotypes, many studies have failed to replicate earlier results, and thus, the strength of this association remains to be established [107,108]. Unlike for *ACTN3* and *ACE* polymorphisms, evidence of an ethnic influence on *VDR* polymorphism frequency is conflicting [109,110]. As with most genetic association studies, much of the research surrounding *VDR* polymorphisms and muscle phenotypes has been conducted using Caucasian subjects. Only nine articles examining *VDR* genotypes were included in this review, seven of which focused on Caucasian individuals [26–28,42,45,62,67]. Furthermore, as with the *ACTN3* and *ACE* genes, limited research has been conducted within an elderly population, further limiting the transferability of findings for older adults.

4.1.4. Other Genes of Interest

Other genes with convincing molecular pathways and findings, that warrant future investigation include the *IGF1/IGFBP3*, *TNFα*, *APOE*, *CNTF/R* and *UCP2/3* genes.

4.1.5. IGF1 and IGFBP3

The *IGF* family of genes encode peptides that are crucial in regulating cell proliferation, apoptosis and differentiation [111]. The mitogenic effect of IGF1 is integral to the facilitation of growth in multiple tissues, including skeletal muscle [112]. Considering that advancing age is associated with a decline in circulating IGF1 levels, the *IGF1* gene is a likely candidate to effect muscle phenotypes among the elderly [113]. The current review found significant associations between *IGF1* variants and skeletal muscle mass and strength. Associations were particularly convincing in longitudinal studies, suggesting that the *IGF1* 192 polymorphism may be particularly influential in the strength-training response of skeletal muscle phenotypes as opposed to baseline measurements.

The function of IGF1 is mediated through interactions with binding proteins, mainly, IGFBP3. Research has demonstrated that IGFBP3 is the most prolific potentiator of IGF1, therefore suggesting its importance in explaining inter-individual variation in muscle phenotypes [114]. While only Yang et al. [75] have investigated the impact of the *IGFBP3* gene in an elderly population, the significant findings of that study combined with the relevant gene mechanisms warrants future research.

4.1.6. TNFα

Like the *IGF* family, the *TNFα* gene aids in the regulation of a multitude of biological processes such as cell proliferation, differentiation and apoptosis, and is thus an important candidate gene for aging skeletal muscle [115]. TNFα is also known to be an integral mediator of the inflammatory response to muscle damage [116]. Considering that inflammation is a vital response to RT in facilitating muscle regeneration, the *TNFα* gene is likely to affect the response of skeletal muscle tissue to RT [117]. This is supported by the findings of Pereira et al. [65] who observed that *TNFα* genotypes associate significantly with TUG performance adaptation. While Tiainen et al. [69] also highlighted significant cross-sectional associations, these were based on self-reported measures and should be interpreted with caution. Thus, longitudinal studies focusing on RT response of skeletal muscle may prove most beneficial in understanding the effect of *TNFα* genotypes on the aging muscle.

4.1.7. APOE

APOE protein encoded by the *APOE* gene, is involved in lipid metabolism and is a well-established risk factor for Alzheimer's disease and various other aging disorders such as cardiovascular disease, atherosclerosis, stroke and impaired cognitive function [118]. Considering the associations between muscle phenotypes such as HG strength and these disorders, research has begun to investigate the relationship between the *APOE* gene and skeletal muscle traits. The gene has three common alleles (e2, e3 and e4), with e2 and e4 carriers having the lowest and highest risk of developing such aging disorders respectively [119]. As a result, much of the research in relation to skeletal muscle has centred around the e4 allele. The e4 allele was consistently associated with unfavourable skeletal muscle traits within this review, and therefore, supports the possibility of *APOE* as a candidate gene for explaining variation in muscle phenotypes with advancing age. Interestingly, like for *ACTN3* and *ACE* genotypes, prevalence of the e4 allele is known to be highly varied among different populations [120]. With only three studies were included in this review, the effect of ethnicity on e4 allele frequency and the resulting association with muscle phenotypes is yet to be confirmed.

4.1.8. CNTF and CNTFR

The *CNTF* and *CNTFR* genes are both mediated through a common signal-transducing component, and thus are often examined in parallel [121]. CNTF, located in glial cells, aids in the promotion of motor neuron survival, and is therefore suggested to limit age-related atrophy of skeletal muscle caused by denervation [122]. The CNTFR is largely expressed in skeletal muscle, promoting research to examine the role of the *CNTF* and *CNTFR* genes in the regulation of muscle phenotypes [123]. To date, however, much of this research has been conducted using rats, with limited research being conducted with human populations. Thus, while the current review has highlighted some significant associations with muscle phenotypes, additional research is required to further understand the mechanisms underpinning this association in humans.

4.1.9. UCP2 and UCP3

Uncoupling proteins (UCPs) are mitochondrial transporters, best known for their involvement in thermogenesis and energy utilisation. As a result, UCPs are most commonly researched in relation to obesity-related phenotypes [124,125]. There is, however, evidence that suggests their importance in regulating muscle phenotypes. UCP2 and UCP3 have both been shown to effect skeletal muscle performance through the inhibition of mitochondrial ATP synthesis [126]. Additionally, *UCP2* and *UCP3* genes serve a key purpose in the protection of cells by attenuating mitochondrial reactive oxygen species (ROS) production, known to exert damaging effects on cells [127]. While loss of skeletal muscle mitochondrial content is known to occur with advancing age [128], evidence suggests UCPs are particularly active in the latter stages of life due to an increase in ROS and the associated rise in mitochondrial superoxide [129]. Therefore, *UCP2* and *UCP3* genes may affect how metabolic function of skeletal muscle is retained during the aging process. While the three studies included in this review found significant associations between *UCP2* and *UCP3* variants and muscle phenotypes, other data from human studies are scarce and as a result, the strength of this association remains to be elucidated.

4.2. Strengths and Limitations

This is the first systematic literature review to explore the genetic association with muscle phenotypes among the elderly. Only healthy subjects were included in the review, allowing for any association to be solely attributed to genotype-phenotype interactions rather than disease. All subjects were over the age of 50 years, ensuring relevance towards developing the understanding of the pathogenesis of sarcopenia. While some methodological weaknesses exist, most studies were well designed and conducted.

Findings within this review were at times conflicting. This incongruity may be partly explained by between-study disparities in methodological aspects such as sample size, subject characteristics and false-positive reporting. Furthermore, not all studies utilised the same measure for each muscle phenotype. For example, muscle strength measured through handgrip or leg extension may lead to different results. Evidently, there is a need for genetic association studies to implement more comprehensive and stringent methodology to maximise the potential of identifying genetic variants relevant to aging muscle phenotypes.

Finally, while not necessarily a limitation of this review itself, the overall lack of research currently available regarding the association between genetic variants and muscle phenotypes within the elderly prevents more definitive inferences to be made. As evidenced in this review, most research to date has focused on European populations, thus limiting the transferability of findings to other ethnic groups. Considering the promising ethnic differences in polymorphism frequency previously highlighted, future genetic studies may benefit from including individuals from a variety of ethnic backgrounds. The distinct lack of GWAS targeting aging muscle phenotypes is also contributive towards the uncertainty surrounding this area. A large body of research has utilised a candidate gene approach. Historically, many candidate gene studies have been statistically underpowered, the replication of findings has been problematic and there has been a suspected bias against publication of negative results, which may lead to conflicting findings [130]. Many of these issues have been overcome by GWAS in large, well characterised cohorts [80,131–133]. Therefore, future GWAS may help to further illuminate the genetic basis of aging muscle phenotypes.

5. Conclusions

The ability to maintain skeletal muscle mass, strength and function with advancing age is essential in preventing sarcopenia. Thus, the elucidation of the genetic variants associated with these phenotypes is of paramount importance. Evidently, skeletal muscle mass, strength and function are multifaceted characteristics that vary widely among the elderly. While heritability studies have highlighted that significant proportions of this inter-individual variability are determined by genetic factors, the specific genes involved remain mostly unknown.

The genetic association with muscle phenotypes is relatively under-researched, with only a limited number of candidate genes being explored to date. This review identified and systematically compiled the key genes shown to be significantly associated with muscle phenotypes within an elderly population. While relatively few genes have been identified which significantly contribute towards variation in muscle phenotypes, promising findings pointing to more extensive associations exist. Evidence is particularly supportive of the *ACTN3*, *ACE* and *VDR* genes, while the *IGF1/IGFBP3*, *TNFα*, *APOE*, *CNTF/R* and *UCP2/3* genes have also been shown to be significantly associated with skeletal muscle phenotypes in two or more studies.

To conclude, the findings from this review helped to further illuminate the genetic basis of sarcopenia. While the molecular genetic pathways are often compelling, the limited volume of research within this field is as yet insufficient to demonstrate a clear genetic basis for sarcopenia. Future GWAS could facilitate the identification of novel genetic variants that may have key regulatory roles in aging muscle phenotypes. Further still, a more extensive exploration of the candidate genes highlighted in this review should provide further insight into the pathogenesis of sarcopenia and further aid in the development of effective prognosis, preventive and treatment protocols to combat the profound consequences of sarcopenia for patients and health systems worldwide.

Author Contributions: Conceptualization, J.P.; Literature search and validation, J.P., G.D.V. and C.B.; Analysis, J.P.; Writing—original draft preparation, J.P.; Writing—review and editing, J.P., G.D.V., C.B., S.E. and A.W.R. All authors have read and agreed to the published version of the manuscript.

References

1.   Rosenburg, I.H. Sarcopenia: Origins and clinical relevance. *J. Nutr.* **1997**, *127*, 990S–S991S. [CrossRef] [PubMed]

2.   Cruz-Jentoft, A.J.; Bahat, G.; Bauer, J.; Boirie, Y.; Bruyère, O.; Cederholm, T.; Cooper, C.; Landi, F.; Rolland, Y.; Sayer, A.A.; et al. Sarcopenia: Revised European consensus on definition and diagnosis. *Age Ageing* **2019**, *48*, 16–31. [CrossRef] [PubMed]

3.   Chin, S.O.; Rhee, S.Y.; Chon, S.; Hwang, Y.C.; Jeong, I.K.; Oh, S.; Ahn, K.J.; Chung, H.Y.; Woo, J.T.; Kim, S.W.; et al. Sarcopenia Is independently associated with cardiovascular disease in older Korean adults: The Korea national health and nutrition examination survey (KNHANES) from 2009. *PLoS ONE* **2013**, *8*, e60119. [CrossRef] [PubMed]

4.   Janssen, I.; Heymsfield, S.B.; Ross, R. Low relative skeletal muscle mass (sarcopenia) in older persons is associated with functional impairment and physical disability. *J. Am. Geriatr. Soc.* **2002**, *50*, 889–896. [CrossRef] [PubMed]

5.   Landi, F.; Liperoti, R.; Russo, A.; Giovannini, S.; Tosato, M.; Capoluongo, E. Sarcopenia as a risk factor for falls in elderly individuals: Results from the ilSIRENTE study. *Clin. Nutr.* **2012**, *31*, 652–658. [CrossRef] [PubMed]
6.   Zhang, X.; Zhang, W.; Wang, C.; Tao, W.; Dou, Q.; Yang, Y. Sarcopenia as a predictor of hospitalization among older people: A systematic review and meta-analysis. *BMC Geriatr.* **2018**, *18*, 188. [CrossRef]
7.   Kim, T.N.; Choi, K.M. The implications of sarcopenia and sarcopenic obesity on cardiometabolic disease. *J. Cell Biochem.* **2015**, *116*, 1171–1178. [CrossRef]
8.   Brown, J.C.; Harhay, M.O.; Harhay, M.N. Sarcopenia and mortality among a population based sample of community-dwelling older adults. *J. Cachexia Sarcopenia Muscle* **2016**, *7*, 290–298. [CrossRef]
9.   Shafiee, G.; Keshtkar, A.; Soltani, A.; Ahadi, Z.; Larijani, B.; Heshmat, R. Prevalence of sarcopenia in the world: A systematic review and meta- analysis of general population studies. *J. Diabetes Metab. Disord.* **2017**, *16*, 16–21. [CrossRef]
10. Melton, L.J.; Khosla, S.; Crowson, C.S.; O'Connor, M.K.; O'Fallon, W.M.; Riggs, B.L. Epidemiology of sarcopenia. *J. Am. Geriatr. Soc.* **2000**, *48*, 625–630. [CrossRef]
11. Ethgen, O.; Beaudart, C.; Buckinx, F.; Bruyère, O.; Reginster, J.Y. The future prevalence of sarcopenia in Europe: A claim for public health action. *Calcif. Tissue Int.* **2017**, *100*, 229–234. [CrossRef] [PubMed]
12. Keller, K.; Engelhardt, M. Strength and muscle mass loss with aging process. Age and strength loss. *Muscles Ligaments Tendons J.* **2014**, *3*, 346–350. [CrossRef] [PubMed]
13. Deschenes, M.R. Effects of aging on muscle fibre type and size. *Sports Med.* **2004**, *34*, 809–824. [CrossRef] [PubMed]
14. Doherty, T.J. The influence of aging and sex on skeletal muscle mass and strength. *Curr. Opin. Clin. Nutr. Metab. Care* **2001**, *4*, 503–508. [CrossRef]
15. Prior, S.J.; Roth, S.M.; Wang, X.; Kammerer, C.; Miljkovic-Gacic, I.; Bunker, C.H.; Wheeler, V.W.; Patrick, A.L.; Zmuda, J.M. Genetic and environmental influences on skeletal muscle phenotypes as a function of age and sex in large, multigenerational families of African heritage. *J. Appl. Physiol.* **2007**, *103*, 1121–1127. [CrossRef]
16. Kemp, G.J.; Birrell, F.; Clegg, P.D.; Cuthbertson, D.J.; De Vito, G.; Van Dieën, J.H.; Del Din, S.; Eastell, R.; Garnero, P.; Goljanek–Whysall, K.; et al. Developing a toolkit for the assessment and monitoring of musculoskeletal ageing. *Age Ageing* **2018**, *47*, 1–19. [CrossRef]
17. Franzke, B.; Neubauer, O.; Cameron-Smith, D.; Wagner, K.H. Dietary protein, muscle and physical function in the very old. *Nutrients* **2018**, *10*, 935. [CrossRef]
18. Buchmann, N.; Spira, D.; Norman, K.; Demuth, I.; Eckardt, R.; Steinhagen-Thiessen, E. Sleep, muscle mass and muscle function in older people. *Dtsch. Arzteblatt Int.* **2016**, *113*, 253–260. [CrossRef]
19. Yoo, J.I.; Ha, Y.C.; Lee, Y.K.; Hana-Choi; Yoo, M.J.; Koo, K.H. High prevalence of sarcopenia among binge drinking elderly women: A nationwide population-based study. *BMC Geriatr.* **2017**, *17*, 114. [CrossRef]
20. Abney, M.; McPeek, M.S.; Ober, C. Broad and narrow heritabilities of quantitative traits in a founder population. *Am. J. Hum. Genet.* **2001**, *68*, 1302–1307. [CrossRef]
21. Zempo, H.; Miyamoto-Mikami, E.; Kikuchi, N.; Fuku, N.; Miyachi, M.; Murakami, H. Heritability estimates of muscle strength-related phenotypes: A systematic review and meta-analysis. *Scand. J. Med. Sci. Sports* **2017**, *27*, 1537–1546. [CrossRef] [PubMed]
22. Zhai, G.; Ding, C.; Stankovich, J.; Cicuttini, F.; Jones, G. The genetic contribution to longitudinal changes in knee structure and muscle strength: A sibpair study. *Arthritis Rheum.* **2005**, *52*, 2830–2834. [CrossRef] [PubMed]
23. Liberati, A.; Altman, D.; Tetzlaff, J.; Mulrow, C.; Gøtzsche, P.; Ioannidis, J.; Clarke, M.; Devereaux, P.; Kleijnen, J.; Moher, D. The PRISMA statement for reporting systematic reviews and meta-analyses of studies that evaluate health care interventions: Explanation and elaboration. *BMJ* **2009**, *339*, b2700. [CrossRef] [PubMed]
24. Sohani, Z.N.; Meyre, D.; de Souza, R.J.; Joseph, P.G.; Gandhi, M.; Dennis, B.B.; Norman, G.; Anand, S.S. Assessing the quality of published genetic association studies in meta-analyses: The quality of genetic studies (Q-Genie) tool. *BMC Genet.* **2015**, *16*, 50. [CrossRef] [PubMed]
25. Arking, D.E.; Fallin, D.M.; Fried, L.P.; Li, T.; Beamer, B.A.; Xue, Q.L.; Chakravarti, A.; Walston, J. Variation in the ciliary neurotrophic factor gene and muscle strength in older Caucasian women. *J. Am. Geriatr. Soc.* **2006**, *54*, 823–826. [CrossRef]

26. Bahat, G.; Saka, B.; Erten, N.; Ozbek, U.; Coskunpinar, E.; Yildiz, S.; Sahinkaya, T.; Karan, M.A. BsmI polymorphism in the vitamin D receptor gene is associated with leg extensor muscle strength in elderly men. *Aging Clin. Exp. Res.* **2010**, *22*, 198–205. [CrossRef]

27. Barr, R.; Macdonald, H.; Stewart, A.; McGuigan, F.; Rogers, A.; Eastell, R.; Felsenberg, D.; Glüer, C.; Roux, C.; Reid, D.M. Association between vitamin D receptor gene polymorphisms, falls, balance and muscle power: Results from two independent studies (APOSS and OPUS). *Osteoporos. Int.* **2010**, *21*, 457–466. [CrossRef]

28. Björk, A.; Ribom, E.; Johansson, G.; Scragg, R.; Mellström, D.; Grundberg, E.; Ohlsson, C.; Karlsson, M.; Ljunggren, Ö.; Kindmark, A. Variations in the vitamin D receptor gene are not associated with measures of muscle strength, physical performance, or falls in elderly men. Data from MrOS Sweden. *J. Steroid Biochem. Mol. Biol.* **2019**, *187*, 160–165. [CrossRef]

29. Buford, T.W.; Hsu, F.C.; Brinkley, T.E.; Carter, C.S.; Church, T.S.; Dodson, J.A.; Goodpaster, B.H.; McDermott, M.M.; Nicklas, B.J.; Yank, V.; et al. Genetic influence on exercise-induced changes in physical function among mobility-limited older adults. *Physiol. Genomics* **2014**, *46*, 149–158. [CrossRef]

30. Bustamante-Ara, N.; Santiago, C.; Verde, Z.; Yvert, T.; Gómez-Gallego, F.; Rodríguez-Romo, G.; González-Gil, P.; Serra-Rexach, J.A.; Ruiz, J.R.; Lucia, A. ACE and ACTN3 genes and muscle phenotypes in nonagenarians. *Int. J. Sports Med.* **2010**, *31*, 221–224. [CrossRef]

31. Charbonneau, D.E.; Hanson, E.D.; Ludlow, A.T.; Delmonico, M.J.; Hurley, B.F.; Roth, S.M. ACE genotype and the muscle hypertrophic and strength responses to strength training. *Med. Sci. Sports Exerc.* **2008**, *40*, 677–683. [CrossRef] [PubMed]

32. Cho, J.; Lee, I.; Kang, H. ACTN3 Gene and susceptibility to sarcopenia and osteoporotic status in older Korean adults. *Biomed. Res. Int.* **2017**, *2017*, 4239648. [CrossRef] [PubMed]

33. Crocco, P.; Montesanto, A.; Passarino, G.; Rose, G. A common polymorphism in the UCP3 promoter influences hand grip strength in elderly people. *Biogerontology* **2011**, *12*, 265–271. [CrossRef] [PubMed]

34. Da Silva, J.R.D.; Freire, I.V.; Ribeiro, Í.J.; dos Santos, C.S.; Casotti, C.A.; dos Santos, D.B.; Barbosa, A.A.L.; Pereira, R. Improving the comprehension of sarcopenic state determinants: An multivariate approach involving hormonal, nutritional, lifestyle and genetic variables. *Mech. Ageing Dev.* **2018**, *173*, 21–28. [CrossRef] [PubMed]

35. Dato, S.; Soerensen, M.; Montesanto, A.; Lagani, V.; Passarino, G.; Christensen, K.; Christiansen, L. UCP3 polymorphisms, hand grip performance and survival at old age: Association analysis in two Danish middle aged and elderly cohorts. *Mech. Ageing Dev.* **2012**, *133*, 530–537. [CrossRef]

36. De Mars, G.; Windelinckx, A.; Beunen, G.; Delecluse, C.; Lefevre, J.; Thomis, M.A. Polymorphisms in the CNTF and CNTF receptor genes are associated with muscle strength in men and women. *J. Appl. Physiol.* **2007**, *102*, 1824–1831. [CrossRef]

37. Delmonico, M.J.; Kostek, M.C.; Doldo, N.A.; Hand, B.D.; Walsh, S.; Conway, J.M.; Carignan, C.R.; Roth, S.M.; Hurley, B.F. Alpha-actinin-3 (ACTN3) R577X polymorphism influences knee extensor peak power response to strength training in older men and women. *J. Gerontol. A Biol. Sci. Med. Sci.* **2007**, *62*, 206–212. [CrossRef]

38. Delmonico, M.J.; Zmuda, J.M.; Taylor, B.C.; Cauley, J.A.; Harris, T.B.; Manini, T.M.; Schwartz, A.; Li, R.; Roth, S.M.; Hurley, B.F.; et al. Association of the ACTN3 genotype and physical functioning with age in older adults. *J. Gerontol. A Biol. Sci. Med. Sci.* **2008**, *63*, 1227–1234. [CrossRef]

39. Garatachea, N.; Fiuza-Luces, C.; Torres-Luque, G.; Yvert, T.; Santiago, C.; Gómez-Gallego, F.; Ruiz, J.R.; Lucia, A. Single and combined influence of ACE and ACTN3 genotypes on muscle phenotypes in octogenarians. *Eur. J. Appl. Physiol.* **2012**, *112*, 2409–2420. [CrossRef]

40. Giaccaglia, V.; Nicklas, B.; Kritchevsky, S.; Mychalecky, J.; Messier, S.; Bleecker, E.; Pahor, M. Interaction between angiotensin converting enzyme insertion/deletion genotype and exercise training on knee extensor strength in older individuals. *Int. J. Sports Med.* **2008**, *29*, 40–44. [CrossRef]

41. González-Freire, M.; Rodríguez-Romo, G.; Santiago, C.; Bustamante-Ara, N.; Yvert, T.; Gómez-Gallego, F.; Rexach, J.A.S.; Ruiz, J.R.; Lucia, A. The K153R variant in the myostatin gene and sarcopenia at the end of the human lifespan. *Age* **2010**, *32*, 405–409. [CrossRef] [PubMed]

42. Gussago, C.; Arosio, B.; Guerini, F.R.; Ferri, E.; Costa, A.S.; Casati, M.; Bollini, E.M.; Ronchetti, F.; Colombo, E.; Bernardelli, G.; et al. Impact of vitamin D receptor polymorphisms in centenarians. *Endocrine* **2016**, *53*, 558–564. [CrossRef] [PubMed]

43. Hand, B.D.; Kostek, M.C.; Ferrell, R.E.; Delmonico, M.J.; Douglass, L.W.; Roth, S.M.; Hagberg, J.M.; Hurley, B.F. Influence of promoter region variants of insulin-like growth factor pathway genes on the strength-training response of muscle phenotypes in older adults. *J. Appl. Physiol.* **2007**, *103*, 1678–1687. [CrossRef] [PubMed]

44. Heckerman, D.; Traynor, B.J.; Picca, A.; Calvani, R.; Marzetti, E.; Hernandez, D.; Nalls, M.; Arepali, S.; Ferrucci, L.; Landi, F. Genetic variants associated with physical performance and anthropometry in old age: A genome-wide association study in the ilSIRENTE cohort. *Sci. Rep.* **2017**, *7*, 15879. [CrossRef] [PubMed]

45. Hopkinson, N.S.; Li, K.W.; Kehoe, A.; Humphries, S.E.; Roughton, M.; Moxham, J.; Montgomery, H.; Polkey, M.I. Vitamin D receptor genotypes influence quadriceps strength in chronic obstructive pulmonary disease. *Am. J. Clin. Nutr.* **2008**, *87*, 385–390. [CrossRef]

46. Judson, R.N.; Wackerhage, H.; Hughes, A.; Mavroeidi, A.; Barr, R.J.; Macdonald, H.M.; Ratkevicius, A.; Reid, D.M.; Hocking, L.J. The functional ACTN3 577X variant increases the risk of falling in older females: Results from two large independent cohort studies. *J. Gerontol. A Biol. Sci. Med. Sci.* **2011**, *66*, 130–135. [CrossRef]

47. Keogh, J.W.L.; Palmer, B.R.; Taylor, D.; Kilding, A.E. ACE and UCP2 gene polymorphisms and their association with baseline and exercise-related changes in the functional performance of older adults. *PeerJ* **2015**, *3*, e980. [CrossRef]

48. Kikuchi, N.; Yoshida, S.; Min, S.K.; Lee, K.; Sakamaki-Sunaga, M.; Okamoto, T.; Nakazato, K. The ACTN3 R577X genotype is associated with muscle function in a Japanese population. *Appl. Physiol. Nutr. Metab.* **2015**, *40*, 316–322. [CrossRef]

49. Klimentidis, Y.C.; Bea, J.W.; Thompson, P.; Klimecki, W.T.; Hu, C.; Wu, G.; Nicholas, S.; Ryckman, K.K.; Chen, Z. Genetic variant in ACVR2B is associated with lean mass. *Med. Sci. Sports Exerc.* **2016**, *48*, 1270–1275. [CrossRef]

50. Kostek, M.C.; Delmonico, M.J.; Reichel, J.B.; Roth, S.M.; Douglass, L.; Ferrell, R.E.; Hurley, B.F. Muscle strength response to strength training is influenced by insulin-like growth factor 1 genotype in older adults. *J. Appl. Physiol.* **2005**, *98*, 2147–2154. [CrossRef]

51. Kostek, M.C.; Devaney, J.M.; Gordish-Dressman, H.; Harris, T.B.; Thompson, P.D.; Clarkson, P.M.; Angelopoulos, T.J.; Gordon, P.M.; Moyna, N.M.; Pescatello, L.S.; et al. A polymorphism near IGF1 is associated with body composition and muscle function in women from the Health, Aging, and Body Composition Study. *Eur. J. Appl. Physiol.* **2010**, *110*, 315–324. [CrossRef] [PubMed]

52. Kritchevsky, S.B.; Nicklas, B.J.; Visser, M.; Simonsick, E.M.; Newman, A.B.; Harris, T.B.; Lange, E.M.; Penninx, B.W.; Goodpaster, B.H.; Satterfield, S.; et al. Angiotensin-converting enzyme insertion/deletion genotype, exercise, and physical decline. *Jama* **2005**, *294*, 691–698. [CrossRef] [PubMed]

53. Li, C.I.; Li, T.C.; Liao, L.N.; Liu, C.S.; Yang, C.W.; Lin, C.H.; Hsiao, J.H.; Meng, N.H.; Lin, W.Y.; Wu, F.Y.; et al. Joint effect of gene-physical activity and the interactions among CRP, TNF-alpha, and LTA polymorphisms on serum CRP, TNF-alpha levels, and handgrip strength in community-dwelling elders in Taiwan-TCHS-E. *Age* **2016**, *38*, 46. [CrossRef] [PubMed]

54. Lima, R.M.; Leite, T.K.; Pereira, R.W.; Rabelo, H.T.; Roth, S.M.; Oliveira, R.J. ACE and ACTN3 genotypes in older women: Muscular phenotypes. *Int. J. Sports Med.* **2011**, *32*, 66–72. [CrossRef] [PubMed]

55. Lin, C.C.; Wu, F.Y.; Liao, L.N.; Li, C.I.; Lin, C.H.; Yang, C.W.; Meng, N.H.; Chang, C.K.; Lin, W.Y.; Liu, C.S.; et al. Association of CRP gene polymorphisms with serum CRP level and handgrip strength in community-dwelling elders in Taiwan: Taichung Community Health Study for Elders (TCHS-E). *Exp. Gerontol.* **2014**, *57*, 141–148. [CrossRef] [PubMed]

56. Lin, C.H.; Lin, C.C.; Tsai, C.W.; Chang, W.S.; Yang, M.D.; Bau, D.T. A novel caveolin-1 biomarker for clinical outcome of sarcopenia. *In Vivo* **2014**, *28*, 383–389.

57. Lunardi, C.C.; Lima, R.M.; Pereira, R.W.; Leite, T.K.; Siqueira, A.B.; Oliveira, R.J. Association between polymorphisms in the TRHR gene, fat-free mass, and muscle strength in older women. *Age* **2013**, *35*, 2477–2483. [CrossRef]

58. Ma, T.; Lu, D.; Zhu, Y.S.; Chu, X.F.; Wang, Y.; Shi, G.P.; Wang, Z.D.; Yu, L.; Jiang, X.Y.; Wang, X.F. ACTN3 genotype and physical function and frailty in an elderly Chinese population: The rugao longevity and ageing study. *Age Ageing* **2018**, *47*, 416–422. [CrossRef]

59. McCauley, T.; Mastana, S.S.; Folland, J.P. ACE I/D and ACTN3 R/X polymorphisms and muscle function and muscularity of older Caucasian men. *Eur. J. Appl. Physiol.* **2010**, *109*, 269–277. [CrossRef]

60. Melzer, D.; Dik, M.G.; van Kamp, G.J.; Jonker, C.; Deeg, D.J. The apolipoprotein E e4 polymorphism is strongly associated with poor mobility performance test results but not self-reported limitation in older people. *J. Gerontol. A Biol. Sci. Med. Sci.* **2005**, *60*, 1319–1323. [CrossRef]

61. Mora, M.; Perales, M.J.; Serra-Prat, M.; Palomera, E.; Buquet, X.; Oriola, J.; Puig-Domingo, M.; Mataró Ageing Study Group. Aging phenotype and its relationship with IGF-I gene promoter polymorphisms in elderly people living in Catalonia. *Growth Horm. IGF Res.* **2011**, *21*, 174–180. [CrossRef] [PubMed]

62. Onder, G.; Capoluongo, E.; Danese, P.; Settanni, S.; Russo, A.; Concolino, P.; Bernabei, R.; Landi, F. Vitamin D receptor polymorphisms and falls among older adults living in the community: Results from the ilSIRENTE study. *J. Bone Miner. Res.* **2008**, *23*, 1031–1036. [CrossRef] [PubMed]

63. Pereira, A.; Costa, A.M.; Izquierdo, M.; Silva, A.J.; Bastos, E.; Marques, M.C. ACE I/D and ACTN3 R/X polymorphisms as potential factors in modulating exercise-related phenotypes in older women in response to a muscle power training stimuli. *Age* **2013**, *35*, 1949–1959. [CrossRef] [PubMed]

64. Pereira, A.; Costa, A.M.; Leitão, J.C.; Monteiro, A.M.; Izquierdo, M.; Silva, A.J.; Bastos, E.; Marques, M.C. The influence of ACE ID and ACTN3 R577X polymorphisms on lower-extremity function in older women in response to high-speed power training. *BMC Geriatr.* **2013**, *13*, 131. [CrossRef]

65. Pereira, D.S.; Mateo, E.C.C.; de Queiroz, B.Z.; Assumpção, A.M.; Miranda, A.S.; Felício, D.C.; Rocha, N.P.; dos Anjos, D.M.D.C.; Pereira, D.A.G.; Teixeira, A.L.; et al. TNF-alpha, IL6, and IL10 polymorphisms and the effect of physical exercise on inflammatory parameters and physical performance in elderly women. *Age* **2013**, *35*, 2455–2463. [CrossRef]

66. Prakash, J.; Herlin, M.; Kumar, J.; Garg, G.; Akesson, K.E.; Grabowski, P.S.; Skerry, T.M.; Richards, G.O.; McGuigan, F.E. Analysis of RAMP3 gene polymorphism with body composition and bone density in young and elderly women. *Gene X* **2019**, *2*, 100009. [CrossRef]

67. Roth, S.M.; Zmuda, J.M.; Cauley, J.A.; Shea, P.R.; Ferrell, R.E. Vitamin D receptor genotype is associated with fat-free mass and sarcopenia in elderly men. *J. Gerontol. A Biol. Sci. Med. Sci.* **2004**, *59*, 10–15. [CrossRef]

68. Skoog, I.; Hörder, H.; Frändin, K.; Johansson, L.; Östling, S.; Blennow, K.; Zetterberg, H.; Zettergren, A. Association between APOE genotype and change in physical function in a population-based swedish cohort of older individuals followed over four years. *Front. Aging Neurosci.* **2016**, *8*, 225. [CrossRef]

69. Tiainen, K.; Thinggaard, M.; Jylha, M.; Bladbjerg, E.; Christensen, K.; Christiansen, L. Associations between inflammatory markers, candidate polymorphisms and physical performance in older Danish twins. *Exp. Gerontol.* **2012**, *47*, 109–115. [CrossRef]

70. Urano, T.; Shiraki, M.; Sasaki, N.; Ouchi, Y.; Inoue, S. Large-scale analysis reveals a functional single-nucleotide polymorphism in the 5'-flanking region of PRDM16 gene associated with lean body mass. *Aging Cell* **2014**, *13*, 739–743. [CrossRef]

71. Verghese, J.; Holtzer, R.; Wang, C.; Katz, M.J.; Barzilai, N.; Lipton, R.B. Role of APOE genotype in gait decline and disability in aging. *J. Gerontol. A Biol. Sci. Med. Sci.* **2013**, *68*, 1395–1401. [CrossRef] [PubMed]

72. Walsh, S.; Zmuda, J.M.; Cauley, J.A.; Shea, P.R.; Metter, E.J.; Hurley, B.F.; Ferrell, R.E.; Roth, S.M. Androgen receptor CAG repeat polymorphism is associated with fat-free mass in men. *J. Appl. Physiol.* **2005**, *98*, 132–137. [CrossRef] [PubMed]

73. Wu, F.Y.; Liu, C.S.; Liao, L.N.; Li, C.I.; Lin, C.H.; Yang, C.W.; Meng, N.H.; Lin, W.Y.; Chang, C.K.; Hsiao, J.H.; et al. Vitamin D receptor variability and physical activity are jointly associated with low handgrip strength and osteoporosis in community-dwelling elderly people in Taiwan: The Taichung Community Health Study for Elders (TCHS-E). *Osteoporos. Int.* **2014**, *25*, 1917–1929. [CrossRef] [PubMed]

74. Xia, Z.; Man, Q.; Li, L.; Song, P.; Jia, S.; Song, S.; Meng, L.; Zhang, J. Vitamin D receptor gene polymorphisms modify the association of serum 25-hydroxyvitamin D levels with handgrip strength in the elderly in Northern China. *Nutrition* **2019**, *57*, 202–207. [CrossRef]

75. Yang, C.W.; Li, T.C.; Li, C.I.; Liu, C.S.; Lin, C.H.; Lin, W.Y.; Lin, C.C. Insulin like growth factor-1 and its binding protein-3 polymorphisms predict circulating IGF-1 level and appendicular skeletal muscle mass in Chinese elderly. *J. Am. Med. Dir. Assoc.* **2015**, *16*, 365–370. [CrossRef]

76. Yoshihara, A.; Tobina, T.; Yamaga, T.; Ayabe, M.; Yoshitake, Y.; Kimura, Y.; Shimada, M.; Nishimuta, M.; Nakagawa, N.; Ohashi, M.; et al. Physical function is weakly associated with angiotensin-converting enzyme gene I/D polymorphism in elderly Japanese subjects. *Gerontology* **2009**, *55*, 387–392. [CrossRef]

77. Zempo, H.; Tanabe, K.; Murakami, H.; Iemitsu, M.; Maeda, S.; Kuno, S. ACTN3 polymorphism affects thigh muscle area. *Int. J. Sports Med.* **2010**, *31*, 138–142. [CrossRef]

78. Zempo, H.; Tanabe, K.; Murakami, H.; Iemitsu, M.; Maeda, S.; Kuno, S. Age differences in the relation between ACTN3 R577X polymorphism and thigh-muscle cross-sectional area in women. *Genet. Test. Mol. Biomark.* **2011**, *15*, 639–643. [CrossRef]

79. Montgomery, H.E.; Marshall, R.; Hemingway, H.; Myerson, S.; Clarkson, P.; Dollery, C.; Hayward, M.; Holliman, D.E.; Jubb, M.; World, M.; et al. Human gene for physical performance. *Nature* **1998**, *393*, 221–222. [CrossRef]

80. Cordero, A.I.H.; Gonzales, N.M.; Parker, C.C.; Sokoloff, G.; Vandenbergh, D.J.; Cheng, R.; Abney, M.; Skol, A.; Douglas, A.; Palmer, A.A.; et al. Genome-wide associations reveal human-mouse genetic convergence and modifiers of myogenesis, CPNE1 and STC2. *Am. J. Hum. Genet.* **2019**, *105*, 1222–1236. [CrossRef]

81. Zillikens, M.C.; Demissie, S.; Hsu, Y.H.; Yerges-Armstrong, L.M.; Chou, W.C.; Stolk, L.; Livshits, G.; Broer, L.; Johnson, T.; Koller, D.L.; et al. Large meta-analysis of genome-wide association studies identifies five loci for lean body mass. *Nat. Commun.* **2017**, *8*, 80. [CrossRef] [PubMed]

82. Houweling, P.J.; North, K.N. Sarcomeric α-actinins and their role in human muscle disease. *Future Neurol.* **2009**, *4*, 731–741. [CrossRef]

83. Blanchard, A.; Ohanian, V.; Critchley, D. The structure and function of α-actinin. *J. Muscle Res. Cell Motil.* **1989**, *10*, 280–289. [CrossRef] [PubMed]

84. North, K.N.; Yang, N.; Wattanasirichaigoon, D.; Mills, M.; Easteal, S.; Beggs, A.H. A common nonsense mutation results in alpha-actinin-3 deficiency in the general population. *Nat. Genet.* **1999**, *21*, 353–354. [CrossRef]

85. Yang, N.; MacArthur, D.G.; Gulbin, J.P.; Hahn, A.G.; Beggs, A.H.; Easteal, S.; North, K. ACTN3 genotype is associated with human elite athletic performance. *Am. J. Hum. Genet.* **2003**, *73*, 627–631. [CrossRef]

86. Druzhevskaya, A.M.; Ahmetov, I.I.; Astratenkova, I.V.; Rogozkin, V.A. Association of the ACTN3 R577X polymorphism with power athlete status in Russians. *Eur. J. Appl. Physiol.* **2008**, *103*, 631–634. [CrossRef]

87. Papadimitriou, I.D.; Lucia, A.; Pitsiladis, Y.P.; Pushkarev, V.P.; Dyatlov, D.A.; Orekhov, E.F.; Artioli, G.G.; Guilherme, J.P.L.; Lancha, A.H.; Ginevičienė, V.; et al. ACTN3 R577X and ACE I/D gene variants influence performance in elite sprinters: A multi-cohort study. *BMC Genomics* **2016**, *17*, 285. [CrossRef]

88. Tieland, M.; Trouwborst, I.; Clark, B.C. Skeletal muscle performance and ageing. *J. Cachexia Sarcopenia Muscle* **2018**, *9*, 3–19. [CrossRef]

89. Pickering, C.; Kiely, J. ACTN3: More than just a gene for speed. *Front. Physiol.* **2017**, *8*, 1080. [CrossRef]

90. Kumagai, H.; Tobina, T.; Ichinoseki-Sekine, N.; Kakigi, R.; Tsuzuki, T.; Zempo, H.; Shiose, K.; Yoshimura, E.; Kumahara, H.; Ayabe, M.; et al. Role of selected polymorphisms in determining muscle fiber composition in Japanese men and women. *J. Appl. Physiol.* **2018**, *124*, 1377–1384. [CrossRef]

91. Nielsen, J.; Christensen, D.L. Glucose intolerance in the West African Diaspora: A skeletal muscle fibre type distribution hypothesis. *Acta Physiol.* **2011**, *202*, 605–616. [CrossRef] [PubMed]

92. Ama, P.F.; Simoneau, J.A.; Boulay, M.R.; Serresse, O.; Thériault, G.; Bouchard, C. Skeletal muscle characteristics in sedentary black and Caucasian males. *J. Appl. Physiol.* **1986**, *61*, 1758–1761. [CrossRef] [PubMed]

93. Jeng, C.; Zhao, L.; Wu, K.; Zhou, Y.; Chen, T.; Deng, H.W. Race and socioeconomic effect on sarcopenia and sarcopenic obesity in the Louisiana Osteoporosis Study (LOS). *JCSM Clin. Rep.* **2018**, *3*, e00027. [CrossRef] [PubMed]

94. Rigat, B.; Hubert, C.; Alhenc-Gelas, F.; Cambien, F.; Corvol, P.; Soubrier, F. An insertion/deletion polymorphism in the angiotensin I-converting enzyme gene accounting for half the variance of serum enzyme levels. *J. Clin. Invest.* **1990**, *86*, 1343–1346. [CrossRef]

95. Gordon, S.E.; Davis, B.S.; Carlson, C.J.; Booth, F.W. ANG II is required for optimal overload-induced skeletal muscle hypertrophy. *Am. J. Physiol. Endocrinol. Metab.* **2001**, *280*, E150–E159. [CrossRef]

96. Danser, A.J.; Schalekamp, M.A.; Bax, W.A.; van den Brink, A.M.; Saxena, P.R.; Riegger, G.A.; Schunkert, H. Angiotensin-converting enzyme in the human heart. Effect of the deletion/insertion polymorphism. *Circulation* **1995**, *92*, 1387–1388. [CrossRef]

97. Tiret, L.; Rigat, B.; Visvikis, S.; Breda, C.; Corvol, P.; Cambien, F.; Soubrier, F. Evidence, from combined segregation and linkage analysis, that a variant of the angiotensin I-converting enzyme (ACE) gene controls plasma ACE levels. *Am. J. Hum. Genet.* **1992**, *51*, 197–205.

98. Williams, A.G.; Day, S.H.; Folland, J.P.; Gohlke, P.; Dhamrait, S.; Montgomery, H.E. Circulating angiotensin converting enzyme activity is correlated with muscle strength. *Med. Sci. Sports Exerc.* **2005**, *37*, 944–948. [CrossRef]

99. Myerson, S.; Hemingway, H.; Budget, R.; Martin, J.; Humphries, S.; Montgomery, H. Human angiotensin I-converting enzyme gene and endurance performance. *J. Appl. Physiol.* **1999**, *87*, 1313–1316. [CrossRef]

100. Puthucheary, Z.; Skipworth, J.R.; Rawal, J.; Loosemore, M.; Van Someren, K.; Montgomery, H.E. The ACE gene and human performance: 12 Years on. *Sports Med.* **2011**, *41*, 433–448. [CrossRef]

101. Al-Hinai, A.T.; Hassan, M.O.; Simsek, M.; Al-Barwani, H.; Bayoumi, R. Genotypes and allele frequencies of angiotensin converting enzyme (ACE) insertion/deletion polymorphism among Omanis. *J. Sci. Res. Med. Sci.* **2002**, *4*, 25–27. [PubMed]

102. Wishart, J.M.; Horowitz, M.; Need, A.G.; Scopacasa, F.; Morris, H.A.; Clifton, P.M. Relations between calcium intake, calcitriol, polymorphisms of the vitamin D receptor gene, and calcium absorption in premenopausal women. *Am. J. Clin. Nutr.* **1997**, *65*, 798–802. [CrossRef] [PubMed]

103. Pfeifer, M.; Begerow, B.; Minne, H.W. Vitamin D and muscle function. *Osteoporos. Int.* **2002**, *13*, 187–194. [CrossRef] [PubMed]

104. Whitfield, G.K.; Remus, L.S.; Jurutka, P.W.; Zitzer, H.; Oza, A.K.; Dang, H.T.; Haussler, C.A.; Galligan, M.A.; Thatcher, M.L.; Dominguez, C.E.; et al. Functionally relevant polymorphisms in the human nuclear vitamin D receptor gene. *Mol. Cell Endocrinol.* **2001**, *177*, 145–159. [CrossRef]

105. Baker, A.R.; McDonnell, D.P.; Hughes, M.; Crisp, T.M.; Mangelsdorf, D.J.; Haussler, M.R.; Pike, J.W.; Shine, J.; O'Malley, B.W. Cloning and expression of full-length cDNA encoding human vitamin D receptor. *Proc. Natl. Acad. Sci. USA* **1988**, *85*, 3294–3298. [CrossRef]

106. Arai, H.; Miyamoto, K.I.; Taketani, Y.; Yamamoto, H.; Iemori, Y.; Morita, K.; Tonai, T.; Nishisho, T.; Mori, S.; Takeda, E. A vitamin D receptor gene polymorphism in the translation initiation codon: Effect on protein activity and relation to bone mineral density in Japanese women. *J. Bone Miner. Res.* **1997**, *12*, 915–921. [CrossRef]

107. Moreno Lima, R.; De Abreu, B.S.; Gentil, P.; de Lima Lins, T.C.; Grattapaglia, D.; Pereira, R.W.; De Oliveira, R.J. Lack of association between vitamin D receptor genotypes and haplotypes with fat-free mass in postmenopausal Brazilian women. *J. Gerontol. A Biol. Sci. Med. Sci.* **2007**, *62*, 966–972. [CrossRef]

108. Iki, M.; Saito, Y.; Dohi, Y.; Kajita, E.; Nishino, H.; Yonemasu, K.; Kusaka, Y. Greater trunk muscle torque reduces postmenopausal bone loss at the spine independently of age, body size, and vitamin D receptor genotype in Japanese women. *Calcif. Tissue Int.* **2002**, *71*, 300–307. [CrossRef]

109. Nelson, D.A.; Vande-Vord, P.J.; Wooley, P.H. Polymorphism in the vitamin D receptor gene and bone mass in African-American and white mothers and children: A preliminary report. *Ann. Rheum. Dis.* **2000**, *59*, 626–630. [CrossRef]

110. Fleet, J.C.; Harris, S.S.; Wood, R.J.; Dawson-Hughes, B. The BsmI vitamin D receptor restriction fragment length polymorphism (BB) predicts low bone density in premenopausal black and white women. *J. Bone Miner. Res.* **1995**, *10*, 985–990. [CrossRef]

111. O'Dell, S.D.; Day, I.N. Insulin-like growth factor II (IGF-II). *Int. J. Biochem. Cell Biol.* **1998**, *30*, 767–771. [CrossRef]

112. Stewart, C.E.; Rotwein, P. Growth, differentiation, and survival: Multiple physiological functions for insulin-like growth factors. *Physiol. Rev.* **1996**, *76*, 1005–1026. [CrossRef] [PubMed]

113. Junnila, R.K.; List, E.O.; Berryman, D.E.; Murrey, J.W.; Kopchick, J.J. The GH/IGF-1 axis in ageing and longevity. *Nat. Rev. Endocrinol.* **2013**, *9*, 366–376. [CrossRef] [PubMed]

114. Jones, J.I.; Clemmons, D.R. Insulin-like growth factors and their binding proteins: Biological actions. *Endocr. Rev.* **1995**, *16*, 3–34. [CrossRef]

115. Baxter, G.T.; Kuo, R.C.; Jupp, O.J.; Vandenabeele, P.; MacEwan, D.J. Tumor necrosis factor-alpha mediates both apoptotic cell death and cell proliferation in a human hematopoietic cell line dependent on mitotic activity and receptor subtype expression. *J. Biol. Chem.* **1999**, *274*, 9539–9547. [CrossRef]

116. Bradley, J.R. TNF-mediated inflammatory disease. *J. Pathol.* **2008**, *214*, 149–160. [CrossRef]

117. Costamagna, D.; Costelli, P.; Sampaolesi, M.; Penna, F. Role of inflammation in muscle homeostasis and myogenesis. *Mediat. Inflamm.* **2015**, *2015*, 805172. [CrossRef]

118. Smith, J.D. Apolipoproteins and aging: Emerging mechanisms. *Ageing Res. Rev.* **2002**, *1*, 345–365. [CrossRef]

119. Bertram, L.; McQueen, M.B.; Mullin, K.; Blacker, D.; Tanzi, R.E. Systematic meta-analyses of Alzheimer disease genetic association studies: The AlzGene database. *Nat. Genet.* **2007**, *39*, 17–23. [CrossRef]

120. Fullerton, S.M.; Clark, A.G.; Weiss, K.M.; Nickerson, D.A.; Taylor, S.L.; Stengård, J.H.; Salomaa, V.; Vartiainen, E.; Perola, M.; Boerwinkle, E.; et al. Apolipoprotein E variation at the sequence haplotype level: Implications for the origin and maintenance of a major human polymorphism. *Am. J. Hum. Genet.* **2000**, *67*, 881–900. [CrossRef]

121. Kami, K.; Morikawa, Y.; Sekimoto, M.; Senba, E. Gene expression of receptors for IL-6, LIF, and CNTF in regenerating skeletal muscles. *J. Histochem. Cytochem.* **2000**, *48*, 1203–1213. [CrossRef] [PubMed]

122. Sendtner, M.; Kreutzberg, G.W.; Thoenen, H. Ciliary neurotrophic factor prevents the degeneration of motor neurons after axotomy. *Nature* **1990**, *345*, 440–441. [CrossRef] [PubMed]

123. Sleeman, M.W.; Anderson, K.D.; Lambert, P.D.; Yancopoulos, G.D.; Wiegand, S.J. The ciliary neurotrophic factor and its receptor, CNTFR alpha. *Pharm. Acta Helv.* **2000**, *74*, 265–272. [CrossRef]

124. Schrauwen, P.; Hesselink, M. UCP2 and UCP3 in muscle controlling body metabolism. *J. Exp. Biol.* **2002**, *205*, 2275–2285.

125. Schrauwen, P.; Hoeks, J.; Hesselink, M.K. Putative function and physiological relevance of the mitochondrial uncoupling protein-3: Involvement in fatty acid metabolism? *Prog. Lipid Res.* **2006**, *45*, 17–41. [CrossRef]

126. Dhamrait, S.S.; Williams, A.G.; Day, S.H.; Skipworth, J.; Payne, J.R.; World, M.; Humphries, S.E.; Montgomery, H.E. Variation in the uncoupling protein 2 and 3 genes and human performance. *J. Appl. Physiol.* **2012**, *112*, 1122–1127. [CrossRef]

127. Brand, M.D.; Pamplona, R.; Portero-Otín, M.; Requena, J.R.; Roebuck, S.J.; Buckingham, J.A.; Clapham, J.C.; Cadenas, S. Oxidative damage and phospholipid fatty acyl composition in skeletal muscle mitochondria from mice underexpressing or overexpressing uncoupling protein 3. *Biochem. J.* **2002**, *368*, 597–603. [CrossRef]

128. Seo, D.Y.; Lee, S.R.; Kim, N.; Ko, K.S.; Rhee, B.D.; Han, J. Age-related changes in skeletal muscle mitochondria: The role of exercise. *Integr. Med. Res.* **2016**, *5*, 182–186. [CrossRef]

129. Brand, M.D.; Affourtit, C.; Esteves, T.C.; Green, K.; Lambert, A.J.; Miwa, S.; Pakay, J.L.; Parker, N. Mitochondrial superoxide: Production, biological effects, and activation of uncoupling proteins. *Free Radic. Biol. Med.* **2004**, *37*, 755–767. [CrossRef]

130. Colhoun, H.M.; McKeigue, P.M.; Smith, D.G. Problems of reporting genetic associations with complex outcomes. *Lancet* **2003**, *361*, 865–872. [CrossRef]

131. Duncan, L.E.; Ostacher, M.; Ballon, J. How genome-wide association studies (GWAS) made traditional candidate gene studies obsolete. *Neuropsychopharmacology* **2019**, *44*, 1518–1523. [CrossRef] [PubMed]

132. Visscher, P.M.; Wray, N.R.; Zhang, Q.; Sklar, P.; McCarthy, M.I.; Brown, M.A.; Yang, J. 10 Years of GWAS discovery: Biology, function, and translation. *Am. J. Hum. Genet.* **2017**, *101*, 5–22. [CrossRef] [PubMed]

133. Sawcer, S. The complex genetics of multiple sclerosis: Pitfalls and prospects. *Brain* **2008**, *131*, 3118–3131. [CrossRef] [PubMed]

10

High-Dimensional Single-Cell Quantitative Profiling of Skeletal Muscle Cell Population Dynamics during Regeneration

Lucia Lisa Petrilli [1,2,†], Filomena Spada [1,†], Alessandro Palma [1], Alessio Reggio [1], Marco Rosina [1], Cesare Gargioli [1], Luisa Castagnoli [1], Claudia Fuoco [1,*] and Gianni Cesareni [1,3]

[1] Department of Biology, University of Rome "Tor Vergata", 00133 Rome, Italy; lucialisa.petrilli@opbg.net (L.L.P.); filomena.spada86@gmail.com (F.S.); alessandro.palma@live.it (A.P.); alessio.reggio@uniroma2.it (A.R.); marco.rosina90@gmail.com (M.R.); Cesare.Gargioli@uniroma2.it (C.G.); castagnoli@uniroma2.it (L.C.); cesareni@uniroma2.it (G.C.)

[2] Department of Onco-hematology, Gene and Cell Therapy—Bambino Gesù Children's Hospital—IRCCS, 00146 Rome, Italy

[3] Fondazione Santa Lucia Istituto di Ricovero e Cura a Carattere Scientifico (IRCCS), 00143 Rome, Italy

*   Correspondence: claudia.fuoco@uniroma2.it;

†   These authors contributed equally to the study.

Abstract: The interstitial space surrounding the skeletal muscle fibers is populated by a variety of mononuclear cell types. Upon acute or chronic insult, these cell populations become activated and initiate finely-orchestrated crosstalk that promotes myofiber repair and regeneration. Mass cytometry is a powerful and highly multiplexed technique for profiling single-cells. Herein, it was used to dissect the dynamics of cell populations in the skeletal muscle in physiological and pathological conditions. Here, we characterized an antibody panel that could be used to identify most of the cell populations in the muscle interstitial space. By exploiting the mass cytometry resolution, we provided a comprehensive picture of the dynamics of the major cell populations that sensed and responded to acute damage in wild type mice and in a mouse model of Duchenne muscular dystrophy. In addition, we revealed the intrinsic heterogeneity of many of these cell populations.

Keywords: single-cell; mass cytometry; skeletal muscle regeneration; skeletal muscle homeostasis; fibro/adipogenic progenitors; myogenic progenitors; muscle populations

1. Introduction

In physiological conditions, the adult skeletal muscle has a relatively low cell turnover [1]. However, physical activity, trauma, or muscle pathologies, undermining tissue integrity, trigger a tightly controlled regeneration process. Although satellite cells (SCs) are the main actors of myofiber regeneration after damage [2–6], successful muscle healing requires the participation of additional cell types that directly or indirectly contribute to this process. In this context, immune cells and fibro/adipogenic progenitors (FAPs) play a prominent role in supporting the clearance of the damaged tissue, while assisting SCs in their regenerative role [7–11]. However, the orchestrated crosstalk of the regeneration machinery gradually fails in patients affected by muscle-related disorders, such as dystrophies [12]. Here, the accumulation of intrinsic cell defects and the changes in the stem cell niche lead to infiltrations of fat and fibrotic deposition, compromising muscle functions [9,13–16].

Over the past decades, the complex cell crosstalk occurring during muscle regeneration has been studied in detail [17–19]. However, to date, most studies have mainly relied on the analysis of bulk cell populations identified by the expression of a few specific markers and sorted for ex vivo analysis.

As a consequence, due to the lack of technologies suitable to address this issue, little is known about muscle cell population heterogeneity. Only recently, the development of technologies to determine the transcriptome of single-cells or their exposed antigen repertoires has permitted to reveal the extent of this heterogeneity and its possible implication in muscle physiology and pathology [20–24]. Moreover, the dynamic changes and the relative abundance of muscle cell populations, upon acute or chronic damage, still remain largely uncharacterized. To fill this gap, we explored, via single-cell mass cytometry, the changes in the multidimensional antigen repertoires of the main players, colonizing the muscle stem cell niche after injury. Here, we described, at single-cell resolution, the time-dependent changes of muscle population dynamics upon myotoxin-induced damage in wild type (wt) and in a mouse model of Duchenne muscular dystrophy (the mdx model).

2. Materials and Methods

2.1. Mouse Strains and Animal Procedures

C57BL/6J (RRID:IMSR_JAX:000664) and C57BL/10ScSn-Dmd^{mdx}/J mice (RRID:IMSR_JAX:001801), hereafter referred to as wt and mdx mice, respectively, were purchased from the Jackson Laboratory.

Mice were bred respecting the standard animal facility procedures, and all the procedures were conducted in accordance with rules of good animal experimentation I.A.C.U.C. n°432 of 12 March 2006 and under ethical approval released on 23/October/2017 from the Italian Ministry of Health, protocol #820/2017-PR.

For muscle injury, 45-day-old wt and mdx mice were anesthetized with an intramuscular injection of saline solution containing ketamine (5 mg/mL) and xylazine (1 mg/mL) prior to the intramuscular administration of 20 µL of 10 µM cardiotoxin solution, isolated from *Naja Pallida* (Latoxan L8102, Portes les valence, France), into *tibialis anterior*, *quadriceps*, and *gastrocnemius* muscles.

2.2. Histological Analysis

Tibialis anterior (TA) muscles were collected, embedded in optimal cutting temperature compound (Killik—O.C.T., Bio Optica, Milan, Italy), and snap-frozen in liquid nitrogen for 10 s. Embedded muscles were stored at −80 °C for transverse cryo-sectioning with a Leica cryostat. Cryosections (10 µm thickness) were collected on Superfrost glass slides (Thermo Fisher Scientific, Monza, Italy), and tissue slides were stained with hematoxylin and eosin (H&E).

For the H&E, cryosections were fixed with 4% paraformaldehyde (PFA, Santa Cruz Biotechnology, D.B.A. Italia S.r.l., Segrate Milan, Italy) for 15 min at room temperature (RT). After washing in 1X PBS, tissue slides were incubated in the hematoxylin solution for 15 min and rinsed for 5 min in tap water. Cryosections were then counterstained with an alcoholic solution of eosin for 30 min. Following the eosin staining, cryosections were dehydrated in increasing concentrations of alcohol, clarified with the histo-clear solution (Agar Scientific Ltd, Stansted, UK), and finally mounted on coverslips, using the resinous Eukitt mounting medium (Electron Microscopy Sciences, Hatfield Township, PA, USA).

H&E images were captured using the Zeiss Lab A1 AX10 microscope at the 20× magnification in the bright field.

2.3. Skeletal Muscle Mononuclear Cell Purification

Isolation of mononuclear cell populations was performed as in Spada et al. [25]. Mice were sacrificed by cervical dislocation, and the hind limbs were washed with 70% ethanol. Mice hind limbs were then dissected and finely minced in Hank's balanced salt solution (HBSS) with calcium and magnesium (Gibco- Thermo Fisher Scientific, Monza, Italy) supplemented with 0.2% bovine serum albumin (BSA) (AppliChem, Cinisello Balsamo, Milan, Italy) and 1% penicillin-streptomycin (P/S) (Life Technologies, Monza, Italy, 10,000 U/mL) (HBSS$^+$) under a sterile hood. The homogenized tissue preparation was centrifuged at 70× *g* for 10 min at 4 °C to separate fat and subjected to enzymatic digestion for 1 h at 37 °C, with gentle mixing in a solution containing 2 µg/µL collagenase A

(Roche- Merck KGaA, Darmstadt, Germany), 2.4 U/mL dispase II (Roche- Merck KGaA, Darmstadt, Germany), and 10 μg/mL DNase I (Roche- Merck KGaA, Darmstadt, Germany) diluted in Dulbecco's phosphate-buffered saline (D-PBS) with calcium and magnesium (Gibco-Thermo Fisher Scientific, Monza, Italy). The reaction was inactivated with HBSS$^+$, and the cell suspension was subjected to three sequential filtrations through 100 μm, 70 μm, and 40 μm cell strainers (BD Falcon, BD Italia, Milan, Italy) and centrifugations at 700× g for 5 min. The lysis of red blood cells was performed by incubating with RBC Lysis Buffer (Santa Cruz Biotechnology, D.B.A. Italia S.r.l., Segrate, Milan, Italy) for 150 s on ice, prior to the 40 μm filtration step.

2.4. Single-Cell Mass Cytometry

For single-cell mass cytometry experiments, 3×10^6 cells were used for each condition. Each time point was analyzed in triplicate, starting from mononuclear cells purified from three different mice. Cells were centrifuged at 600× g for 5 min and washed in D-PBS w/o calcium and magnesium (BioWest-VWR INTERNATIONAL PBI S.r.l., Milan, Italy). To minimize the inter-sample antibody staining variation, we applied a mass-tag barcoding protocol on fixed cells. Cells were fixed with 1 mL of Fix I Buffer (Fluidigm, South San Francisco, CA, USA) and then incubated for 10 min at RT. The fixation was quenched with Barcode Perm Buffer (Fluidigm, South San Francisco, CA, USA). The different samples were barcoded by individually incubating the cell suspensions with the appropriate combination of palladium isotopes from the Cell-ID^{TM} 20-Plex Pd Barcoding Kit (Fluidigm, South San Francisco, CA, USA) in Barcode Perm Buffer for 30 min at RT. The staining was quenched with MaxPar Cell Staining Buffer (Fluidigm, South San Francisco, CA, USA).

The antibody staining with metal-tagged antibodies that target surface and intracellular antigens was performed on the samples pooled after mass-tag barcoding. Samples were collected in a single tube, and the surface antibody staining protocol was performed according to manufacturers' instructions for 30 min at RT. Surface-stained cells were then washed twice with MaxPar Cell Staining Buffer (Fluidigm South San Francisco, CA, USA) and permeabilized with ice-cold methanol for 10 min on ice. Membrane-permeabilized cells were washed twice with MaxPar Cell Staining Buffer (Fluidigm, South San Francisco, CA, USA) and incubated with antibodies against intracellular antigens for 30 min at RT according to manufacturers' instructions. The full list of antibodies is detailed in Table 1. All the antibodies listed were purchased from Fluidigm (South San Francisco, CA, USA). After intracellular antibody staining, cells were washed twice with MaxPar Cell Staining Buffer and stained for 1 h at RT with the intercalation solution, composed of Cell-ID Intercalator-Ir (191Ir and 193Ir, Fluidigm South San Francisco, CA, USA) in MaxPar Fix and Perm Buffer (Fluidigm, South San Francisco, CA, USA) at a final concentration of 125 nM. Cells were washed twice with MaxPar Cell Staining Buffer and MaxPar Water.

For mass cytometry analysis, cells were resuspended at the final concentration of 2.5×10^5 cells/mL in MaxPar Water containing 10% of EQ^{TM} Four Element Calibration Beads (Fluidigm, South San Francisco, CA, USA) and filtered through a 30-μm filter-cap FACS tube. Samples were kept on ice prior to the acquisition by using the mass cytometry platform CyTOF2 System (Fluidigm, South San Francisco, CA, USA).

Table 1. List of the metal-tagged antibodies used in the mass cytometry experiments.

Antibody	Metal
Anti-mouse CD45	147Sm
Anti-mouse Ly-6A/E (SCA1)	164Dy
Anti-mouse CD90.2 (Thy-1.2)	156Gd
Anti-mouse CD146	141Pr
Anti-mouse F4/80	146Nd
Anti-mouse CD140α	148Nd
Anti-mouse CD140β	151Eu
Anti-mouse α7-integrin	161Dy
Anti-mouse CD206	169Tm
Anti-mouse CD34	144Nd
Anti-mouse CXCR4	159Tb
Anti-mouse CD4	172Yb
Anti-mouse CD25 (IL-2R)	150Nd
Anti-vimentin	154Sm
Anti-CD31 (PECAM-1)	165Ho
Anti-pan-actin	175Lu
Anti-mouse interleukin-6 (IL-6)	167Er
Anti-phospho-Akt (S473)	152Sm
Anti-phospho-Stat1 (Y701)	153Eu
Anti-phospho-Erk1/2 (T202/Y204)	171Yb
Anti-phospho-Stat3 (Y705)	158Gd
Anti-cleaved caspase3	142Nd
Anti-phospho-Creb	176Yb

CD: Cluster Differentiation; SCA1: Stem Cell Antigen1; CXCR4: C-X-C Motif Chemokine Receptor 4; PECAM-1: Platelet Endothelial Cell adhesion-1; Akt: RAC alpha serine/threonine-protein kinase; Stat1: Signal Transducer and activator of transcription 1; Erk1/2: Extracellular signal-regulated kinases 1, 2; Stat3: Signal transducer and activator of transcription 3; cleaved caspase3: cysteine-aspartic proteases; Creb: cAMP response element-binding protein.

2.5. CyTOF Data Analysis

Following data acquisition, channel intensity was normalized using calibration beads [26], and the normalized *fcs* file was de-barcoded by using the Debarcoder software (Fluidigm, South San Francisco, CA, USA). Data have been pre-processed using the Cytobank software platform [27]. Cells were manually gated from debris on the basis of DNA content monitored by the incorporation of the iridium (Ir) intercalator. Doublets were then excluded according to the event length parameter, and single live cells were finally manually gated by using the cisplatin (Pt) intercalator signal. Manually gated singlet ($191Ir^+$ $193Ir^+$), viable ($195Pt^-$) events were imported into Cytofkit for further analysis [28]. Cytofkit [28] parameters were set as follows: 14 biomarkers were included for clustering all the detected live cells per sample ("all" merge method); transformation method: cytofAsinh; FlowSOM was used as clustering algorithm with $k = 15$, tSNE perplexity set to 30; 2000 iterations and seed: 42.

Data were analyzed with Cytofkit shiny app [28] https://github.com/JinmiaoChenLab/cytofkit) and R scripts. Gating for marker-positive cells was performed by setting the mean +/- standard deviation as a threshold, depending on the expression value distribution of the specific marker.

2.6. Statistical Analysis

The experiments were performed at least in biological triplicates, that is, from at least 3 independent mononuclear cell preparations for each experiment. Only for the time point at day 5 in the wild type time series, we had just two biological repeats. Results were presented as mean ± SEM unless otherwise mentioned. Statistical evaluation was done by using One-way or Two-way ANOVA. Comparisons were considered statistically significant at * $p < 0.05$; ** $p < 0.01$; *** $p < 0.001$; **** $p < 0.0001$. All statistical analysis was performed using Prism 6 (GraphPad, San Diego, CA, USA).

3. Results

3.1. Histological Profiling of Skeletal Muscle Tissue from wt and mdx Muscles Following Acute Damage

To gain insights into the skeletal muscle repair process, we aimed at describing the dynamics of muscle cell populations following acute damage. To induce muscle injury, we used a well-established protocol based on the injection of the snake (*Naja pallida*) myotoxin (cardiotoxin, CTX) into the hind limb muscles of wt and mdx dystrophic mice (Figure 1A) [29,30]. Cardiotoxin, by inhibiting protein kinase C (PKC), induced the increase of cytosolic calcium, causing myofiber myolysis that, in turn, triggers regeneration [31–33]. First, we monitored, by hematoxylin and eosin staining, the changes in the skeletal muscle architecture at five different time points that were chosen to monitor the key events of the muscle healing process after damage: necrosis, inflammation, regeneration, and remodeling (Figure 1B,C).

Sections of uninjured wt muscles were characterized by polygonal fibers of uniform size containing peripheral nuclei (Figure 1B) [34]. Upon CTX injection, the skeletal muscle underwent degeneration, setting in motion the regeneration process. The degeneration of the muscle architecture was clearly observable at day 1 after injury, while interstitial cells, either resident cell populations [8] or infiltrating immune cells [35], became conspicuous at day 3 after damage. The regeneration process was completed after 20 days, as highlighted by the presence of multinucleated regenerated myofibers.

The mdx skeletal muscle, on the other hand, even in the absence of acute insult, was characterized by infiltrating inflammatory interstitial cells and centrally nucleated myofibers of different sizes, hallmarks of the dystrophic pathology (Figure 1C) [12,36,37]. Following CTX injection, the injured tissue underwent a regeneration process, without being apparently impacted further by extensive necrosis. If anything, the mdx muscle seemed to be more resilient to the myotoxin-induced damage and did not undergo the massive structural damage that was observed early after cardiotoxin injection in the wt muscle. Altogether, the histological analysis showed that the muscles from the two genetic backgrounds responded differently to CTX-induced injury.

3.2. Single-Cell Quantitative Profiling of Skeletal Muscle Populations Following Myotoxin-Induced Injury

Next, we sought to characterize the different mononuclear cell populations in the two mouse models and monitor their abundance changes during the regeneration process. To this end, we resorted to using mass cytometry [8].

In wt muscles, the number of isolated mononuclear cells increased after damage and peaked at day 3 to return to almost baseline levels at day 10 (Figure 1D). In contrast, consistent with the resilience of the mdx muscle observed in the histological analysis, this response was not detected in the injured muscles of mdx mice, where the mononuclear cell number remained constant over the whole regeneration process (Figure 1E).

The mononuclear cell samples from both animal models were separately barcoded and labeled with a panel of 23 metal-tagged antibodies (Table 1) targeting antigens expressed by muscle resident cells and/or by cell populations from the hematopoietic compartment. Mononuclear cells were purified from the uninjured and injured muscles at five time-points and, after barcoding and labeling, analyzed with a CyTOF2 mass cytometer in a single-run experiment [38]. Signals were debarcoded, and live cells were identified using the cisplatin (Pt) intercalator signal. Live/dead cell analysis highlighted that dead wt cells significantly increased at day 3 (Figure S1A), while for mdx muscles, the live/dead cell ratio remained constant (Figure S1B).

Single-cell data were analyzed by applying, as a dimensionality reduction method, the t-distributed stochastic neighbor embedding (t-SNE) algorithm implemented in Cytofkit [28,39].

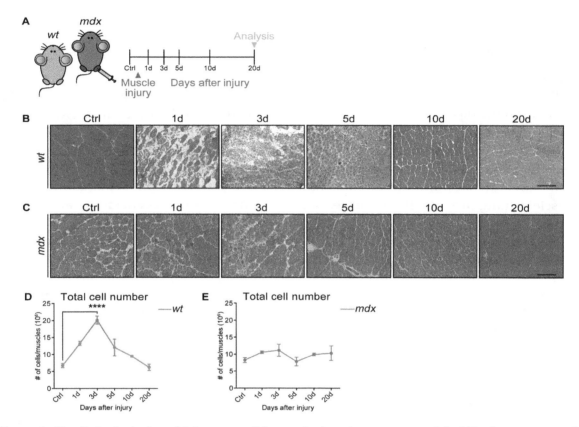

Figure 1. Cardiotoxin-induced injury on wild type (wt) and a mouse model of Duchenne muscular dystrophy (mdx) skeletal muscle tissue. (**A**) Experimental procedure. 45-day-old wt and mdx mice were injected intramuscularly with cardiotoxin (CTX) (10 μM), and the skeletal muscles were analyzed 1, 3, 5, 10, and 20 days (d) after injury. (**B**) Representative hematoxylin and eosin staining of uninjured wt *tibialis anterior* (TA) muscles and regenerating wt TA muscles at 1, 3, 5, 10, and 20 days after intramuscular CTX injection. Regenerating muscles were characterized by centrally located nuclei at day 5, but reconstituted multinucleated myofibers by day 10. (**C**) Representative hematoxylin and eosin staining on histological sections of uninjured and regenerating mdx TA muscles at 1, 3, 5, 10, and 20 days after intramuscular CTX injection. All along the considered time points, mdx muscles were characterized by infiltrating inflammatory interstitial cells and centrally nucleated myofibers of different sizes. (**D,E**) The number of cells (in millions) extracted from uninjured and CTX-injured wt (**D**) and mdx (**E**) mice (n=3; for 5d wt time point, n=2). All data were represented as mean ± SEM, and the statistical significance was estimated by two-way ANOVA (**** $p < 0.0001$). (**B,C**) 20× magnification; scale bar: 100 μm.

As the readouts of phospho-antibodies were barely above the background signal, albeit cell-specific (Figure S2), they were not considered in this analysis. The readouts of the 14 antigens in Figure 2A were used as input for the t-SNE algorithm. This approach yielded a two-dimensional map of the antigenic expression profiles of mononuclear cell populations in the wt skeletal muscle (Figure 2A) and led to the identification of 15 different cell clusters (Figure 2B).

The 15 identified clusters (Figure 2B) were further grouped into eight cell types by matching their expression profile to that of cell types already described in the literature [20,40]. More specifically, we were able to identify populations expressing antigens typical of immune cells (CD45$^+$) (clusters 7, 8, 12, 13, 14, and 15), macrophages (CD45$^+$ and F4/80$^+$) (clusters 7, 13, and 14), myogenic progenitors (MPs) (α7-integrin$^+$) (cluster 1), fibro/adipogenic progenitors (FAPs) (SCA1$^+$, CD34$^+$, CD140α^+, CD90.2$^+$, and vimentin$^+$) (cluster 10), endothelial progenitor cells (CD31$^+$) (clusters 3 and 4), pericyte-like cells (CD146$^+$ and CD140β^+) (cluster 11), and mesenchymal-like cells (CD90.2$^+$) (cluster 5). The expression profiles of three remaining non-abundant clusters (clusters 2, 6, and 9) could not be matched to any of the already described muscle cell types and were collectively dubbed "others" (Figure 2B,C).

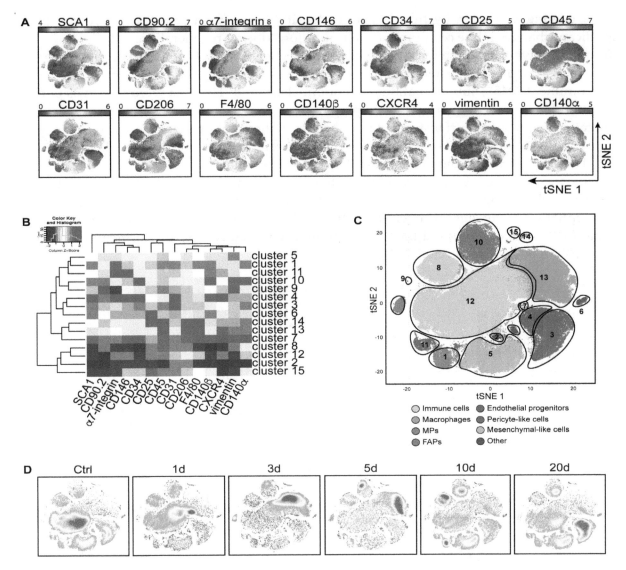

Figure 2. Dynamic changes of mononuclear cell subpopulations in wt muscles during regeneration. (**A**) The different mononuclear cell samples from uninjured and CTX-injured wt hind limb muscles were merged to create a single t-distributed stochastic neighbor embedding (t-SNE) map; colored according to expression levels of SCA1, CD90.2, α7-integrin, CD146, CD34, CD25, CD45, CD31, CD206, F4/80, CD140β, CXCR4, vimentin, and CD140α (blue: low expression; red: high expression of the selected marker). (**B**) FlowSOM heatmap of column normalized (Z-score) marker expression for each of the 15 identified clusters. Colors varied according to the expression level of the considered marker in a blue to red scale, indicating low to high expression, respectively. (**C**) Cell clusters defined by the FlowSOM analysis were assigned to arbitrary colors (yellow: immune cells; light blue: macrophages; pink: myogenic progenitors (MPs); dark green: fibro/adipogenic progenitors (FAPs); red: endothelial progenitors; blue: pericyte-like cells; light green: mesenchymal-like cells; purple: other). (**D**) Time course of the variation in cell subpopulation abundance upon CTX-induced injury. The dynamic changes were illustrated by density plots, colored according to cell density (blue: low density; red: high density).

As we analyzed samples at different time points, we could also monitor the dynamic of cell populations after CTX damage. The picture in Figure 2C, in fact, was not static as the relative abundance of the different cell populations changed along the regeneration process. These could be best appreciated by comparing the bidimensional t-SNE maps at different time points (Figure 2D). Here the colors, relating to cell density, from blue (low density) to red (high density), allowed to appreciate the significant changes in the cell population proportions during regeneration.

To quantitatively describe the dynamics of these changes, we first classified the observed cell populations into two main clusters according to CD45 expression: (i) the immune (CD45$^+$) and the (ii) non-immune (CD45$^-$) subpopulations of mononuclear cells. The data were shown as population relative abundance in the mononuclear cell preparations analyzed in the CyTOF. However, this data representation could be easily transformed into changes in the absolute numbers of each cell population in the mouse muscle as the total number of mononuclear cells in each condition was known (Figures S3 and S4). The curve trends in the two representations were similar.

We first focused on CD45$^+$ hematopoietic cells as they play a critical role in the regeneration process by sending regulatory signals by removing the damaged-fiber debris and by stimulating proliferation and differentiation of myogenic progenitors [19,41–45]. In a homeostatic muscle, approximately 60% of the mononuclear cells exposed the CD45 antigen. This cell compartment increased in number, after damage, to peak at days 1 and 3 (Figure 3A).

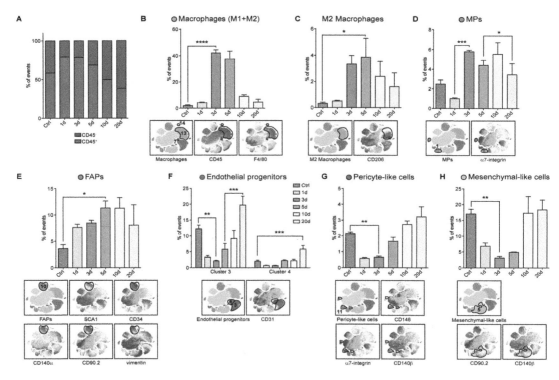

Figure 3. Characterization of the cell-population density rearrangements induced by CTX in the wt skeletal muscle after 1, 3, 5, 10, 20 days. (**A**) Bar plots, showing the CD45$^-$ (blue) / CD45$^+$ (red) ratio in mononuclear cells from wt skeletal muscles at different time points after CTX injury. Data were represented as mean, while the statistical significance was estimated by two-way ANOVA. (**B–H**) Identification in the t-SNE maps of mononuclear cell populations. The different plots were color-coded according to the expression of surface antigens that characterize the relevant cell types. The bar plots quantitated the variation in population abundance in the wt limb muscles at different times during regeneration. Cell percentages were assessed on the total number of cells in each sample (n = 3; for 5d wt time point, n = 2). The statistical significance was estimated by one-way ANOVA. All data were represented as mean ± SEM, and the statistical significance was defined as * $p < 0.05$; ** $p < 0.01$; *** $p < 0.001$; **** $p < 0.0001$.

In physiological conditions, a fraction of the hematopoietic cells, less than 2% of the total recorded events, also expressed the F4/80$^+$ antigen, a pan-macrophage marker (Figure 3B). However, already 3 days after injury, the macrophage population significantly increased, reaching a maximum of approximately 40%. At later times, macrophage abundance gradually decreased, returning close to baseline levels at day 20. The macrophage population is not homogeneous as it contains pro-inflammatory (M1) and anti-inflammatory (M2) macrophages that differ in the expression of the CD206 antigen and play a different role in muscle regeneration [46,47].

Noteworthy, CD206$^+$ M2 macrophages, which are responsible for the resolution of the inflammatory response [48–50], increased significantly on day 5 at the expense of inflammatory macrophages M1 that peaked at day 3 (Figure 3B,C).

We next focused on the cell populations that did not express the CD45 antigen. This group included the two main players of the regeneration process: myogenic progenitors (MPs) and fibro/adipogenic progenitors (FAPs) [5,6,8,51,52]. Our single-cell analysis revealed that both cell types more than doubled in number from day 3 to 10 (Figure 3D,E).

We could not obtain mass cytometry grade antibodies, specifically recognizing the paired box protein PAX7 antigen, which labels satellite cells. Thus, we resorted to using the α7-integrin antigen as a marker of the myogenic progenitor (MP) cluster (Figure 3D), including both satellite cells and myoblasts. Within the population expressing α7-integrin, we could identify two smaller clusters expressing different levels of vimentin (Figure S1C). During regeneration, the MP cell population, after an initial decrease, became more populated (Figure 3D). The relative abundance of the two subpopulations changed in time with the vimentin expressing MP, significantly increasing in number at day 3 (Figure S1C). At day 3 post-injury, the MPs accounted for about 6% of the total recorded cell events.

The FAP compartment was defined in our t-SNE map by a cluster of cells expressing SCA1, CD34, CD140α, CD90.2, and vimentin. Similar to the MP population, albeit with a different trend, the FAP population became more numerous as the regeneration process progressed, reaching the maximum expansion between 5–10 days after CTX injury (about 11.3% of total events), to return to almost control levels at day 20 (Figure 3E).

Our analysis also allowed us to characterize the kinetic of vessel-associated populations during regeneration [53,54]. These were identified, among CD45 negative cells, as they expressed the CD31 antigen. We were able to distinguish two subpopulations of cells expressing additional markers of endothelial populations at different levels (SCA1, CD146, and CD34) (Figure S1D). CD31 cluster 4 was considered a myoendothelial cell subpopulation, containing cells that also express high levels of the α7-integrin antigen [55]. Overall, we observed that the whole endothelial progenitor pool followed a kinetic that was different from the populations examined so far. They decreased significantly in number in the first few days after damage and then increased over the homeostatic level toward the end of the regeneration process (Figure 3F).

We also considered a population of cells whose expression profile was reminiscent of that of pericytes [56,57]. They were characterized by the expression of CD146, CD140β, and α7-integrin (Figure 3G). These pericyte-like cells followed a trend that was very similar to that of endothelial cells, with a sharp decrease early after damage and a rapid increase in the late regeneration phase, when vascularization took place (Figure 3G). We also looked at a cluster of cells that we were not able to match to any of the cell types described so far. We dubbed this population as mesenchymal-like cells, as they were highly positive for CD90.2 and CD140β markers. The abundance of this population followed a kinetic that seemed to be governed by the regeneration process and was also very similar to that of the classical endothelial cells (Figure 3H).

3.3. Single-Cell Profiling of the mdx Muscle

We further aimed at characterizing the response to acute damage and the ensuing regeneration process in the mdx dystrophic muscle. Mononuclear cells were isolated from the uninjured and CTX-injured skeletal muscles of mdx mice, following the same procedure described for the wt in the previous section (Figure 4A–D). Mononuclear cells were separated from muscle fibers, barcoded, labeled with the same antibody panel, and prepared for mass cytometry. The resulting single-cell antigen expression profile was processed, as described for the wt cells, in order to obtain a two-dimensional representation of antigen expression in the different cell types. As the wt and mdx mass cytometry analyses were performed at different times, the resulting t-SNE maps could not be directly compared (Figures 2A and 4A). However, by comparing the antigen expression profiles in the different clusters, we were able to associate each cluster to one of the main muscle mononuclear cell types and match it to those observed in the wt (Figure 4B,C). As observed in injured-recovering wt muscles, the relative numerosity of the different cell populations also changed after damage and during regeneration in the mdx model (Figure 4D).

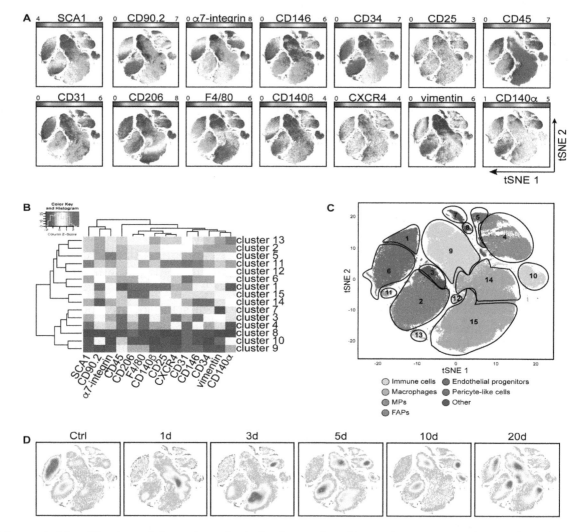

Figure 4. Identification of the main mdx skeletal muscle cell populations upon CTX-induced injury. (**A**) A mononuclear cell suspension was purified from uninjured and CTX-injured mdx hind limb muscles. The different samples were combined, barcoded, and analyzed to create a single t-SNE map colored according to SCA1, CD90.2, α7-integrin, CD146, CD34, CD25, CD45, CD31, CD206, F4/80, CD140β, CXCR4, vimentin, and CD140α expression levels (blue: low expression; high expression of the selected marker). (**B**) FlowSOM heatmap of column normalized (Z-score) marker expression for each of the 15 clusters identified by Cytofkit analysis. Colors varied according to the expression level of each considered marker in a blue to red scale, indicating low and high expression, respectively. (**C**) Cell population clusters defined by overlapping the expression for each of the different analyzed antigens were projected onto t-SNE space and assigned to specific colors (yellow: immune cells; light blue: macrophages; pink: myogenic progenitors (MPs); dark green: fibro/adipogenic progenitors (FAPs); red: endothelial progenitors; blue: pericyte-like cells; purple: other). (**D**) Density plots colored by density (blue: low density; red: high density), showing cell abundance variations at different times during the regeneration process.

The number of cells in the CD45$^+$ compartment (clusters 9, 10, 11, 12, 13, 14, and 15), as a whole, did not change significantly along the regeneration process (Figure 5A). However, the distribution of cells in the different populations in the compartment was found to be highly dynamic. In particular, macrophages (clusters 11, 14, and 15), which were already abundant in the mdx muscle before acute damage, increased significantly in the early days after CTX treatment, as observed in the wt model, to return to mdx baseline levels, approximately 30% of total mononuclear cells, at day 20 (Figure 5B). M2 macrophages, on the other hand, remained rather constant early after an injury to increase only late in the regeneration process (Figure 5C).

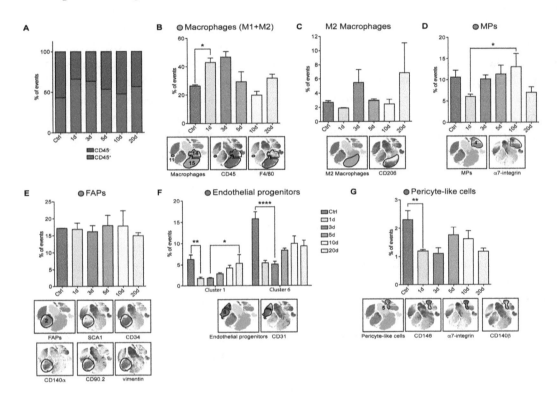

Figure 5. Characterization of the population dynamics induced by CTX injury in the mdx skeletal muscle at day 1, 3, 5, 10, 20 after injury. (**A**) Bar plots, showing the CD45$^-$ (blue) / CD45$^+$ (red) ratio in the mdx mononuclear cells at different time points after CTX injury. Data were represented as mean, and the statistical significance was estimated by two-way ANOVA. (**B**) t-SNE maps, showing the population gated as macrophage, colored for CD45 and F4/80 expression (red: high expression; blue: low expression) together with the macrophage trend observed in uninjured and CTX-injured mdx hind limb muscles. (**C**) M2 macrophages, expressing the CD206 antigen. (**D**) t-SNE maps of the myogenic progenitor (MP) population colored according to the levels of α7-integrin expression (red: high expression) and MP population dynamics during regeneration. (**E**) t-SNE maps, representing fibro/adipogenic progenitors (FAPs) identified among uninjured and CTX-injured mdx hind limb muscles, colored according to the expression of SCA1, CD34, CD140α, CD90.2, and vimentin (red: high expression; blue: low expression). The bar plot illustrated the population dynamics during regeneration. (**F**) Bar plots, showing the abundance of two different subclusters (cluster 1 and cluster 6) of endothelial progenitor cells at different time points. (**G**) t-SNE maps of pericyte-like cells identified in uninjured and CTX-injured mdx hind limb cell populations. Cell clusters were colored according to the expression of CD146, α7-integrin, and CD140β (red: high expression; blue: low expression). The bar plot illustrated the population dynamics during regeneration. Population abundance was assessed by calculating the percentage of cells in any given population over the total number of mononuclear cells in each sample (n = 3). The statistical significance was estimated by one-way ANOVA. All data were represented as mean $\pm$ SEM, and the statistical significance was defined as * $p < 0.05$; ** $p < 0.01$; **** $p < 0.001$.

When compared to wt, myogenic progenitors (MPs) (cluster 4) and fibro/adipogenic progenitors (FAPs) (cluster 2) followed a different trend. As the mdx muscle was under chronic stress, we observed that both progenitor cell populations were more populated in the absence of acute damage. However, while MPs decreased in number as early as one day after acute damage to return to unperturbed levels at later times, FAPs remained at a constant high level along the whole regeneration process (Figure 5D,E).

As already observed for the wt, also for the mdx mouse model, the CD31 expressing cells (clusters 1 and 6), defining endothelial progenitors, comprised two sub-populations differing for the expression of α7-integrin and other markers (CD90.2, CD140β, and CXCR4) (Figure S1E). The population expressing higher levels of α7-integrin was twice as abundant as the other. Nevertheless, both sub-populations reacted similarly to acute damage and first dropped in abundance by a factor of approximately three, to recover at the late stages of the regeneration process (Figure 5F). However, consistently, the cluster enriched in α7-integrin expressing cells (cluster 6) had not fully recovered at day 20, suggesting that the vascularization was still ongoing at times when histology seemed to indicate completion of the regeneration process. This differed from what was observed in the wt. Consistent with this consideration, and differently from what observed in the wt, also the pericyte-like population (cluster 5) behaved similarly, dropping in abundance immediately after damage and then slowly recovering without, however, reaching full recovery at day 20 (Figure 5G).

4. Discussion

The skeletal muscle has a remarkable capacity to self-repair if damaged [7–10,49,58]. However, this healing process may fail, owing to excessive damage, aging, or genetic disorders [12,59–62]. As a consequence of this failure in the repair process, as in muscle dystrophies, the tissue undergoes degeneration, leading to progressive muscle wasting and weakness characterized by chronic inflammation and, at later stages, fat and fibrotic tissue infiltrations [9,13,14].

Here, we exploited the resolution power of mass cytometry to characterize the modulation of the profile of the mononuclear cell population following chronic or acute damage [63–65]. To this end, we assembled a panel of 23 metal-tagged antibodies and characterized, at the single-cell level, the dynamics of muscle mononuclear cell populations after acute damage in wild type (wt) and in a mouse model of Duchenne muscular dystrophy (mdx). The regeneration process was monitored by examining samples of muscle mononuclear cells at 1, 3, 5, 10, and 20 days after cardiotoxin injection in wt or mdx mice [29,30].

This approach yielded a reach multiparametric dataset, disclosing the details of how the composition and heterogeneity of mononuclear cell populations changed in time as the muscle healing process proceeded. By applying a dimensionality reduction technique, such as the t-distributed stochastic neighbor embedding (t-SNE) algorithm, we generated bidimensional maps, providing a visual description of the regeneration process. Furthermore, this representation contributed to revealing subtle differences in the expression of specific markers in subpopulations within the major clusters that identified "classical" muscle populations. This population heterogeneity could not be only explained by experimental variability, even if any functional implication in muscle physiology or pathology remains to be established. In this report, we only dwelt upon a few of these t-SNE map features, while the dataset remains as a resource for additional analysis for the community.

A time-dependent variation in the abundance of muscle mononuclear cells was observed in wt mice, starting at day 1, indicating that the system sensed the damage and promptly responded to restore muscle tissue homeostasis. Inflammatory cells were the predominant population 3 days after the injury, accounting for over 40% of the total mononuclear cells. The activation of the inflammatory compartment was limited to the first few days after the injury as macrophages returned to baseline levels after 10 days.

Fibro/adipogenic progenitors (FAPs), here identified as SCA1$^+$, CD34$^+$, CD140α^+, CD90.2$^+$, and vimentin$^+$ [66], stimulate satellite cell activation and differentiation, thus playing a positive role in muscle regeneration [8]. FAPs are quiescent in intact muscles, while they proliferate in response to injury [8,67,68]. Consistently, we observed that FAPs, after CTX injection, rapidly expanded, in wt muscles, reaching a peak between days 5 and 10, to return eventually to baseline level, having accomplished their function of providing a transient production of pro-differentiation signals and of depositing extracellular matrix for muscle remodeling.

In response to the secreted inflammatory and fibro/adipogenic stimulating signals, the myogenic compartment also promptly activated at day 3, as confirmed by vimentin expression, which marked activated MPs or myoblasts [69]. After an initial drop in concentration, α7-integrin$^+$ MPs, including satellite cells and myoblasts, expanded on day 3, still remaining high on day 10, when they started to decrease.

Different kinetics was observed for endothelial progenitor cells, here, characterized as CD31, SCA1, CD34, and CD146 expressing cells, and for pericyte-like cells, mainly identified as CD146 and CD140β-positive cells. The endothelial and pericyte-like cell contribution to skeletal muscle recovery only took place at the end of the regeneration process; once the inflammatory cells were removed, FAPs decreased in number, and MPs differentiated.

Due to the incomplete nature of our panel, some cell clusters in our t-SNE maps remained loosely defined. One cluster included cells with an antigen repertoire reminiscent of mesenchymal cells, as they were positive for the mesenchymal markers CD90.2 and CD140β [70]. This population had a clear kinetic, suggesting a late intervention of the mesenchymal population in the muscle regeneration process.

We also investigated the response to acute injury of a muscle environment that was already chronically perturbed as in the mdx mice. Mononuclear cells extracted from the muscle of mdx mice did not experience any significant increase in number following cardiotoxin injury. However, by looking into the details of the population profiles at each time point, we observed a significant modulation of the population distributions as the increase in the number of the cells in one population was counterbalanced by the decrease in another one. For instance, while we observed that the cells in the inflammatory compartment, essentially macrophages, expanded early after damage, the endothelial and pericyte-like clusters dropped in numerosity to recover the initial values only late in the process. On the other hand, differently from wt, the myogenic and fibro/adipogenic compartments, the two main players in muscle regeneration, showed little variation during the regeneration process, probably because they were already chronically activated.

Overall, our multiparametric analysis offered a comprehensive description of both muscle tissue homeostasis and the rearrangements induced in the mononuclear cell population profile by a perturbation of the muscle system, be it a chronic condition, as in the case of mdx mice, or acute stress, as that triggered by cardiotoxin injection.

Author Contributions: Conceptualization, L.L.P., F.S., C.G., L.C., C.F., and G.C.; methodology, L.L.P., F.S., A.P., A.R., M.R., C.G., and C.F.; software, L.L.P., F.S., and A.P.; validation, L.L.P., F.S., A.P., A.R., M.R., C.G., and C.F.; formal analysis, L.L.P., F.S., A.P., A.R., and M.R.; investigation, L.L.P., F.S., A.P., A.R., and M.R; resources, C.G., L.C., C.F., and G.C.; data curation, L.L.P., F.S., and A.P.; writing—original draft preparation, L.L.P. and F.S.; writing—review and editing, L.L.P., F.S., C.G., L.C., C.F., and G.C.; visualization, L.L.P., F.S., C.G., L.C., C.F., and G.C.; supervision, C.G, L.C., C.F., and G.C.; project administration, L.C., C.F., and G.C.; funding acquisition, G.C. All authors have read and agreed to the published version of the manuscript.

Acknowledgments: We acknowledge the Umberto Veronesi Foundation for awarding C. Fuoco with post-doctoral fellowship 2019.

References

1. Decary, S.; Mouly, V.; Hamida, C.B.; Sautet, A.; Barbet, J.P.; Butler-Browne, G.S. Replicative potential and telomere length in human skeletal muscle: Implications for satellite cell-mediated gene therapy. *Hum. Gene Ther.* **1997**, *8*, 1429–1438. [CrossRef] [PubMed]

2. Mauro, A. Satellite cell of skeletal muscle fibers. *J. Biophys. Biochem. Cytol.* **1961**, *9*, 493–495. [CrossRef] [PubMed]

3. Yin, H.; Price, F.; Rudnicki, M.A. Satellite cells and the muscle stem cell niche. *Physiol. Rev.* **2013**, *93*, 23–67. [CrossRef]

4. Lepper, C.; Partridge, T.A.; Fan, C.-M. An absolute requirement for Pax7-positive satellite cells in acute injury-induced skeletal muscle regeneration. *Development* **2011**, *138*, 3639–3646. [CrossRef] [PubMed]

5. Sambasivan, R.; Yao, R.; Kissenpfennig, A.; Van Wittenberghe, L.; Paldi, A.; Gayraud-Morel, B.; Guenou, H.; Malissen, B.; Tajbakhsh, S.; Galy, A. Pax7-expressing satellite cells are indispensable for adult skeletal muscle regeneration. *Development* **2011**, *138*, 3647–3656. [CrossRef]

6. Seale, P.; Sabourin, L.A.; Girgis-Gabardo, A.; Mansouri, A.; Gruss, P.; Rudnicki, M.A. Pax7 is required for the specification of myogenic satellite cells. *Cell* **2000**, *102*, 777–786. [CrossRef]

7. Heredia, J.E.; Mukundan, L.; Chen, F.M.; Mueller, A.A.; Deo, R.C.; Locksley, R.M.; Rando, T.A.; Chawla, A. Type 2 innate signals stimulate fibro/adipogenic progenitors to facilitate muscle regeneration. *Cell* **2013**, *153*, 376–388. [CrossRef]

8. Joe, A.W.B.; Yi, L.; Natarajan, A.; Le Grand, F.; So, L.; Wang, J.; Rudnicki, M.A.; Rossi, F.M.V. Muscle injury activates resident fibro/adipogenic progenitors that facilitate myogenesis. *Nat. Cell Biol.* **2010**, *12*, 153–163. [CrossRef]

9. Uezumi, A.; Ito, T.; Morikawa, D.; Shimizu, N.; Yoneda, T.; Segawa, M.; Yamaguchi, M.; Ogawa, R.; Matev, M.M.; Miyagoe-Suzuki, Y.; et al. Fibrosis and adipogenesis originate from a common mesenchymal progenitor in skeletal muscle. *J. Cell Sci.* **2011**, *124*, 3654–3664. [CrossRef]

10. Murphy, M.M.; Lawson, J.A.; Mathew, S.J.; Hutcheson, D.A.; Kardon, G. Satellite cells, connective tissue fibroblasts and their interactions are crucial for muscle regeneration. *Development* **2011**, *138*, 3625–3637. [CrossRef]

11. Malecova, B.; Gatto, S.; Etxaniz, U.; Passafaro, M.; Cortez, A.; Nicoletti, C.; Giordani, L.; Torcinaro, A.; Bardi, M.; Bicciato, S.; et al. Dynamics of cellular states of fibro-adipogenic progenitors during myogenesis and muscular dystrophy. *Nat. Commun.* **2018**, *9*, 1–12. [CrossRef] [PubMed]

12. Emery, A.E.H. The muscular dystrophies. *Lancet* **2002**, *359*, 687–695. [CrossRef]

13. 1Marden, F.A.; Connolly, A.M.; Siegel, M.J.; Rubin, D.A. Compositional analysis of muscle in boys with Duchenne muscular dystrophy using MR imaging. *Skelet. Radiol.* **2004**, *34*, 140–148. [CrossRef]

14. Contreras, O.; Rebolledo, D.L.; Oyarzún, J.E.; Olguin, H.C.; Brandan, E. Connective tissue cells expressing fibro/adipogenic progenitor markers increase under chronic damage: Relevance in fibroblast-myofibroblast differentiation and skeletal muscle fibrosis. *Cell Tissue Res.* **2016**, *364*, 647–660. [CrossRef] [PubMed]

15. Hogarth, M.W.; Defour, A.; Lazarski, C.; Gallardo, E.; Diaz-Manera, J.; Partridge, T.A.; Nagaraju, K.; Jaiswal, J.K. Fibroadipogenic progenitors are responsible for muscle loss in limb girdle muscular dystrophy 2B. *Nat. Commun.* **2019**, *10*, 1–13. [CrossRef]

16. Madaro, L.; Passafaro, M.; Sala, D.; Etxaniz, U.; Lugarini, F.; Proietti, D.; Alfonsi, M.V.; Nicoletti, C.; Gatto, S.; De Bardi, M.; et al. Denervation-activated STAT3-IL-6 signalling in fibro-adipogenic progenitors promotes myofibres atrophy and fibrosis. *Nat. Cell Biol.* **2018**, *20*, 917–927. [CrossRef] [PubMed]

17. Sirabella, D.; De Angelis, L.; Berghella, L. Sources for skeletal muscle repair: From satellite cells to reprogramming. *J. Cachexia Sarcopenia Muscle* **2013**, *4*, 125–136. [CrossRef]

18. Dey, D.; Goldhamer, D.J.; Yu, P.B. Contributions of muscle-resident progenitor cells to homeostasis and disease. *Curr. Mol. Biol. Rep.* **2015**, *1*, 175–188. [CrossRef]

19. Pillon, N.J.; Bilan, P.J.; Fink, L.N.; Klip, A. Cross-talk between skeletal muscle and immune cells: Muscle-derived mediators and metabolic implications. *Am. J. Physiol. Endocrinol. Metab.* **2013**, *304*, E453–E465. [CrossRef]

20. Giordani, L.; He, G.J.; Negroni, E.; Sakai, H.; Law, J.Y.C.; Siu, M.M.; Wan, R.; Corneau, A.; Tajbakhsh, S.; Cheung, T.H.; et al. High-dimensional single-cell cartography reveals novel skeletal muscle-resident cell populations. *Mol. Cell* **2019**, *74*, 609–621.e6. [CrossRef]

21. Gatto, S.; Puri, P.L.; Malecova, B. Single cell gene expression profiling of skeletal muscle-derived cells. *Methods Mol. Biol.* **2017**, *1556*, 191–219. [PubMed]

22. Rubenstein, A.B.; Smith, G.R.; Raue, U.; Begue, G.; Minchev, K.; Ruf-Zamojski, F.; Nair, V.D.; Wang, X.; Zhou, L.; Zaslavsky, E.; et al. Single-cell transcriptional profiles in human skeletal muscle. *Nat. Publ. Group* **2020**, *10*, 229. [CrossRef]

23. Dell'Orso, S.; Juan, A.H.; Ko, K.-D.; Naz, F.; Perovanovic, J.; Gutierrez-Cruz, G.; Feng, X.; Sartorelli, V. Single cell analysis of adult mouse skeletal muscle stem cells in homeostatic and regenerative conditions. *Development* **2019**, *146*, dev174177. [CrossRef] [PubMed]

24. Marinkovic, M.; Fuoco, C.; Sacco, F.; Cerquone Perpetuini, A.; Giuliani, G.; Micarelli, E.; Pavlidou, T.; Petrilli, L.L.; Reggio, A.; Riccio, F.; et al. Fibro-adipogenic progenitors of dystrophic mice are insensitive to NOTCH regulation of adipogenesis. *Life Sci. Alliance* **2019**, *2*, e201900437. [CrossRef] [PubMed]

25. Spada, F.; Fuoco, C.; Pirrò, S.; Paoluzi, S.; Castagnoli, L.; Gargioli, C.; Cesareni, G. Characterization by mass cytometry of different methods for the preparation of muscle mononuclear cells. *New Biotechnol.* **2016**, *33*, 514–523. [CrossRef]

26. Finck, R.; Simonds, E.F.; Jager, A.; Krishnaswamy, S.; Sachs, K.; Fantl, W.; Pe'er, D.; Nolan, G.P.; Bendall, S.C. Normalization of mass cytometry data with bead standards. *Cytom. Part* **2013**, *83*, 483–494. [CrossRef]

27. Kotecha, N.; Krutzik, P.O.; Irish, J.M. Web-based analysis and publication of flow cytometry experiments. *Curr. Protoc. Cytom.* **2010**. [CrossRef]

28. Chen, H.; Lau, M.C.; Wong, M.T.; Newell, E.W.; Chen, J. Cytofkit: A bioconductor package for an integrated mass cytometry data analysis pipeline. *PLoS Comput. Biol.* **2016**, *12*, e1005112. [CrossRef]

29. Ramadasan-Nair, R.; Gayathri, N.; Mishra, S.; Sunitha, B.; Mythri, R.B.; Nalini, A.; Subbannayya, Y.; Harsha, H.C.; Kolthur-Seetharam, U.; Srinivas Bharath, M.M. Mitochondrial alterations and oxidative stress in an acute transient mouse model of muscle degeneration: Implications for muscular dystrophy and related muscle pathologies. *J. Biol. Chem.* **2014**, *289*, 485–509. [CrossRef]

30. Duchen, L.W.; Excell, B.J.; Patel, R.; Smith, B. Changes in motor end-plates resulting from muscle fibre necrosis and regeneration. A light and electron microscopic study of the effects of the depolarizing fraction (cardiotoxin) of Dendroaspis jamesoni venom. *J. Neurol. Sci.* **1974**, *21*, 391–417. [CrossRef]

31. Wang, H.-X.; Lau, S.-Y.; Huang, S.-J.; Kwan, C.-Y.; Wong, T.-M. Cobra venom cardiotoxin induces perturbations of cytosolic calcium homeostasis and hypercontracture in adult rat ventricular myocytes. *J. Mol. Cell. Cardiol.* **1997**, *29*, 2759–2770. [CrossRef] [PubMed]

32. Raynor, R.L.; Zheng, B.; Kuo, J.F. Membrane interactions of amphiphilic polypeptides mastoparan, melittin, polymyxin B, and cardiotoxin. Differential inhibition of protein kinase C, Ca2+/calmodulin-dependent protein kinase II and synaptosomal membrane Na,K-ATPase, and Na+ pump and differentiation of HL60 cells. *J. Biol. Chem.* **1991**, *266*, 2753–2758. [PubMed]

33. Suh, B.C.; Song, S.K.; Kim, Y.K.; Kim, K.T. Induction of cytosolic Ca2+ elevation mediated by Mas-7 occurs through membrane pore formation. *J. Biol. Chem.* **1996**, *271*, 32753–32759. [CrossRef]

34. Bentzinger, C.F.; Wang, Y.X.; Dumont, N.A.; Rudnicki, M.A. Cellular dynamics in the muscle satellite cell niche. *EMBO Rep.* **2013**, *14*, 1062–1072. [CrossRef] [PubMed]

35. St Pierre, B.A.; Tidball, J.G. Differential response of macrophage subpopulations to soleus muscle reloading after rat hindlimb suspension. *J. Appl. Physiol.* **1994**, *77*, 290–297. [CrossRef]

36. Sacco, A.; Mourkioti, F.; Tran, R.; Choi, J.; Llewellyn, M.; Kraft, P.; Shkreli, M.; Delp, S.; Pomerantz, J.H.; Artandi, S.E.; et al. Short telomeres and stem cell exhaustion model Duchenne muscular dystrophy in mdx/mTR mice. *Cell* **2010**, *143*, 1059–1071. [CrossRef]

37. Anderson, J.E.; Ovalle, W.K.; Bressler, B.H. Electron microscopic and autoradiographic characterization of hindlimb muscle regeneration in the mdx mouse. *Anat. Rec.* **1987**, *219*, 243–257. [CrossRef]

38. Zunder, E.R.; Finck, R.; Behbehani, G.K.; Amir, E.-A.D.; Krishnaswamy, S.; Gonzalez, V.D.; Lorang, C.G.; Bjornson, Z.; Spitzer, M.H.; Bodenmiller, B.; et al. Palladium-based mass tag cell barcoding with a doublet-filtering scheme and single-cell deconvolution algorithm. *Nat. Protoc.* **2015**, *10*, 316–333. [CrossRef]

39. Amir, E.-A.D.; Davis, K.L.; Tadmor, M.D.; Simonds, E.F.; Levine, J.H.; Bendall, S.C.; Shenfeld, D.K.; Krishnaswamy, S.; Nolan, G.P.; Pe'er, D. VISNE enables visualization of high dimensional single-cell data and reveals phenotypic heterogeneity of leukemia. *Nat. Biotechnol.* **2013**, *31*, 545–552. [CrossRef]

40. Palma, A.; Cerquone Perpetuini, A.; Ferrentino, F.; Fuoco, C.; Gargioli, C.; Giuliani, G.; Iannuccelli, M.; Licata, L.; Micarelli, E.; Paoluzi, S.; et al. Myo-REG: A portal for signaling interactions in muscle regeneration. *Front. Physiol.* **2019**, *10*, 1216. [CrossRef]

41. Arnold, L.; Henry, A.; Poron, F.; Baba-Amer, Y.; Van Rooijen, N.; Plonquet, A.; Gherardi, R.K.; Chazaud, B. Inflammatory monocytes recruited after skeletal muscle injury switch into antiinflammatory macrophages to support myogenesis. *J. Exp. Med.* **2007**, *204*, 1057–1069. [CrossRef] [PubMed]

42. McLennan, I.S. Degenerating and regenerating skeletal muscles contain several subpopulations of macrophages with distinct spatial and temporal distributions. *J. Anat.* **1996**, *188*, 17–28.

43. Lolmede, K.; Campana, L.; Vezzoli, M.; Bosurgi, L.; Tonlorenzi, R.; Clementi, E.; Bianchi, M.E.; Cossu, G.; Manfredi, A.A.; Brunelli, S.; et al. Inflammatory and alternatively activated human macrophages attract vessel-associated stem cells, relying on separate HMGB1- and MMP-9-dependent pathways. *J. Leukoc. Biol.* **2009**, *85*, 779–787. [CrossRef]

44. Chazaud, B.; Sonnet, C.; Lafuste, P.; Bassez, G.; Rimaniol, A.-C.; Poron, F.; Authier, F.-J.; Dreyfus, P.A.; Gherardi, R.K. Satellite cells attract monocytes and use macrophages as a support to escape apoptosis and enhance muscle growth. *J. Cell Biol.* **2003**, *163*, 1133–1143. [CrossRef] [PubMed]

45. Dumont, N.; Frenette, J. Macrophages protect against muscle atrophy and promote muscle recovery in vivo and in vitro: A mechanism partly dependent on the insulin-like growth factor-1 signaling molecule. *Am. J. Pathol.* **2010**, *176*, 2228–2235. [CrossRef] [PubMed]

46. Martinez, F.O.; Gordon, S. The M1 and M2 paradigm of macrophage activation: Time for reassessment. *F1000Prime Rep.* **2014**, *6*, 13. [CrossRef] [PubMed]

47. Kharraz, Y.; Guerra, J.; Mann, C.J.; Serrano, A.L.; Muñoz-Cánoves, P. Macrophage plasticity and the role of inflammation in skeletal muscle repair. *Mediat. Inflamm.* **2013**. [CrossRef] [PubMed]

48. Mantovani, A.; Biswas, S.K.; Galdiero, M.R.; Sica, A.; Locati, M. Macrophage plasticity and polarization in tissue repair and remodelling. *J. Pathol.* **2013**, *229*, 176–185. [CrossRef] [PubMed]

49. Saclier, M.; Yacoub-Youssef, H.; Mackey, A.L.; Arnold, L.; Ardjoune, H.; Magnan, M.; Sailhan, F.; Chelly, J.; Pavlath, G.K.; Mounier, R.; et al. Differentially activated macrophages orchestrate myogenic precursor cell fate during human skeletal muscle regeneration. *Stem Cells* **2013**, *31*, 384–396. [CrossRef] [PubMed]

50. Stout, R.D.; Jiang, C.; Matta, B.; Tietzel, I.; Watkins, S.K.; Suttles, J. Macrophages sequentially change their functional phenotype in response to changes in microenvironmental influences. *J. Immunol.* **2005**, *175*, 342–349. [CrossRef]

51. Fu, X.; Wang, H.; Hu, P. Stem cell activation in skeletal muscle regeneration. *Cell. Mol. Life Sci.* **2015**, *72*, 1663–1677. [CrossRef]

52. Nguyen, H.X.; Tidball, J.G. Interactions between neutrophils and macrophages promote macrophage killing of rat muscle cells in vitro. *J. Physiol. (Lond.)* **2003**, *547*, 125–132. [CrossRef] [PubMed]

53. Musarò, A. The basis of muscle regeneration. *Adv. Biol.* **2014**, *2014*, 1–16. [CrossRef]

54. Hansen-Smith, F.M.; Hudlicka, O.; Egginton, S. In vivo angiogenesis in adult rat skeletal muscle: Early changes in capillary network architecture and ultrastructure. *Cell Tissue Res.* **1996**, *286*, 123–136. [CrossRef] [PubMed]

55. Zheng, B.; Cao, B.; Crisan, M.; Sun, B.; Li, G.; Logar, A.; Yap, S.; Pollett, J.B.; Drowley, L.; Cassino, T.; et al. Prospective identification of myogenic endothelial cells in human skeletal muscle. *Nat. Biotechnol.* **2007**, *25*, 1025–1034. [CrossRef] [PubMed]

56. Dellavalle, A.; Sampaolesi, M.; Tonlorenzi, R.; Tagliafico, E.; Sacchetti, B.; Perani, L.; Innocenzi, A.; Galvez, B.G.; Messina, G.; Morosetti, R.; et al. Pericytes of human skeletal muscle are myogenic precursors distinct from satellite cells. *Nat. Cell Biol.* **2007**, *9*, 255–267. [CrossRef] [PubMed]

57. Birbrair, A.; Zhang, T.; Wang, Z.-M.; Messi, M.L.; Enikolopov, G.N.; Mintz, A.; Delbono, O. Role of pericytes in skeletal muscle regeneration and fat accumulation. *Stem Cells Dev.* **2013**, *22*, 2298–2314. [CrossRef] [PubMed]

58. Christov, C.; Chrétien, F.; Abou-Khalil, R.; Bassez, G.; Vallet, G.; Authier, F.-J.; Bassaglia, Y.; Shinin, V.; Tajbakhsh, S.; Chazaud, B.; et al. Muscle satellite cells and endothelial cells: Close neighbors and privileged partners. *Mol. Biol. Cell* **2007**, *18*, 1397–1409. [CrossRef] [PubMed]

59. Almada, A.E.; Wagers, A.J. Molecular circuitry of stem cell fate in skeletal muscle regeneration, ageing and disease. *Nat. Rev. Mol. Cell Biol.* **2016**, *17*, 267–279. [CrossRef]

60. Blau, H.M.; Cosgrove, B.D.; Ho, A.T.V. The central role of muscle stem cells in regenerative failure with aging. *Nat. Med.* **2015**, *21*, 854–862. [CrossRef]

61. Kuswanto, W.; Burzyn, D.; Panduro, M.; Wang, K.K.; Jang, Y.C.; Wagers, A.J.; Benoist, C.; Mathis, D. Poor repair of skeletal muscle in aging mice reflects a defect in local, interleukin-33-dependent accumulation of regulatory T cells. *Immunity* **2016**, *44*, 355–367. [CrossRef]

62. Pastoret, C.; Sebille, A. Age-related differences in regeneration of dystrophic (mdx) and normal muscle in the mouse. *Muscle Nerve* **1995**, *18*, 1147–1154. [CrossRef] [PubMed]

63. Ornatsky, O.; Bandura, D.; Baranov, V.; Nitz, M.; Winnik, M.A.; Tanner, S. Highly multiparametric analysis by mass cytometry. *J. Immunol. Methods* **2010**, *361*, 1–20. [CrossRef] [PubMed]

64. Bendall, S.C.; Nolan, G.P.; Roederer, M.; Chattopadhyay, P.K. A deep profiler's guide to cytometry. *Trends Immunol.* **2012**, *33*, 323–332. [CrossRef] [PubMed]

65. Bandura, D.R.; Baranov, V.I.; Ornatsky, O.I.; Antonov, A.; Kinach, R.; Lou, X.; Pavlov, S.; Vorobiev, S.; Dick, J.E.; Tanner, S.D. Mass cytometry: Technique for real time single cell multitarget immunoassay based on inductively coupled plasma time-of-flight mass spectrometry. *Anal. Chem.* **2009**, *81*, 6813–6822. [CrossRef] [PubMed]

66. Reggio, A.; Rosina, M.; Palma, A.; Cerquone Perpetuini, A.; Petrilli, L.L.; Gargioli, C.; Fuoco, C.; Micarelli, E.; Giuliani, G.; Cerretani, M.; et al. Adipogenesis of skeletal muscle fibro/adipogenic progenitors is affected by the WNT5a/GSK3/β-catenin axis. *Cell Death Differ.* **2020**, *108*, 1–21. [CrossRef] [PubMed]

67. Uezumi, A.; Fukada, S.-I.; Yamamoto, N.; Takeda, S.; Tsuchida, K. Mesenchymal progenitors distinct from satellite cells contribute to ectopic fat cell formation in skeletal muscle. *Nat. Cell Biol.* **2010**, *12*, 143–152. [CrossRef]

68. Lemos, D.R.; Babaeijandaghi, F.; Low, M.; Chang, C.-K.; Lee, S.T.; Fiore, D.; Zhang, R.-H.; Natarajan, A.; Nedospasov, S.A.; Rossi, F.M.V. Nilotinib reduces muscle fibrosis in chronic muscle injury by promoting TNF-mediated apoptosis of fibro/ adipogenic progenitors. *Nat. Med.* **2015**, *21*, 1–11. [CrossRef]

69. Vater, R.; Cullen, M.J.; Harris, J.B. The expression of vimentin in satellite cells of regenerating skeletal muscle in vivo. *Histochem. J.* **1994**, *26*, 916–928. [CrossRef]

70. Chirieleison, S.M.; Feduska, J.M.; Schugar, R.C.; Askew, Y.; Deasy, B.M. Human muscle-derived cell populations isolated by differential adhesion rates: Phenotype and contribution to skeletal muscle regeneration in Mdx/SCID mice. *Tissue Eng. Part* **2012**, *18*, 232–241. [CrossRef]

Permissions

All chapters in this book were first published by MDPI; hereby published with permission under the Creative Commons Attribution License or equivalent. Every chapter published in this book has been scrutinized by our experts. Their significance has been extensively debated. The topics covered herein carry significant findings which will fuel the growth of the discipline. They may even be implemented as practical applications or may be referred to as a beginning point for another development.

The contributors of this book come from diverse backgrounds, making this book a truly international effort. This book will bring forth new frontiers with its revolutionizing research information and detailed analysis of the nascent developments around the world.

We would like to thank all the contributing authors for lending their expertise to make the book truly unique. They have played a crucial role in the development of this book. Without their invaluable contributions this book wouldn't have been possible. They have made vital efforts to compile up to date information on the varied aspects of this subject to make this book a valuable addition to the collection of many professionals and students.

This book was conceptualized with the vision of imparting up-to-date information and advanced data in this field. To ensure the same, a matchless editorial board was set up. Every individual on the board went through rigorous rounds of assessment to prove their worth. After which they invested a large part of their time researching and compiling the most relevant data for our readers.

The editorial board has been involved in producing this book since its inception. They have spent rigorous hours researching and exploring the diverse topics which have resulted in the successful publishing of this book. They have passed on their knowledge of decades through this book. To expedite this challenging task, the publisher supported the team at every step. A small team of assistant editors was also appointed to further simplify the editing procedure and attain best results for the readers.

Apart from the editorial board, the designing team has also invested a significant amount of their time in understanding the subject and creating the most relevant covers. They scrutinized every image to scout for the most suitable representation of the subject and create an appropriate cover for the book.

The publishing team has been an ardent support to the editorial, designing and production team. Their endless efforts to recruit the best for this project, has resulted in the accomplishment of this book. They are a veteran in the field of academics and their pool of knowledge is as vast as their experience in printing. Their expertise and guidance has proved useful at every step. Their uncompromising quality standards have made this book an exceptional effort. Their encouragement from time to time has been an inspiration for everyone.

The publisher and the editorial board hope that this book will prove to be a valuable piece of knowledge for researchers, students, practitioners and scholars across the globe.

List of Contributors

Ester Casanova, Josepa Salvadó and Albert Gibert-Ramos
Nutrigenomics Research Group, Department of Biochemistry and Biotechnology, Universitat Rovira I Virgili (URV), Campus Sescelades, 43007 Tarragona, Spain

Anna Crescenti
Technological Unit of Nutrition and Health, EURECAT-Technology Centre of Catalonia, Avinguda Universitat 1, 43204 Reus, Spain

Iwona Grabowska, Malgorzata Zimowska, Karolina Maciejewska, Zuzanna Jablonska, Anna Bazga, Michal Ozieblo, Wladyslawa Streminska, Joanna Bem, Maria A. Ciemerych, Bartosz Mierzejewski and Edyta Brzóska
Department of Cytology, Faculty of Biology, University of Warsaw, Miecznikowa 1 St, 02-096 Warsaw, Poland

Casper Soendenbroe
Institute of Sports Medicine Copenhagen, Department of Orthopedic Surgery M, Bispebjerg Hospital, Building 8, Nielsine Nielsens vej 11, 2400 Copenhagen NV, Denmark
Xlab, Department of Biomedical Sciences, Faculty of Health and Medical Sciences, University of Copenhagen, Blegdamsvej 3, 2200 Copenhagen N, Denmark

Cecilie J. L. Bechshøft, Peter Schjerling, Anders Karlsen, Michael Kjaer and Jesper L. Andersen
Institute of Sports Medicine Copenhagen, Department of Orthopedic Surgery M, Bispebjerg Hospital, Building 8, Nielsine Nielsens vej 11, 2400 Copenhagen NV, Denmark
Center for Healthy Aging, Faculty of Health and Medical Sciences, University of Copenhagen, Blegdamsvej 3, 2200 Copenhagen N, Denmark

Mette F. Heisterberg, Simon M. Jensen and Emma Bomme
Institute of Sports Medicine Copenhagen, Department of Orthopedic Surgery M, Bispebjerg Hospital, Building 8, Nielsine Nielsens vej 11, 2400 Copenhagen NV, Denmark

Abigail L. Mackey
Institute of Sports Medicine Copenhagen, Department of Orthopedic Surgery M, Bispebjerg Hospital, Building 8, Nielsine Nielsens vej 11, 2400 Copenhagen NV, Denmark

Xlab, Department of Biomedical Sciences, Faculty of Health and Medical Sciences, University of Copenhagen, Blegdamsvej 3, 2200 Copenhagen N, Denmark
Center for Healthy Aging, Faculty of Health and Medical Sciences, University of Copenhagen, Blegdamsvej 3, 2200 Copenhagen N, Denmark

Letizia Zullo
Istituto Italiano di Tecnologia, Center for Micro-BioRobotics & Center for Synaptic Neuroscience and Technology (NSYN), 16132 Genova, Italy
IRCCS Ospedale Policlinico San Martino, 16132 Genova, Italy

Matteo Bozzo, Simona Candiani, Alon Daya, Nir Nesher and Tal Shomrat
Laboratory of Developmental Neurobiology, Department of Earth, Environment and Life Sciences, University of Genova, Viale Benedetto XV 5, 16132 Genova, Italy

Alessio Di Clemente
Istituto Italiano di Tecnologia, Center for Micro-BioRobotics & Center for Synaptic Neuroscience and Technology (NSYN), 16132 Genova, Italy
Department of Experimental Medicine, University of Genova, Viale Benedetto XV, 3, 16132 Genova, Italy

Francesco Paolo Mancini and Alberto Zullo
Department of Science and Technology, University of Sannio, 82100 Benevento, Italy

Aram Megighian
Department of Biomedical Sciences, University of Padova, 35131 Padova, Italy
Padova Neuroscience Center, University of Padova, 35131 Padova, Italy

Eric Röttinger
Institute for Research on Cancer and Aging (IRCAN), Université Côte d'Azur, CNRS, INSERM, 06107 Nice, France

Stefano Tiozzo
Laboratoire de Biologie du Développement de Villefranche-sur-Mer (LBDV), Sorbonne Université, CNRS, 06230 Paris, France

Fabio Maiullari
Gemelli Molise Hospital, 86100 Campobasso, Italy

Denisa Baci
Institute of Biochemistry and Cell Biology, National Research Council, 00015 Rome, Italy
Department of Biotechnology and Life Sciences, University of Insubria, 21100 Varese, Italy

Maila Chirivì, Valentina Pace, Marika Milan, Andrea Rampin and Dario Presutti
Institute of Biochemistry and Cell Biology, National Research Council, 00015 Rome, Italy

Paolo Somma
Flow Cytometry Core, Humanitas Clinical and Research Center, 20089 Milan, Italy

Silvia Garavelli
Institute for Endocrinology and Oncology "Gaetano Salvatore", National Research Council, 80131 Naples, Italy

Antonino Bruno
IRCCS MultiMedica, 20138 Milan, Italy

Roberto Rizzi and Chiara Lanzuolo
Institute of Biomedical Technologies, National Research Council, 20090 Milan, Italy
Fondazione Istituto Nazionale di Genetica Molecolare, 20122 Milan, Italy

Claudia Bearzi
Institute of Biochemistry and Cell Biology, National Research Council, 00015 Rome, Italy
Fondazione Istituto Nazionale di Genetica Molecolare, 20122 Milan, Italy

Preethi Poovathumkadavil and Krzysztof Jagla
Institute of Genetics Reproduction and Development, iGReD, INSERM U1103, CNRS UMR6293, University of Clermont Auvergne, 28 Place Henri Dunant, 63000 Clermont-Ferrand, France

Debora Libetti, Andrea Bernardini, Sarah Sertic, Graziella Messina, Diletta Dolfini and Roberto Mantovani
Dipartimento di Bioscienze, Università degli Studi di Milano, Via Celoria 26, 20133 Milano, Italy

Łukasz Pulik and Paweł Łęgosz
Department of Orthopaedics and Traumatology, Medical University of Warsaw, Lindley 4 St, 02-005 Warsaw, Poland

Jedd Pratt
Institute for Sport and Health, University College Dublin, Dublin, Ireland
Genomics Medicine Ireland, Dublin, Ireland

Colin Boreham
Institute for Sport and Health, University College Dublin, Dublin, Ireland

Sean Ennis
Genomics Medicine Ireland, Dublin, Ireland
UCD ACoRD, Academic Centre on Rare Diseases, University College Dublin, Dublin, Ireland

Anthony W. Ryan
Genomics Medicine Ireland, Dublin, Ireland

Giuseppe De Vito
Institute for Sport and Health, University College Dublin, Dublin, Ireland
Department of Biomedical Sciences, University of Padova, Via F. Marzolo 3, 35131 Padova, Italy

Lucia Lisa Petrilli
Department of Biology, University of Rome "Tor Vergata", 00133 Rome, Italy
Department of Onco-hematology, Gene and Cell Therapy — Bambino Gesù Children's Hospital — IRCCS, 00146 Rome, Italy
Filomena Spada, Alessandro Palma, Alessio Reggio, Marco Rosina, Cesare Gargioli, Luisa Castagnoli, Stefano Cannata and Claudia Fuoco
Department of Biology, University of Rome "Tor Vergata", 00133 Rome, Italy

Gianni Cesareni
Department of Biology, University of Rome "Tor Vergata", 00133 Rome, Italy
Fondazione Santa Lucia Istituto di Ricovero e Cura a Carattere Scientifico (IRCCS), 00143 Rome, Italy

Index

Printed in the USA
CPSIA information can be obtained
at www.ICGtesting.com
JSHW051513050324
58622JS00005B/53